PERIMENOPAUSE

Second Edition

Changes in Women's Health After 35

James E. Huston, M.D. & L. Darlene Lanka, M.D.
Foreword by Lois Jovanovic, M.D.

New Harbinger Publications, Inc.

Publisher's Note

Care has been taken to confirm the accuracy of the information presented and to describe generally accepted practices. However, the authors, editors, and publisher are not responsible for errors or omissions or for any consequences from application of the information in this book and make no warranty, express or implied, with respect to the contents of the publication.

The authors, editors, and publisher have exerted every effort to ensure that any drug selection and dosage set forth in this text are in accordance with current recommendations and practice at the time of publication. However, in view of ongoing research, changes in government regulations, and the constant flow of information relating to drug therapy and drug reactions, the reader is urged to check the package insert for each drug for any change in indications and dosage and for added warnings and precautions. This is particularly important when the recommended agent is a new or infrequently employed drug.

Some drugs and medical devices presented in this publication may have Food and Drug Administration (FDA) clearance for limited use in restricted research settings. It is the responsibility of the health care provider to ascertain the FDA status of each drug or device planned for use in their clinical practice.

Distributed in Canada by Raincoast Books

Copyright © 2001   James E. Huston and Darlene Lanka
New Harbinger Publications, Inc.
5674 Shattuck Avenue
Oakland, CA 94609

Cover design by SHELBY DESIGNS AND ILLUSTRATES
Edited by Clancy Drake
Text design by Michele Waters

ISBN-10 1-57224-234-5
ISBN-13 978-1-57224-234-0

Printed in the United States of America

New Harbinger Publication's Web site address: www.newharbinger.com

08   07   06

15   14   13   12   11   10   9   8   7   6

Contents

Why Should You Have a Hysterectomy? • Types of Hysterectomy • Hysterectomy Complications • Elective Removal of Ovaries as Part of the Hysterectomy • The Bottom Line • Elective Hysterectomy Accompanying Removal of the Ovaries • You Needed That Hysterectomy and You Don't Miss Your Uterus—So Why Are You So Sad? • Summary of Treatment for Abnormal Uterine Bleeding • Ovarian Cysts • Functional Ovarian Cysts • Nonfunctional Ovarian Cysts • Endometriomas • Summary of Ovarian Cysts • Ectopic (Tubal) Pregnancy • Diagnosis of Ectopic Pregnancy • Medical Treatment of Ectopic Pregnancy • Surgical Treatment of Ectopic Pregnancy • Urinary Incontinence • The Genito-Urinary System • Continence—the Way It Ought to Be • Types of Incontinence • Surgical Options for Incontinence • The Estrogen Connection • Summary

Foreword

"Oh, no! Not another book on menopause. Hey, wait a minute, Lois, do not be so quick to dismiss this book. Take another look and you will see it is exactly what the doctor ordered!" These words were the exact conversation I had with myself when I was asked to write a Foreword for this book. Writing the Foreword did not seem to be the chore, but reading another book on menopause was not what I really wanted to do for a weekend. Wow, once I settled into the first few sentences I was glued for the entire piece. Rather than writing a Foreword to another "me, too" book for others to read, I was asked to write the Foreword to a wonderful, gentle introduction to the next phase of my life. Although I have actually written two books on the menopause, perhaps I, too, was struggling with the notion that one day I would experience all the ups and downs of menopause. So I wrote the books as though I was writing about a different species and that all that was in store really did not apply to me. In fact, when I was asked to market the books, I politely declined. I did not want to be known as "Miss Menopause." The power of my denial is not at all uncommon, as I learned from the beginning of this book. I am among over thirty-one million women who are part of the "mighty baby boomer generation" and thus are facing the perimenopausal years. Rather that preparing and correcting my deviations from healthy attitudes, I just chalked up my mood swings, weight gain, hair, skin, and nail changes to "stress." If an endocrinologist, trained in the care of postmenopausal women, could deny the perimenopausal changes so obviously happening, then how could a general doctor, let alone the general woman on the street, properly prepare for the rest of her life? This book struck a harmonious chord in my musical shift to a minor key. Now discordant sounds can be placed in a rhythmic pattern to produce a beautiful, melodious result. Thank you, Drs. Lanka and Huston!

From the first chapter on what changes to expect, I almost skipped past important information, but the good doctors knew that I might be cheating and caught me page turning. I laughed out loud when they told me not to cut past this chapter. How did they know? They seem to know a lot of other very personal things about me, too. Such as the subtle changes in my menstrual cycle, my irritability and my concern about the few extra pounds which seemed to come out of the air. How could I be so dumb? Perhaps it was because I never really thought about the perimenopausal state as being part of life and a part of my life which I had control over. After the astute introduction which had me "hooked," I passionately read every word, searching for "truth and justice." Each and every chapter then taught me a thing or two which definitely will make me a better physician for my female patients. Such things as changes in fertility, premenstrual syndrome in these transition years, prevention strategies to minimize the complications of cardiovascular disease and osteoporosis, a new look at thyroid disease as "a masquerader" of menopause (a notion which I really had not thought of before, and if I haven't thought of it, imagine how many other physicians have also been amiss . . .).

Thank goodness the good Drs. Lanka and Huston offer ways to change the odds. Rather than merely pointing out to the reader the changes of the perimenopause, and what's in store for the future, this book provides concrete, bona fide therapies to make a difference for the rest of our lives. Yes, I did know most of the literature on hormonal replacement therapy; after all I am an endocrinologist. However, the stuff on alternative medical disciplines was an eye-opener for me. I guarantee you, even the best medical school in the Bronx (I am an Einstein alum) did not teach me one whit about Chinese medicine, herbs, acupuncture, homeopathic remedies, and mind/body exercises. My savvy patients ask me about these alternatives all the time. Previously, I just dismissed the conversation, hiding behind my ignorance; now I am prepared to advise, guide, and succeed in helping to incorporate these alternatives into a plan to change the odds.

Although I have a good background in nutrition, I did not know of a good reference for my patients to read. Thus, I would find myself trying to provide a makeshift educational piece on this very important area of care. This book is now mandatory for all my female patients. After all, we are what we eat, but more importantly, we will be what we eat! Because this book has the expertise of a great gynecological surgeon, the section on gynecological surgery and cosmetic surgery is a wonderful reference for any or all of my patients who are faced with the news that they need a hysterectomy. This section is informative and written with a comforting, loving perspective of "you needed that hysterectomy and you don't miss your uterus—so why are you so sad?"

As a grand finale, the authors leave us taking charge of our destiny. What started as a drudgery and a tremendous resistance to accepting that I too am aging and needing a bit of guidance through this phase of my life, ended in an invigorated response to work on my lack of attention to important things in my life. Better than a New Year's resolution, this book has given me the rationale and thus empowered me to stick to a healthier diet, to increase my exercise program, and to try techniques to minimize the stresses and episodes of depression. Yes, this book has made me wiser, and one weekend older, but it also has made me a better physician and given me the strategies to be a better me, despite the perimenopause!

Lois Jovanovic, M.D.
Sansum Medical Research Foundation
Santa Barbara, California

Preface

Authors' Note

The second edition of this book has been written in the same spirit as the first. Both authors remain dedicated to educating women about perimenopause, a watershed era after age thirty-five when significant bodily changes occur. Much has been published about menopause, but the literature concerning perimenopause remains rather sparse.

Since publication of this book's first edition in 1997, research in women's health concerns has continued to escalate in quantity and quality. As a result, a huge amount of new information has become available, which we have used to update the sections on heart disease, osteoporosis, breast cancer, and hormone replacement. Newer principles for nutrition, weight control, and exercise have been included. Birth control methods and infertility management have also changed. Information on the latest in surgical treatment of various problems common to the perimenopausal transition is in this edition. With the public's increasing interest in alternative medical care and the scientific community's stepped-up research efforts, we have expanded the chapter on this topic.

We continue to believe that this isn't a dress rehearsal you're going through. It's an authentic life, and we want you to live it that way. Our fondest hope for you as our reader is that the contents of our book will increase your fund of knowledge about perimenopause, and enable you to stay focused on the overarching goal of living your life in wellness.

James E. Huston, M.D.
L. Darlene Lanka, M.D.

Section I

The Changes

1

What Changes? An Overview

We can almost hear what you're thinking: "Changes? You mean I'm already changing, and I'm only thirty-seven?" Yes, it's true. "Is this the Change of Life?" No, it's not menopause. "What's causing it?" Your female hormones are declining. "I can stop it though, right?" Not a chance. "What should I do?" Read this book from cover to cover.

Change is what life is about. Whether for good or for ill, all of us continually change as time passes. Males change in a steady, slow fashion. Females are rhythmic. The gender difference is mediated by hormones. Every month your uterus builds a new lining and then, if a pregnancy is not begun, sheds it. Every month your breasts change in concert with this rhythm. Think of the other patterns of change you experience on a rhythmic basis in your appetite, skin, mood, sexual desire, and energy, among many others aspects of your life.

Then there are the macrohormone changes of puberty, pregnancy, and menopause. The engine of the rhythmic pattern of change is female hormone production. It follows, then, that a change in hormone output will alter your rhythms. In this book you will learn about the changes that occur in your body and in your life as a result of fluctuating and decreasing hormone levels. A transition is gradually taking place that you can prepare for and influence in a positive fashion. This book is a guide to maintaining good health during these transition years. It will teach you how to prepare for the best half of your life.

Let's Talk Hormones

Estrogen and progesterone are the female hormones that regulate many of the changes we've mentioned. These two hormones are "behind the scenes" support players, somewhat akin to the stagehands in a play. They aren't visible to the audience or actors during the performance, but the show functions smoothly only as long as the stagehands are doing their job. Estrogen and progesterone are like those unheralded stagehands: You don't appreciate all they do for you until they stop doing it.

Of these two hormones, estrogen is the most influential in causing the changes we will be discussing in this book. A woman's lifetime peak of estrogen production is reached at age twenty-seven to twenty-eight. Then a faintly declining plateau is maintained until about thirty-five. Although there is a slight decline in the plateau years, there is always sufficient estrogen to fully support your body. After age thirty-five, though, the average amount of estrogen production per menstrual cycle begins to decline sufficiently to produce subtle changes in your body. Each of these changes makes its individual appearance without relation to the others. Figure 1.1 shows the approximate timeline for the appearance of various perimenopausal symptoms.

Ultimately, there may be more than one such change taking place simultaneously. For the most part they are individually manageable; but for some women (perhaps 20 percent), the sum of the changes can make coping with them very difficult. These women's symptoms are severe enough to disrupt their everyday functioning in important spheres such as marriage, occupation, and relationships with children, parents, coworkers, and friends.

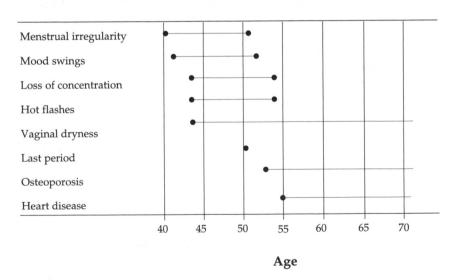

Age

Adapted from: Nancy Lee Teaff and Kim Wright. 1996. *Perimenopause: Preparing for the Change*. Rocklin, Calif.: Prima Publishing

Figure 1.1. Approximate Timeline for Perimenopausal Symptoms

Figure 1.2 demonstrates your estrogen level at various ages. It first declines in only the second half of your cycle, after ovulation (Eskin 1995). But estrogen output in the first half of your cycle remains sufficient to cause ovulation for many more years. The decline is not a landslide. You will not suddenly (nor need you ever) become the stereotypic "little old lady." In your forties, estrogen production fluctuates, but the overall pattern is one of accelerating decline. By ages fifty-one to fifty-two, female hormone output is minimal. This book is about those fifteen years from age thirty-five to fifty, and a few years beyond.

Boomers Are Perimenopausal

You are not alone in this period of life. You are part of the mighty "baby boomer" generation born after World War II, between 1946 and 1964. Seventy-six million babies were born in the United States during those years, 38 million of you are women, and about 30 million of you are perimenopausal. According to a widely reported 1995 study by the National Council on the Aging (Graham 1995), the first "boomer" turned fifty on January 1, 1996. The youngest of your generation turned thirty-five in 1999. Your boomer cohorts are entering and completing their transitional years at the rate of about 2 million women per year. Not only is yours the largest group of American women ever to pass through this stage of life, it is also the most inquisitive, the most energetic, and the most vocal.

Your generation is not content to accept things as they are simply because that's the way they have always been. For example, you changed birthing methods in the U.S. by advocating natural childbirth with fathers in attendance, making it a family event. Our culture has come to understand that you will demand and expect to receive accurate information about

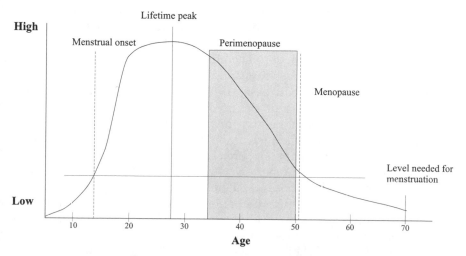

Figure 1.2. Estrogen Levels by Age

whatever interests you or confronts you. For this reason, the expectation is that you will more likely change your transitional years than be changed by them. As always, you first need up-to-date, accurate information about your potential changes; then you can unleash your collective imagination and energy to deal with these changes in innovative ways. If this book furthers that ability, it will have been wildly successful.

An Overview of Change

This chapter provides you with a general description of what happens during these years, how it happens, and the role of hormone diminution in causing changes. This is a normal process in every woman—no exceptions. There is plenty you can do, however, to control these changes. The medical term for these transitional years is perimenopause, which means the period of time leading up to, and the period of time just after, menopause. Menopause itself refers to a point in time: the first anniversary of your last menstrual period. Postmenopause refers to the years of life following menopause.

Perimenopausal symptoms and the effects of declining hormones begin in your mid-thirties. The changes, mostly after age forty, include irregular menstrual cycles, menstrual flow variability, hot flashes, fragmented sleep, mood swings, short-term memory loss, unexplained fatigue, diminished sexual desire, and others. These symptoms develop gradually—they don't suddenly grab you one morning as you step out of the shower. If you are attuned to your body rhythms, you may be able to detect the very subtle changes that are taking place.

What is the significance of these changed body rhythms and feelings, and what should you do about them? Your initial response might be to ignore them or to deny the possibility that they are a result of hormone decline. If you do seek advice, you may find that your doctor knows little more than you about these changes; and, if you are still having menstrual periods, your doctor may not recognize that your hot flashes, fatigue, and sleep disruptions might be from hormone depletion. Therefore your responsibility is to educate yourself about the transitional years and the biological markers you may experience. The more you do, the easier it will be to find a health-care adviser who can help you during this phase of your life. Then, you and your doctor can work together to smooth the way for your transitional years.

Postmenopause is now known as the time when women become vulnerable to heart disease, osteoporosis, breast cancer, mental decline, and other conditions. A burgeoning number of methods for relieving symptoms of estrogen loss and reducing the associated health risks have burst upon the scene in the past decade. Drug companies, supplement manufacturers, and researchers of all stripes are working overtime to provide new approaches. The question for you as a transitional woman is: "Which method is best—or best for me?" The list of choices is a lengthy one, but it certainly begins with estrogen. We cover most of the other choices later in the book.

The Ovary Connection

To help you better understand the topics covered in this book, let's take a look at some anatomy and a little physiology. (Wait! Don't slam the book shut. It will be in plain language, and it won't take long.)

The Anatomy

By the time a female fetus is twenty weeks old, her ovaries contain about 7 million egg follicles (Speroff 1989). Over the remainder of intrauterine life, the growing ovaries gradually push the surface follicles out of the ovaries into the abdominal cavity, and they disintegrate. At birth, a baby girl has about 2 million follicles left. This number continues to diminish so that at puberty, about 400,000 remain. Does it worry you that this may not be enough? It turns out that it's plenty. The rate of loss slows from an average of 250,000 follicles per week during fetal life to about 2,500 per week in childhood, and after puberty it is less than 1,000 per month. A woman ovulates only 400 to 500 times during the childbearing years, so the numbers work out okay.

Each month, several hundred follicles are readied to release an egg. Usually only one is released at ovulation, and the rest of the follicles shrink away. Occasionally, of course, multiple ovulations take place, producing a multiple pregnancy. Humans are not well designed for litters, however, and single egg release is the usual result. By the mid-thirties and beyond, the number of follicles will have diminished sufficiently to result in a decreased ability to produce estrogen and progesterone, the female sex hormones. As this process continues, perimenopausal changes begin and the ability to achieve a successful pregnancy declines.

Menopause is ultimately reached by about age fifty-one, at which time the childbearing years of life are concluded. Clearly, it is not a sudden process. In fact, in light of the inexorable decrease of ovarian follicles culminating in menopause, one might make the case that the approach to menopause begins in fetal life!

The Physiology

Alphabet Soup	
GnRH	Gonadotropin releasing hormone
FSH	Follicle stimulating hormone
LH	Leuteinizing hormone (LH)

To understand the changes of perimenopause, it is important to know how the ovarian cycle, or menstrual cycle, works. Then it becomes easier to understand what happens when it doesn't work. The cycle is really sort of a daisy chain, as you can see in Figure 1.3. The chain involves three hormone-producing glands:

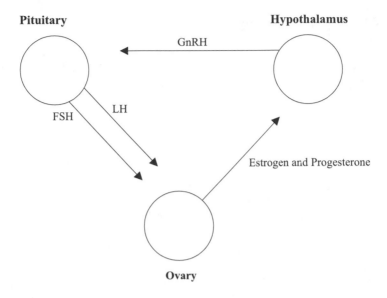

Figure 1.3. Ovarian Cycle

- The hypothalamus, in the brain

- The pituitary, in the brain

- The ovaries, in the pelvis

These glands work in concert with each other. Each produces hormones that are recognized by the other two. The hormones act as chemical messengers that are carried to their targets by your bloodstream. Some of these hormones influence the ovarian cycle.

We need to start our discussion somewhere in the cycle, so let's enter it at the end of a menstrual period, after the uterine lining has been shed. At this point, your ovaries are producing low levels of estrogen and progesterone, as the chart shown in Figure 1.4 demonstrates. The hypothalamus detects this and sends a hormone called gonadotropin releasing hormone (GnRH) to the pituitary. In response, the pituitary releases two hormones that target the ovaries: follicle stimulating hormone (FSH) and leuteinizing hormone (LH). FSH stimulates the ovaries to do two things: start producing more estrogen (which, among other things, rebuilds the lining of the uterus) and get some follicles ready for ovulation. At midcycle, estrogen reaches a critical level, which triggers a sudden surge of LH from the pituitary; this causes ovulation.

After the follicle has released its egg, it turns into a structure called the corpus luteum, which manufactures progesterone. Progesterone increases the blood supply in the uterine lining and fills the glands of the lining with glycogen (a sugar). This prepares the lining of the uterus for receiving and nourishing a fertilized egg.

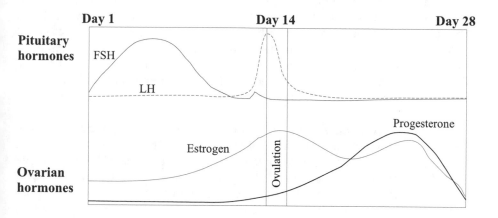

Figure 1.4. Hormone Levels in Menstrual Cycle

At this point, the bloodstream contains high levels of estrogen and pro-gesterone. In response, the hypothalamus reduces the GnRH level, signaling the pituitary to cut back on FSH and LH. This in turn causes the ovaries to de-crease estrogen and progesterone production. The net result is that, once again, the bloodstream contains a low level of female hormones. The lining of the uterus is no longer supported by hormones, and it is shed—in other words, a menstrual period occurs. Then the cycle, which usually takes about four weeks, begins again.

Diagnosis of Perimenopause

As we mentioned earlier in this chapter, if you are still having menstrual peri-ods, you may find it hard to believe that hormone depletion may be causing the symptoms you've been having (hot flashes, moodiness, short-term mem-ory loss, vaginal dryness)—and equally hard to have this confirmed by a doc-tor. There are steps you can take, though, to ensure proper diagnosis and treatment of the symptoms you experience during the transitional years.

Get Smart: Educate Yourself

Health care in the U.S. today is less personalized than it used to be, and it has become increasingly important for people to become more personally involved in maintaining their own wellness. The responsibility for initiating certain procedures, such as screening exams, falls more and more into the in-dividual's own hands.

Diagnosing perimenopause (or any other altered body state, for that matter) is a process that you can actually initiate by becoming aware that a change has taken place in your body. We're not talking about an occasional change in menstrual flow or timing, occasionally tender breasts, excess fluid retention, or an increase in skin blemishes; variations of this type are normal. What we are talking about is an awareness of a persistent and recurring change—you can look back over recent cycles and realize that they are different from those in prior years.

The more you know about your body, the better able you are to observe these changes. An important aspect of educating yourself is becoming aware of your personal risk factors for particular health problems. How you live your life, what foods you eat, how well you exercise, the toxins to which you are exposed, preexisting conditions, and in some cases inheritance, can play major roles in your current and future health. For example, if you are a smoker, then cancer, heart disease, and osteoporosis may all be part of your future. Also, try to find out as much as you can about your family's health history, which can provide further clues to your own risk factors. The risk factors you identify for yourself can help decide the kinds of screening tests you might need, and their frequency. The goal, of course, is to avoid illness or to treat it early. (Specific risk factors for heart disease, osteoporosis, and cancer are covered in Chapters 4 and 6).

Arrange for a complete physical exam, which is also important to helping you understand your body. The exam should include your height, weight, blood pressure, head (including eyes, mouth, throat, ears), neck (including thyroid, lymph glands, blood vessels), chest, breasts, armpits with lymph glands, heart, abdomen, pelvic exam with rectal, extremities, pulses, skin, and neurological. A complete exam is a must for your first visit to the doctor you choose; but if you are in good health in your transitional years, it isn't necessary to have a complete exam every year.

Testing Hormone Levels

Until recently, doctors often tested women for follicle stimulating hormone (FSH) to determine whether their ovaries were producing enough estrogen. FSH testing was based on the knowledge that in menopausal women, the FSH level is high because of low production of estrogen. The pituitary gland is sending out high levels of FSH in an effort to get the failing ovaries to produce more estrogen. The problem with FSH testing in perimenopausal women, however, is that estrogen production may wax and wane from one month to the next, so consistent results are not possible. For this reason, most doctors no longer rely on FSH blood levels to diagnose perimenopause. What other options are there?

One option, advocated by leading experts in the field, is to do a clinical test: to give you a trial dose of a hormone supplement. If your perimenopausal symptoms are improved, you are on the right track. If not, you and your doctor need to look elsewhere for a cause of the changes you are experiencing, such as thyroid abnormalities, ovarian disease, or perhaps stressful events in your life. Some women are now opting to use low-dose birth control pills during their entire perimenopause. In this way, they can control perimenopausal symptoms, help prevent long-term problems such as heart disease and osteoporosis, and prevent pregnancy.

CAUTION! If you have abnormal uterine bleeding, it must not be treated with hormones unless it is clearly established that you do not have uterine disease. (Chapter 14 covers this topic in detail.)

Biological Markers of Perimenopause

Let's take a look at the changes in body function and behavior, as well as the cognitive changes, that may arise for you in the transitional years. There is enormous variation among women in terms of which of these symptoms they experience, and to what degree. Some of them may seem unpleasant, and some of them can even be threatening to your health. Throughout this book, you'll find ways of managing the troublesome changes.

Ovarian Slowdown

At birth, a female infant has all the eggs (ova) she will ever have. (This is in contrast to males, who manufacture new sperm throughout life.) Each egg in the ovary is contained in a structure called a follicle. Female sex hormones, estrogen and progesterone, are produced by the cells of the follicle walls. As egg release (ovulation) takes place on a monthly basis, your follicles gradually diminish in number. This reduction begins to be noticeable after age thirty-five in a measurable decrease in average monthly hormone production (Eskin 1995). The reduction proceeds over about fifteen years to an eventual point at which not enough hormones are produced to cause menstrual periods; they cease entirely (menopause). Menopause doesn't just pop up at age fifty-one or so. It is a process that has its beginnings in the mid-thirties as the result of the natural aging of the reproductive system. The reduced estrogen availability has an enormous influence on your body and the way it functions. For example, a woman forty years old may have difficulty becoming pregnant because the eggs her ovaries supply are also forty years old and may have lost some of their reproductive efficacy.

Menstrual Cycle and Menstrual Period Changes

Changes in your menstrual cycle and menstrual period can vary tremendously. Cycles may become longer or shorter or fall into a "no pattern" pattern. Menstrual bleeding may be heavier or lighter, more prolonged or shorter, or entirely absent. Variable and declining hormone production is the cause.

TIP! Keeping a menstrual calendar is a great help in determining what may be happening to your cycles. Just mark each day you have bleeding with an L, N, or H for light, normal, or heavy, and S for spotting.

CAUTION! A menstrual pattern in which the cycle is shortened to fewer than twenty days from the first day of one period to the first day of the next is abnormal and may signal a disease in your endometrium (the lining of your uterus). In this situation, an endometrial biopsy should be done—an office procedure in which a thin, flexible canula (hollow tube) is inserted into the uterus to remove a sample of tissue for microscopic examination. Menstrual abnormalities are discussed in detail in Chapter 14.

Hot Flashes

Decreased estrogen availability changes the heat release and heat conservation mechanisms in your body. This results in flushing in your upper body, head, and neck. Doctors call it a flush and professors call it vasomotor instability; but women with this symptom call it like it is: a hot flash! You may hear yourself making comments like these: "My makeup felt like it was raised about an inch off my face." "The first course was cold gazpacho, and yet there I sat sweating like I had jogged to the dinner party." Yes, they're hot flashes, and hot flash is the term we use in this book.

About 75 percent of American women experience hot flashes in the perimenopausal-postmenopausal years (Kronenberg 1994). They can start as early as the late thirties for some, but they are more common after the mid-forties. Following menopause, hot flashes recede in three to four years to infrequent occurrences, although the duration in years of hot flashes varies widely.

What Is a Hot Flash, Anyway?

Hot flashes occur when the blood vessels in your skin dilate and bring large amounts of blood to the surface. This makes your skin red during a hot flash. Your body has a heat release and heat conservation mechanism. For example, in cold weather, when you are in a heat conservation mode, these surface vessels constrict to keep blood deeper inside your body, and your skin looks paler; in hot weather, your vessels dilate to help get rid of the heat. A hot flash occurs when this conservation/release system gets off-kilter and the vessels dilate even though it isn't necessary to get rid of any heat. Everyone else around you may be quite comfortable, but you are sweating buckets.

A typical hot flash lasts thirty seconds to several minutes. It is preceded by an aura of about a minute—you may experience a sense of anxiety or dread, plus a stepped-up heart rate and a feeling of weakness. This phase is caused by a release of adrenaline. The aura is soon followed by sudden dilation of your skin's surface vessels over your upper body, head, and neck. The increased blood flow may raise skin temperature (not body temperature) by up to 7 degrees. This is when the skin becomes reddened. Then comes profuse sweating, which can melt your hairstyle, run your eyeliner, and ruin your new sheer blouse. Air movement across your skin (such as fanning yourself with the menu or rolling down the car window) starts evaporation of the abundant skin moisture. Evaporation itself is a cooling process, and now you may actually get a chill. Complete recovery can take up to half an hour.

What Causes Hot Flashes?

The hypothalamus, introduced earlier in this chapter, is your body's thermostat. It is aided by the autonomic nervous system (ANS), which controls blood vessel dilation and constriction. The hypothalamus requires estrogen to function properly. Scientists believe the lack of estrogen disturbs the usual smooth coordination between the hypothalamus and the ANS, the two temperature regulators. In the absence of adequate estrogen, the hypothalamus changes its set point, and this signals the ANS to throw open those surface blood vessels and release some heat. It may not be the right time for you to be a heat exchanger, but the hypothalamus did not receive its estrogen "fix," and that made it get crazy. Well, there you are. It's estrogen again.

How Bad or Frequent Are Hot Flashes?

For most women, hot flashes are, at worst, unpleasant, inconvenient, and easily tolerated. However, as Kronenberg reported in 1993, 10 to 15 percent of women find hot flashes to be a debilitating influence on their lives. The intensity and frequency of hot flashes devastate these women.

Hot flashes can range in frequency from one to four per day or night. As a matter of fact, hot flashes most commonly occur at night. This seems to be related to the fact that the hypothalamus is involved in fewer regulatory functions during sleep. With less estrogen available and some free time, it seems to start fiddling with the thermostat, permitting the ANS to cause a hot flash. Guess what that does to your sleep? You may wake up with your hair wet, your pillow soaked, the covers thrown back, and your partner wondering what the devil all the thrashing around is about. Chronic sleep deprivation from nighttime hot flashes is widely regarded as the primary cause of irritability, moodiness, fatigue, short-term memory loss, and other common perimenopausal changes.

TIP! If you are on HRT (hormone replacement therapy), try taking your estrogen at bedtime. Many women find that the improved estrogen level during sleep prevents or substantially diminishes their hot flashes. You can call this a "hot tip."

Hot Flashes and Brain Function

Hot flashes may harm your brain by permanently damaging neurons (brain cells). A study by Phillips and Sherman looked at women who had a hysterectomy and removal of both ovaries (Phillips 1992). They found a 60 percent decrease in verbal memory and learning test scores in those women who suffered severe hot flashes, which could not be explained by postoperative depression, anxiety, or insomnia. It is hypothesized that loss of estrogen results in a decrease in the transport of glucose into the hippocampus area of the brain, where memory function resides. Your brain uses more glucose (sugar) than any other organ.

Another study found that women who took estrogen for hot flashes for more than one year experienced a dramatic delay in the onset of Alzheimer's disease. This was true even though estrogen use had been twenty to thirty years earlier. This further suggests that severe hot flashes may permanently damage neurons (Tang 1996).

What Can You Do about Hot Flashes?

Many things can help you control hot flashes, including:

- Replacing the estrogen

- Exercising

- Using alternative medical remedies

- Avoiding trigger situations

The simplest and quickest solution is to go after the basic cause: replace the estrogen you lack. Estrogen replacement reliably relieves hot flashes in one to four weeks. (See Chapter 7 for a full discussion of the various estrogen preparations and their routes of administration.)

Exercise helps control hot flashes. A brisk walk can be helpful during a hot flash. This isn't a particularly convenient means to deal with it if it's 3:00 A.M. when your hot flash engulfs you, so regular aerobic exercise for thirty to forty-five minutes, three to four times weekly, is a more sensible routine. (See Chapter 9 for a discussion of effective exercise techniques.)

Many women are reporting favorable results from alternative medical remedies. These include homeopathic remedies, herbs, acupuncture, mind/body techniques, and holistic approaches. (See Chapter 8 for details.)

Avoiding situations that trigger hot flashes can be helpful. A big meal is a common source, because digestion brings large amounts of blood into the abdomen. This raises your core body temperature, and your hypothalamus reacts accordingly. Other situations to consider are hot weather, overheated rooms, overdressing, too many blankets, hot tubs, hot drinks, spicy foods, alcohol, and stress. If you are underweight, you may have more hot flashes. This is because a weak form of estrogen, called estrone, is made from body fat.

Reduced Stamina

It is most commonly women who are not fit to begin with who experience reduced stamina in the transitional years. A decrease in muscle tone and strength bears a direct relationship to a woman's diet and how much she exercises.

Changes in the Skin, Vagina, and Hair

The most common time for changes in the skin, vagina, and hair is after the mid-forties. With lessened estrogen, natural secretions diminish, and tissues become thinner and drier than they had been. Atrophy is the medical term for these changes; it refers to the loss of tissue in any part of the body as a result of diminished tissue nutrition. In the transitional years, the tissues most likely to show atrophic change are the skin and mucous membranes, including the face, neck, chest, hair, vagina, and bladder. Diminished natural secretions result in thinning and drying of these tissues, causing wrinkles, loss of luster in hair, lessened vaginal lubrication, and urinary tract infections. Eighty percent of skin damage occurs from sun exposure before you are eighteen years old, but estrogen loss and smoking also accelerate wrinkling. Chapter 13 deals with skin changes.

Premenstrual Syndrome (PMS) May Worsen

If PMS symptoms worsen, it is usually in the late thirties and early forties. Some women develop PMS for the first time in their late forties. PMS usually disappears about the time of menopause. Chapter 3 presents a full discussion of perimenopausal PMS.

Cognitive Changes

Estrogen receptors exist throughout the brain. A receptor site is much like a lock-and-key arrangement. An estrogen molecule (the key) fits only into a receptor site (the lock) that is specifically designed for it. When an estrogen molecule is plugged into a cell receptor site, it directs the cell to perform certain metabolic functions that benefit you. If these receptors don't get their regular supply of estrogen, they can cause wide swings in emotional responses, including transitory episodes of moodiness, short-term memory loss, unexplained sadness, decreased sexual desire, and lessened ability to concentrate. To understand how these symptoms occur, let's take a look at how the brain works.

Neurotransmitters

Brain cells are called neurons. Each neuron is capable of receiving messages from millions upon millions of other cells The messages, or electrical impulses, travel along the nerve fiber of a neuron to its end point, or synapse. A synapse is the connecting point with other nerves. It's like a junction. For the message to cross the synapse to an adjacent neuron and continue along its way, neurotransmitter chemicals are necessary. There are many neurotransmitters, but the main three are norepinephrine, dopamine, and serotonin. Each of them is produced in the neuron and is stored inside the neuron near the synapse. When your brain is sending a message (such as "Take your finger off that hot stove"), a nerve cell generates the impulse and releases a neurotransmitter to transport the impulse across the synapse. On the other side of the synapse, the neurotransmitter molecule plugs into a receptor on the next nerve cell and passes the impulse along. This process continues from nerve cell to nerve cell until the message gets to its destination (in this example, your hand, and you move that toasty finger). Every cell has multiple receptors, so one cell can receive and transmit multiple impulses. After the message has been sent, the neurotransmitter is reabsorbed by the brain cell to await the next transmission job.

By their presence or absence, certain chemicals, including hormones like estrogen, can influence the ability of the receiving cell to pick up the message being sent. The message can get garbled if estrogen receptors on the cell are not well supplied. Do you see where this is leading? If your brain doesn't get its normal allotment of estrogen, it's going to be out of sorts and start sending some strange messages, or maybe no messages at all. This changes brain function, and especially mood.

Moods

During perimenopause, you may feel helpless to control your mood swings. It's as though someone else is inside you pulling the levers and you can do nothing but watch yourself respond in out-of-character ways. Perhaps you burst into tears when the paper deliverer throws the newspaper into the birdbath again, or you cancel an entire appointment because it's going to start ten minutes late. These changes from your usual demeanor can be frustrating and embarrassing. Fortunately, changes like these are not a constant, everyday thing; they come and go. For many, the fluctuations are not severe at all. Perhaps you simply feel on edge and have a sense that you are not coping as well as you used to. Don't worry—none of these are signs of mental illness.

TIP! Your moods, and the frequency of their changes, are not entirely in your control. Hormonal fluctuation is at the root of it. Talk to your family and others close to you about your mood swings. You can ask them not to confront you with divisive issues when one of these moods is upon you, but to wait until your equanimity has returned. Then a productive discussion will be possible.

Memory

In her landmark book *The Silent Passage*, Gail Sheehy put it well when she said, "At forty you can't read the numbers in the phone book. At fifty you can't remember them." Short-term memory loss isn't a disaster. You won't need to start wearing a wristband with your address on it so someone can take you home. It's little things that get away from you, like forgetting your point halfway through a scintillating conversation. Vocabulary selection becomes labored as you struggle to bring just the right word to your narrative. Thinking gets slower, logic gets fuzzy, and if it isn't on your list of things to do, it doesn't get done. Dr. Barbara Sherwin published a study showing that estrogen deficiency is linked to changes in memory, as well as mood and sexual function (1996). Disturbed sleep resulting from nighttime hot flashes may be a major contributor to short-term memory loss. Campbell and Whitehead reported in an elegant study (1977) that hot flashes caused sleep disruption, and sleep deprivation triggered short-term memory loss, fatigue, irritability, diminished sexual desire, and mood swings. When estrogen was supplemented, the hot flashes disappeared, sleep improved, and a domino effect took over, with improvement in all the other parameters of change. Campbell and Whitehead found that taking estrogen at night was most beneficial in controlling hot flashes.

There are other steps you can take to enhance your memory:

- Eat a balanced diet in smaller meals and at regular intervals. This keeps a steadier flow of nutrients to your brain.

- Do aerobic exercise four to five times per week. Several studies have demonstrated that exercise improves memory and learning ability in all age groups. This is especially true if the activity involves complex movement, such as aerobic dancing as opposed to aerobic walking, but both work.

- Stop smoking. Brain oxygenation will be improved. (Smoking can also cause an earlier menopause and therefore an earlier perimenopause.)

- Eliminate or reduce alcohol. Ever had so much you couldn't remember how much you had?

- Get enough sleep, and don't use sleeping pills. (You may need to wean yourself from a sleeping pill habit.)

- Challenge your brain by learning a new skill or examining new ideas. Brain exercise with new learning has been shown to increase the actual number of connections between nerve cells.

Osteoporosis

Loss of bone mineral density, and therefore bone strength, is a well-proven result of estrogen loss. Other factors, such as a poor diet, lack of exercise, and smoking, also contribute to a deteriorating skeleton, but the cornerstone for prevention is estrogen supplementation. Osteoporosis tends to be a postmenopausal event. Nonetheless, developing a sturdy skeleton before you reach midlife may prevent this crippling and potentially life-threatening problem. (Chapter 4 deals with the prevention of osteoporosis.)

Cardiovascular Disease (CVD)

It is important to point out that heart disease is the number one cause of death for women between the ages of fifty and seventy-five. It may surprise you to learn that heart attack deaths are twelve times more common than breast cancer deaths (American Heart Association 1997). A major goal for you in the transitional years of life is to find out how to maintain cardiovascular fitness. (See Chapter 4 for a complete discussion of heart disease.)

Thyroid Problems

The thyroid requires estrogen to function normally. A lack of estrogen can lead to underactive thyroid hormone production (hypothyroidism). This condition can leave you feeling weak and lethargic, depressed and moody. If your thyroid is found to be sluggish and you are transitional, your estrogen production may be at the root of it. (Chapter 5 discusses thyroid diseases in detail.)

Decreased Sexual Desire

Decreased sexual desire can occur during the transitional years. The good news is that you may not experience any loss of sexual desire The bad news is that you might. Sexuality is a complex issue with diverse origins and influences. Changes in any of them are capable of altering your sexual desire, including relationship problems, lifestyle excesses, self-esteem issues, and hormone loss.

Sexuality is also influenced by the responsiveness of your genital anatomy. Inadequate sexual lubrication, a chronically dry vagina, and diminished clitoral sensitivity all have a dampening effect on sexual activity. These changes are a direct result of inadequate estrogen and respond well to estrogen replacement. Vaginal dryness with painful sex and clitoral insensitivity typically make their appearance late in your transitional years but you may notice diminished sexual lubrication in your early forties. (See Chapter 12 for a full discussion of sexual issues during the transitional years.)

Urinary Incontinence

Involuntary loss of urine is a common problem during the transition. Somebody tells a devastatingly funny joke, and there you are laughing like the others, but with wet pants. You urge your partner to stop the car at the very next available restroom because you really "gotta go," but you can feel urine leaking out as you scurry across the parking lot. How frustrating. You have just emptied your bladder; but upon returning to your guests and sitting down on the couch, some more urine squirts out! Doctors call these three conditions stress incontinence, urge incontinence, and intrinsic sphincter deficiency incontinence. Each has its own root cause, but a contributing factor they all have in common is loss of estrogen. (They are covered in Chapter 14.)

Your Hormones Are Down a Little—Should You Worry?

You may be wondering why generations of women before yours didn't worry about perimenopausal symptoms. One reason was that relatively little was known about menopause, and the term perimenopause was not even used until the late 1970s or early 1980s. Menopause was neither a topic of conversation nor a subject of research.

Another reason is that prior to the twentieth century, women often did not live very long after the childbearing years. In the last hundred years or so, though, women have been living longer, thanks to improvements in childbirth safety. Better nutrition, sanitation, medical care, housing, clothing, work savers, and accident prevention have all contributed, but surviving childbirth has been the real reason women are living longer. The current life expectancy for American women is just over eighty years.

What hasn't changed, however, is the age at which female hormones decline. It has been happening in a woman's forties for many centuries, and it still is. For American women, the average age of menopause is 51.4. (The age differs in other cultures.) The simple arithmetic is that women now live more than one-third of their lives after their childbearing role is completed. For many, this is a forty-year span. Staying healthy during these years takes some advance planning and preparation.

Planning and Preparation

During the transitional years of perimenopause, you have a good shot at keeping the balance of your life healthy and enjoyable. If you don't have to have hot flashes, moodiness, and short-term memory loss, why put up with them? Granted, these symptoms are not life threats, and they will subside in a few years even if you do nothing. Still, controlling or eliminating these symptoms can improve your quality of life. In addition, you now have an opportunity to prevent or modify your risk for a few more ominous problems that can plague significant portions of the second half of your life.

With the help of your health consultant, you can follow a proactive program of prevention ranging from hormone replacement, to lifestyle changes, to use of alternative medical remedies, to more aggressive preventive care, including screening techniques and a fitness program. Life is a journey, so why not enjoy the trip?

Table 1.1. Symptoms and Signs of Estrogen Loss	
Irregular periods	Hot flashes
Mood swings	Fragmented sleep
Short-term memory loss	Difficulty concentrating
Irritability	Anxiety
Minor depression	Skin dryness
Wrinkling	Reduced sexual lubrication
Vaginal dryness	Decreased sexual desire
Reduced muscle tone	Reduced stamina
Constipation	Recurrent urinary tract infection
Breast sag	Eye dryness
Underactive thyroid	Osteoporosis
Rise in cholesterol	Beginning risk of heart disease

Hormone Replacement—The Easy Part

If the primary cause of perimenopausal change is fluctuating and decreased estrogen production, hormone replacement therapy (HRT) is a logical option for dealing with it. There has been much debate in recent years on the appropriateness of this form of management. Certainly, there are risks in using HRT, but there are also risks in failing to do so. Take a look at Table 1.1, which lists the changes caused by estrogen loss through the transitional years and beyond. This a daunting list of potential problems, but you may experience few or none of them. The point of Table 1.1 is to demonstrate that estrogen is widely utilized throughout your body, and that HRT is not recommended solely for the relief of symptoms that are not health threats. Estrogen levels affect your entire body, and reduction of this hormone changes the way your body looks and operates.

Be aware that a variety of not-as-yet mainstream alternative treatment modalities other than HRT are available for perimenopausal changes. Some, like Chinese herbal medicine, predate Western medicine by many centuries. Many perimenopausal changes are considerably helped by these alternative remedies, but unfortunately, there is a scarcity of information from the scientific community as to their safety and effectiveness. Homeopathy, Chinese herbal medicine, acupuncture, holistic medicine, and mind/body medicine are discussed in Chapter 8.

Lifestyle Changes—The Hard Part

You might think at this point that all you need is to load up on hormone replacement and go merrily on with your life. Alas, there is much more to maintaining good health and vitality than HRT. These are the major issues:

- **Fitness:** Becoming fit has been embraced by boomers as by no other generation of Americans. In Chapter 9 you will learn about diet and exercise, the two major components of fitness—be sure not to skip that chapter!

- **Stress management:** In our culture of busy individuals and two-income families, stress management is of signal importance to us all. Stress may be magnified during your perimenopausal transition, so it is helpful for you to know how to deal with it. When poorly controlled, stress takes a serious toll on relationships important to you—those with your partner, children, coworkers, relatives, and friends—and it takes its toll on your body as well. Chapter 11 provides a discussion on a variety of ways to manage stress.

- **Alcohol, tobacco, and other deleterious drugs:** Lifestyle choices that include use of harmful drugs may contribute to many of the adverse perimenopausal changes. Chapter 10 takes a look at why these substances can harm you.

Summary

Consider carefully the forty or so years ahead of you. How well you prepare for the second half of life may be the most important quality-of-life consideration you will ever undertake. The balance of this book is devoted to showing you how to prepare yourself.

○ ○ ○ ○

2

Changes in Fertility: Pregnancy, Infertility, and Contraception

This chapter is about pregnancy. It's for those of you who will, those of you who won't, and those of you who can't have children during the transitional years. First we take a look at the special risks of having a baby when you are over thirty-five and what you can do to eliminate or minimize these risks. Then we talk about why you may not be able to get pregnant as you approach the end of your reproductive life. We examine the causes of difficulty in conceiving and the variety of fertility aids available when you can't get pregnant. The final part of the chapter is for women who don't want to have babies during the transitional years. We discuss the contraceptive methods now available, as well as the pros and cons of choosing each.

Alphabet Soup	
CVS	Chorionic villus sampling
FAS	Fetal alcohol syndrome
HBV	Hepatitis B virus
NTD	Neural tube defect
STD	Sexually transmitted disease

Pregnancy

Twenty years ago a new mother of thirty-five would be encouraged to have her tubes tied, especially if the delivery was a cesarean. Today, attitudes have changed and many women over thirty-five are choosing to have children.

They delay marriage and then establish their careers before considering a family. Some don't finish their families until they are in their early forties. What has happened that makes being pregnant at thirty-five okay today, when it was not okay twenty years ago?

The major difference today is the safety and reliability of fetal diagnosis (Rose 1994). The chances of your having an abnormal child today are the same as they were fifty years ago (Cuckle 1987). The difference is that now doctors can diagnose most of these abnormalities during pregnancy, and you can make a decision about whether to continue the pregnancy. These choices give women freedom that wasn't possible in their parents' day.

Abnormal Pregnancies

Every year you age increases the risk of an abnormal pregnancy. For example, if you are over forty, the chance of miscarriage increases to almost 50 percent (Asch 1993). The risk of bearing a child with trisomy (Down syndrome, which we explain in a moment) also increases. An abnormal egg usually causes these abnormalities. Every cell in your body except your eggs contains forty-six chromosomes (the components of the cell nucleus that contain genes). Genes determine your various body characteristics, such as eye and hair color. Your forty-six chromosomes are pairs, with twenty-three from your father's sperm cell and twenty-three from your mother's egg. The chromosomes are separate until ovulation occurs. Then the chromosomes from your parents intertwine, exchanging genetic material before splitting apart. An egg cell begins with forty-six chromosomes, but at ovulation, it discards twenty-three of them. The twenty-three remaining chromosomes contain genes from both your mother and your father. Your egg is now ready to receive the sperm, which has gone through a similar process of discarding twenty-three of its chromosomes. As you age, though, variations can occur, resulting in an egg with an extra chromosome (twenty-four instead of twenty-three), and the fertilized egg develops into an embryo with forty-seven chromosomes. This condition is called trisomy. Trisomy is always due to an extra chromosome from the egg. Sperm containing more than twenty-three chromosomes can't swim, and if they can't swim, they can't penetrate an egg.

Most trisomies are incompatible with life. An exception, and the best known of these conditions, is trisomy 21, or Down syndrome. Down syndrome occurs in younger mothers when extra genes from chromosome 21 attach to another chromosome. In older women, two number 21 chromosomes in the egg combine with one 21 chromosome in the sperm cell. The child born with this syndrome has mental retardation, a sweet personality, and a distinctive facial structure, as well as heart and bowel problems. As you get older, your risk of bearing a child with Down syndrome increases, as you can see in Table 2.1 (Cuckle 1987, Palomali 1995). Eighty percent of Down syndrome babies are born to women under age thirty-five (American College of

Obstetricians and Gynecologists 1991), while women over thirty-five account for fewer than 10 percent of all pregnancies. However, they account for 20 percent of all cases of Down syndrome.

Table 2.1 Risk of Down Syndrome By Age	
Age	**Risk**
20	1 in 1,353
25	1 in 1,196
30	1 in 802
35	1 in 340
40	1 in 99
42	1 in 57
44	1 in 33
45	1 in 25
46	1 in 18
48	1 in 9
50	1 in 5

Adapted from: Cuckle 1987; Palomali 1995

Single Gene Abnormalities

Unlike trisomies, most single gene abnormalities, such as hemophilia, cannot be detected before birth. Rarely, a specific family history will alert doctors to a possible single gene abnormality. Then the geneticist looks for a specific fetal chemical change to make the diagnosis. Trisomy has been linked to older mothers, but single gene abnormalities have been linked to older fathers. (Finally, there is something they can't blame on women!)

Abnormal Pregnancies Not Related to Age

Abnormal pregnancies in women of all ages can also result from neural tube defects (NTDs), viral infections, and other conditions. Starting prenatal vitamins containing 0.4 to 0.8 milligrams of folic acid before you get pregnant markedly reduces your risk of having a baby with a neural tube defect (Centers for Disease Control 1997; Perlow 1999). The risk of these abnormalities does not appear to increase in perimenopause.

Testing for Abnormal Pregnancies

Let's take a look at some tests your doctor can perform to diagnose an abnormal pregnancy.

Amniocentesis and Chorionic Villus Sampling (CVS)

Trisomies may be diagnosed through an amniocentesis, which involves testing the amniotic fluid (the liquid surrounding the growing fetus). Or a chorionic villus sampling (CVS), which examines placental tissue. Both tests are offered to women who will be thirty-five or older when they give birth.

In an amniocentesis, a thin needle is passed through the abdominal wall, into the uterus, and into the amniotic sac containing the fetus. A small amount of amniotic fluid is sent to a laboratory, where the fetal cells are cultured for Down syndrome, other chromosomal abnormalities, and NTDs. These abnormalities can almost always be detected by an amniocentesis. Amniocentesis is done between the fifteenth and twentieth weeks of pregnancy. Pregnancy loss from the procedure is about 1 in 200.

An amniocentesis is not recommended until after age thirty-five, when the risk for giving birth to a baby with Down syndrome exceeds the risk of the test. An amniocentesis costs between $1,000 and $1,500, but most insurance policies pay for the test (California Department of Health Services 1995).

CVS is done between the tenth and twelfth weeks of pregnancy, and the placental cells are obtained by passing a needle through the lower abdomen or through the cervix. The placental cells, which have the same chromosomal makeup as the fetus, are then grown and examined for abnormalities. With CVS, Down syndrome can be detected 98 percent of the time, but CVS cannot detect neural tube defects. Women who choose CVS must also have an AFP blood test (see the next section) between the fifteenth and eighteenth weeks of pregnancy to screen for neural tube defects. The advantage of CVS over amniocentesis is an earlier diagnosis and an earlier choice for women who would choose to not carry an abnormal fetus. The disadvantage is a higher miscarriage rate of about 1 percent. The cost of CVS is between $1,200 and $1,800. Not all insurance companies pay for this test.

Triple Marker

A combination of three blood tests, called the *triple marker*, screens for neural tube defects and the risk of Down syndrome, as well as other abnormalities. These tests are maternal blood tests, so they avoid invasion of the pregnancy and risk of fetal damage.

A mother's blood is tested for three substances: alpha-fetoprotein (AFP), human chorionic gonadotropin (HCG), and unconjugated estriol (UE). The test can be done between the fifteenth and twentieth weeks of pregnancy, but the most accurate results are between the sixteenth and seventeenth weeks. The triple marker doesn't make a diagnosis, but it gives the percentage of risk for the possible abnormalities. If this risk is low, nothing more needs to be done. If it is high, further testing may be done, including an ultrasound and possibly an amniocentesis.

Handling the Test Results

The purpose of all these tests is to see whether the baby you are carrying is normal. If your decision will be to keep the baby regardless of any abnormality, knowing in advance can help you prepare yourself and your family emotionally—though this must be weighed against the tests' risks to the fetus. Preparation includes seeking the resources available to help your child. Support groups can help you understand and cope with raising a child with Down syndrome. People with Down syndrome live well into middle age, and early intervention, within the first six months to a year, has helped them join mainstream society (Connolly 1993).

Other Factors to Consider

In this section we examine some other factors you should consider before becoming pregnant that can help decrease the chance of fetal abnormalities.

"High Risk" Pregnancies Over Age Thirty-Five

Traditionally, pregnant women over thirty-five have been regarded as being "high risk" in terms of their own health. Two recent studies supply even more support for this point of view. In both studies, women with abnormal babies were excluded. Edge and Laros (1993) studied over 800 women having their first pregnancy at age thirty-five or older. They found no increase in chronic diseases, such as high blood pressure, but did find an increased rate of pregnancy complications, resulting in a higher cesarean rate. Gilbert (1999) studied 24,000 women over forty. While the babies were just as big and healthy as the babies of younger mothers, they found a significant increase in the rate of cesarean section, chronic illness, and virtually every complication of pregnancy. The increased risks were even higher when the mothers were having their first baby over forty.

Extra Care for Chronic Diseases

Some women have medical conditions that require special care before, during, and sometimes after pregnancy. A pregnancy puts increased demands on the body. A health problem that was well controlled before pregnancy might be more troublesome once pregnancy occurs. For example, if you have high blood pressure, your antihypertensive medication may need to be changed prior to conception to a drug that is safe for a developing baby. If you are diabetic, it's important to have your blood sugars at target range and take 4 milligrams of folic acid daily before conception to ensure a normal baby. If you have thyroid disease, be sure your thyroid levels are monitored. (There is a high incidence of thyroid problems occurring for the first time in the initial three months after your baby is born. See Chapter 5 for a more detailed discussion of this subject.)

Known Familial Diseases

If your family has a history of a particular disease or diseases, be sure to discuss this issue with your doctor before conception. That way, you can make informed decisions as to the best way to have a healthy pregnancy.

Stopping Birth Control Pills

Birth control pills regulate your menstrual periods. When you decide to get pregnant and quit taking them, your menstrual periods may become irregular for a while. If you become pregnant before your periods are regular again, it makes establishing the duration of your pregnancy more difficult. Your endometrium will have been thinned during your years of taking birth control pills. It needs time to develop into the lush, sugar-filled glandular tissue needed to support an embryo. Therefore, it is a good idea to stop taking the Pill several months before getting pregnant. However, using birth control pills before you become pregnant does *not* cause birth defects, regardless of how close to pregnancy you stop taking them.

Herbal Remedies

The use of over-the-counter herbal remedies may impair fertility or damage a developing embryo. St.-John's-wort, echinacea, palmetto, and ginkgo biloba have been found to have harmful effects on sperm and eggs in laboratory animals (Ondrizek 1999). Since there can be long-lasting effects from any herb, you should not take over-the-counter remedies while trying to get pregnant or during your pregnancy.

Cigarettes, Alcohol, and Drugs

Tobacco, alcohol, and social drugs have adverse effects on a developing baby. This is true both during the time the organs are forming and throughout fetal life. Let's take a look at what can happen.

Smoking is associated with low–birth weight babies, an increase in fetal death, and an increase in crib death called sudden infant death syndrome (SIDS) (Jauniaux 1999). Children raised in a house of smokers have a 50 percent increase in their lifetime chance of developing cancer (Stjernfeldt 1986; John 1991). Quitting smoking helps you and your baby.

Fetal alcohol syndrome (FAS) occurs when a woman drinks heavily during her pregnancy. This syndrome results in abnormal facial features and mental retardation. The amount of alcohol needed to cause FAS varies from person to person. As few as two drinks a day can cause this syndrome, but most children with FAS are born to women who drink considerably more. It doesn't matter whether you drink wine, beer, or hard liquor; they all cause fetal alcohol syndrome (Dorris 1990). If you are trying to get pregnant, it is a good idea to abstain from drinking. In the event of an unplanned pregnancy, stop drinking immediately. If you think you might have a problem with alcohol abuse, get help before you try to get pregnant.

In case you haven't heard, using cocaine, crack cocaine, or heroin while pregnant will seriously damage—if not kill—a fetus. "Crack babies" have short attention spans, are irritable and hyperactive, and have trouble learning. More information will no doubt be forthcoming on the continuing negative effects of maternal drug use during pregnancy as these children grow up, and the picture won't be a pretty one.

It takes time to quit a habit. According to research in human learning, it takes six weeks to six months for nerves to shrivel and new neural pathways to form in their place (Soares 1996). Don't be embarrassed if you have a habit that is difficult to quit. Ask your health-care provider for support and medical advice. The decision to quit may be one of the most difficult things you've ever done, but one of the most worthwhile.

Viral Infections

Infections with measles, mumps, chicken pox, and rubella (German measles) during your pregnancy can cause serious birth defects or illness in your baby. Vaccination against these viral infections can prevent them. Find out if you are immune to these diseases prior to pregnancy. If not, get vaccinated and then pregnant, but in that order.

Hepatitis B (HBV), a viral infection, is the most common cause of hepatitis in the United States (U.S. Department of Health, Education, and Welfare 1977). It results in 300,000 new cases of acute hepatitis yearly. If you are a carrier of this virus, you can give it to your infant during birth or immediately afterwards. Over 16,000 babies are at risk each year. A baby that becomes infected may become a chronic carrier. Twenty-five percent of chronic carriers eventually develop cancer or cirrhosis of the liver. As a result, when you first become pregnant, your doctor will test to see whether you are an HBV carrier. If you aren't but are in a high-risk group, you should be immunized to prevent the disease. If you are in a high-risk group, you should be tested before you get pregnant and then immunized as soon as possible. Your risk for being an HBV carrier is increased if you:

- Are originally from Asia or Oceania, or are Inuit

- Use illicit drugs

- Have acute or chronic liver disease

- Have had a blood transfusion

- Are a health-care worker

- Have multiple sex partners

- Have had any sexually transmitted diseases

If you are identified as a carrier, your baby will be given HBV prophylaxis immediately after birth to prevent its becoming infected with this disease. It is common practice to immunize babies after birth, but if you are diagnosed before the baby is born, your baby get hyperimmune gamma globulin as well to help prevent infection.

Hepatitis C is a sexually transmitted viral infection of the liver similar to hepatitis B. Although the infection is less acute than either hepatitis A (a food-borne, self-limiting infection without permanent liver damage) or hepatitis B, the death rate is higher. Half of those who become infected with hepatitis C will develop liver failure or primary liver cancer. Unlike hepatitis A and B, there is no vaccine available. Hepatitis C can be transmitted to your unborn child. If you have any of the risk factors for hepatitis B, you are at increased risk for hepatitis C as well, and you should be tested for it prior to pregnancy.

Sexually Transmitted Diseases (STDs)

Diseases you can get through sexual contact include gonorrhea, chlamydia, genital herpes, syphilis, venereal warts (human papilloma virus or HPV), hepatitis B and C, and HIV/AIDS. Not only can these diseases adversely affect your ability to get pregnant, they can infect and harm your baby. Certain contraceptive methods, such as condoms and spermicides (contraceptive foams or creams), lower your risk of contracting an STD. Once you are trying to get pregnant, however, you obviously stop using these methods. This places you at a higher risk for contracting an STD. If you think you or your partner has a sexually transmitted disease, see your health-care provider right away and get treatment. Then abstain from sex until both of you have completed treatment and been rechecked.

Infertility

Perhaps you have delayed your first pregnancy until your career is set and you have bought your first home. You have started prenatal vitamins, you've seen your health-care provider, and you're healthy. You may have even stopped your birth control pills three months ago. You are ready to get pregnant, but nothing happens. You find this pregnancy business isn't going the way you had planned. Well, you are not alone. More than 14 percent of couples are infertile (Silva 1999). You have probably heard stories of women who tried to get pregnant for years but became pregnant only after they had stopped trying. Actually, that sort of pregnancy doesn't happen very often. Most of the time, if you are having trouble getting pregnant on your own, you need help from your health-care provider. There are numerous causes for infertility. In this section we will explore some of them. (Note: It is estimated that 40 percent of all infertility is caused by the male factor [Jaffe 1991]. If you are having infertility problems, make sure your partner is not warming his scrotum [warm sperm are sluggish] by wearing tight underwear, jeans, or padded bicycle shorts, or taking hot showers.)

- **Ovulation:** After the age of thirty-five, your ovaries have fewer eggs and gradually produce less and less estrogen and progesterone. (See the next section for a full discussion of ovarian issues.) Less estrogen and progesterone, fewer eggs, and more abnormal eggs reduce your chances of conception. Figure 2.1 illustrates the relationship between pregnancies and age. If progesterone levels fall too much, the endometrium does not produce enough sugar (glycogen) to support a little embryo. As a result, even when you conceive normally, you have an increased miscarriage risk.

- **Tubal disease:** Twenty percent of all infertility is due to tubal or uterine disease. Several factors contribute to this high rate. Contemporary women are delaying their childbearing and face a greater cumulative risk of STDs such as gonorrhea and chlamydia. These STDs damage the fallopian tubes and affect fertility.

- **Thyroid disease:** Thyroid hormone, either too much or too little, can cause infertility. Chapter 5 is devoted to this issue.

- **Weight:** Either too much or too little body fat greatly reduces pregnancy rates due to ovulation failure, and also increases pregnancy complications (Silva 1999).

- **Frequency of sex:** Couples have sex less often as they age for a variety of reasons. Once you are in your late thirties, you will have intercourse half as often as you did when you were younger (Menken 1986).

- **Age of partner:** As you age, so does your partner; as his interest in having sex decreases, so does the pregnancy rate.

- **Postponement of childbearing:** If you chose a career outside of the home, you probably went to college, found a job, got established, and then decided to have children. All of this takes time and each year you wait, you have fewer fresh, grade AA eggs left to be fertilized.

Ovarian Problems and Infertility

As you reach perimenopause, you're getting older, and so are your eggs. Even if you are lucky enough to ovulate a grade AA egg, the follicle from which the egg emerged may not make enough progesterone in the luteal phase (the two weeks after ovulation) to sustain an embryo. Production of progesterone must be constant during the luteal phase to prepare the endometrium for pregnancy. When your progesterone level begins to fall before the two weeks are over, you have a luteal phase deficiency. The embryo can't implant in your uterus, and a miscarriage results.

Your doctor can diagnose a short luteal phase by "dating" your endometrium. A biopsy of the endometrial lining is taken, usually two or

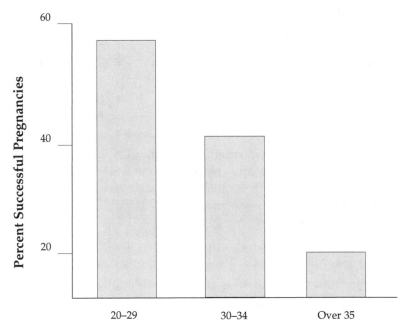

Adapted from: R. T. Scott et al. 1995

Figure 2.1.   Percent of Pregnancies vs. Age

three days before your next period is due. A pathologist looks at the endometrial lining and "dates" it—that is, determines from the size and character of your endometrial lining when your next period is due. If you don't have your period within the time predicted by the pathologist, you have a luteal phase deficiency. You are not making enough progesterone to support a pregnancy. (Note: Your doctor can also order a blood test to tell you whether you are making enough progesterone [Jaffe 1991]. A blood test is less painful than an endometrial biopsy, but your doctor cannot as accurately diagnose a luteal phase deficiency by a blood test.)

The usual treatment for a shortened luteal phase is progesterone gel (marketed as Crinone Gel), which is inserted vaginally. Progesterone shots are also available, but they don't work as well as the gel.

Assisted Reproductive Technologies

Pregnancy rates decrease with age. There are many reasons for this decline but the main reason is fewer normal eggs. Remember, you only produce one egg per month. If there is a defect in your egg, it is less likely to be fertilized. The incidence of these defects increases with age (Palomali 1995). To increase your chance of pregnancy, your doctor may recommend a fertility-enhancing drug (clomiphene citrate, human menopausal gonadotropins, human chorionic gonadotropins) to help you produce more than one egg per month. Multiple eggs increase the likelihood that one or more of them will be successfully fertilized and you will be on your way to motherhood.

Fertility-enhancing drugs don't always work. When they don't, a number of assisted reproductive technologies (ARTs) are available for women trying to conceive. The main treatment is in vitro fertilization (IVF), or fertilization in a laboratory dish or test tube, as illustrated in Figure 2.2. Assisted hatching is an enhancement of IVF in which the cells around the fertilized egg are removed to help the fertilized egg implant in the uterus. The placement of a single sperm into a single egg is called intracytoplasmic sperm injection (ICSI) and is used frequently.

If you are under forty, your success rate with IVF in any given month compares favorably with the natural pregnancy rate of the general fertile population (33.6 percent per cycle) (Society for Assisted Reproductive Technology 1996). Routinely, only three fertilized eggs are inserted in your uterus; all others are frozen for future use. If you are thirty-five to thirty-nine, your cumulative live birth rate is very high; 69 percent over four cycles of a combination of NF and frozen embryo transfer (thawing, then placing the frozen embryo in the uterus). If you are over forty and have healthy ovaries, your chance of having a successful pregnancy is about 52 percent over four cycles incorporating IVF, frozen embryos, and assisted hatching (Lurie 2000). This high rate incorporates ICSI and assisted hatching.

When fertility enhancing drugs and assisted reproductive technologies don't work, an egg donor can be considered. This may seem very radical, but remember that donor sperm have been used for thirty years with wonderful success rates. With a donor-egg pregnancy, the sperm comes from your partner, the egg comes from a younger woman, and you carry the pregnancy. The advantage of this over surrogate pregnancy, where another woman carries the baby to term, is that you are in control of the food, drugs, and alcohol to which your baby is exposed. You carry the baby to term, and your maternal gene (recently discovered in humans) is turned on (Brown 1996).

Contraception—If You Would Rather Be Forty Than Pregnant

During the perimenopause, your cycles often lose their regularity. If you've used the rhythm method, be careful: Your cycles are no longer rhythmic!

Some women nearing the end of reproductive life spot a little blood when they ovulate. This can last for several days. If this happens to you, don't be fooled into assuming this is the beginning of your menstrual period (especially if it is overdue). Continue using contraception to be sure of avoiding pregnancy.

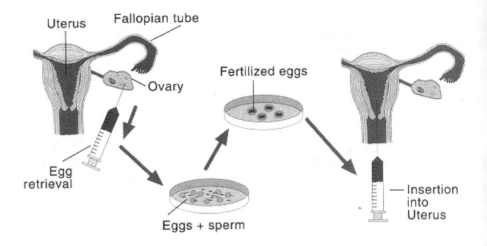

Figure 2.2.   In Vitro Fertilization

Contraception in Perimenopause

A variety of contraceptive methods are available for use by women. (This discussion doesn't include the topic of vasectomy, a surgical procedure performed on men.)

Barrier Methods—Foam, Condoms, and Diaphragms Work Well

Once you are perimenopausal, barrier methods work better than ever before. This is because you are less fertile. You aren't infertile, though, so use your diaphragm, cervical cap, condom, contraceptive foam, or cream all the time. Even if you think you are having your menstrual period, don't take chances. If properly used, the barrier methods are nearly foolproof at this age. They include:

- **Condoms:** This is an effective method, but not if you use a torn condom. Your vagina lubricates more slowly than it used to, and a lack of adequate lubrication makes a condom more likely to tear. For this reason, use a contraceptive jelly or foam as an adjunct to the condom.

- **Diaphragm:** Women who use a diaphragm as their birth control method are more than twice as likely to contract a bladder infection. The spermicidal jelly used with the diaphragm kills normal bacteria in the vagina, but allows infection-causing bacteria to survive and get into the bladder. If you have a history of recurrent bladder infections, you shouldn't use a diaphragm.

- **Cervical cap:** This variation on the diaphragm fits over the mouth of the womb (the cervix) and can be worn for several days at a time, which allows greater spontaneity in lovemaking. As with the diaphragm, there is a potential risk of increased bladder infections.

- **Spermicides:** Spermicides are a very safe method of birth control. If the method fails, there is no increased risk of birth defects. Also, when used alone or with a condom the spermicide doesn't increase the risk of bladder infection (Grimes 1997).

- **Contraceptive sponge:** This method is easy to use and is an effective method for women who have never had a child, but much less so for women with children, because the cervical opening is larger.

- **Female condom:** This is the first totally woman-controlled method that prevents pregnancy and sexually transmitted diseases. However, the pregnancy rate for this method is 12 percent over six months, which suggests the female condom is used inconsistently (Grimes 1997).

Intrauterine Device (IUD)—Safe and Effective, but with a Bad Reputation

The intrauterine device (IUD) is a great method of birth control. Unfortunately, because of the serious problems that occurred in women using the Dalkon Shield, the IUD has been blamed for infertility. It has been estimated that, during the 1980s, over 300,000 women worldwide were injured by infections caused by the Dalkon Shield (Grimes 1997). Other, safe IUDs were judged guilty by association and were taken off the market.

Gradually, the truth about infection and IUDs became known: The number of sex partners a woman has, not the IUD, is responsible for pelvic infection and subsequent sterility (Fortney 1999). The risk of significant infection from the IUD insertion occurs only in the first month after insertion and, for the most part, can be prevented by giving prophylactic antibiotics (Grimes 1997).

There are three types of IUDs on the American market. All three are made from plastic and are T-shaped. They are all small and easy to insert, and act as a spermicide so pregnancy doesn't occur in the uterus or fallopian tubes. Each of the three differs from the others in its active ingredients, its effect on menstrual flow and cramps, and its useful life. One is the "Copper T," which can stay in place for ten years. Menstrual flow is heavier with the Copper T, but can be controlled with the use of a nonsteroidal anti-inflammatory medication (NSAID), such as ibuprofen or naproxen. Another type of IUD contains progesterone instead of copper as its active ingredient. It reduces your endometrial lining, thickens your cervical mucus (which acts as a barrier to sperm migration), and decreases your menstrual flow and cramps, but it must be replaced each year. The third T-shaped IUD contains a synthetic progestin and is good for seven years. It has an even lower failure rate than the other two and a greater reduction in menstrual flow by as much as 94 percent (Irvine 1998). It significantly reduces cramps and pelvic pain but has some increased systemic effects. FDA approval of this IUD is expected in late 2000. The World Health Organization has concluded that "today's copper and hormone-bearing devices are among the safest and most effective reversible methods of contraception in the world" (Grimes 1997).

CAUTION! Neither of the progesterone IUDs should be used if you have had an ectopic pregnancy in the past, because both carry an increased risk of tubal pregnancy.

The latest IUD in clinical trials is a bodiless copper IUD. It has a monofilament string and six copper bands, but there is no body onto which the copper is mounted. (The body in other IUDs is what causes cramping.) Another prototype being considered has very pliable arms that point downward to prevent its expulsion. No one knows which will get the FDA nod, but it is encouraging to see advances being made in this important area of contraception (Grimes 1997).

Birth Control Pills—Now?

Birth control pills are an excellent option during perimenopause. Doctors prescribe them for perimenopausal women who experience heavy or irregular bleeding, including women who have had their tubes tied. For many women, taking the pill during perimenopause is multipurpose: It serves as a method of birth control, bleeding control, and perimenopausal symptom control.

There is, unfortunately, a large group of women who cannot use the Pill safely after age thirty-five. They include women with the following health issues:

- **Smoking:** If you smoke, your risk of having a heart attack while on the Pill is twenty times higher than for women not taking the Pill (Croft 1989). This statistic is for all women. It only becomes a significant risk to you, though, once you are over thirty-five, when the risk of heart disease begins to rise for all women (Darney 1996). There is no increased risk of heart attack in women over thirty-five who take the Pill and do not smoke (Darney 2000).

- **Diabetes:** Older forms of birth control pills (Loestrin, Triphasil, Ovcon, and Ortho-Novum 7-7-7, to name a few) make management of diabetes more difficult. For insulin-dependent diabetics, fasting blood sugars are raised and insulin dose regulation gets tricky. If you take oral antidiabetic pills or use diet to control your diabetes, the older varieties of birth control pills may also make management of your blood sugar a bit of a problem. Newer birth control pills (such as Desogen, Ortho Tri-Cyclen, and Mircette), however, will not affect your blood sugar at all. The insulin dose regulation that you normally require from time to time is easy when you are on the new pill (Burkman 1992).

CAUTION! Metformin, an oral agent for treating diabetes, may negate the contraceptive effects of the birth control pill. Don't count on any birth control pill, new or old, to protect you if you start this medication.

- **Family history of blood clots in veins:** Eight percent of northern European women carry V Leiden factor, which greatly increases their likelihood of having a blood clot when pregnant or taking birth control pills (Darney 2000). Women with protein S, protein C, or antithrombin III deficiencies are at even greater risk of having this problem. If you have a strong family history of venous blood clots, you can be tested for these blood factors before you go on birth control pills.

- **Cancer:** Women with a history of breast or uterine cancer should not take birth control pills. However, birth control pills do not increase your risk of developing breast cancer, and there is growing evidence that prolonged use of birth control pills decreases your risk of developing ovarian or uterine cancer (Darney 2000).

- **Hypertension:** Women with high blood pressure are cautioned *not* to take the Pill. Birth control pills raise blood pressure in susceptible people (Physician's Desk Reference 1997). The one exception is Yasmin, the new drospirenone-containing birth control pill, which was FDA approved in 2000. It has no effect on blood pressure (Oelkers 1995). Uncontrolled hypertension can lead to stroke and kidney failure. It is a silent illness, diagnosed only by blood pressure tests.

- **Fibroid tumors:** Fibroids are muscle tumors of the uterus. They tend to start growing in a woman's early forties. They can cause severe bleeding, as well as bladder and back problems. The engine for fibroid growth is estrogen, and birth control pills raise estrogen levels. If you have fibroids, these higher levels of estrogen may make them grow, causing more problems than you had to begin with.

- **Antitubercular and anticonvulsive drugs:** Rifampin (Rifater), phenobarbital, phenytoin sodium (Dilantin), and other anticonvulsive drugs activate liver enzymes that destroy the hormones in birth control pills, as well as the hormones in Norplant (described in the next section). The only safe birth control methods for you are the IUD, Depo-Provera (also described in the next section), and barrier methods (Darney 1996; Grimes 1997).

- **Classic migraine headache:** Birth control pills may aggravate the symptoms of a migraine, or they may improve them. In any case, there is no increased risk of stroke in women using birth control pills that contain 35 micrograms or less of ethinyl estradiol (University of Minnesota 1997). If your migraines become more frequent after beginning birth control pills, or they occur for the first time after you begin them, however, you should consider a different form of contraception (Silberstein 1992).

If you are not affected by any of the factors described above, the birth control pill may be ideal for you. It regulates your periods, may decrease your PMS, protects you from getting pregnant, and delays your risk of osteoporosis. Many women continue to take birth control pills into the first five years or so of menopause itself, as their drug of choice for hormone replacement therapy. The Pill has little or no effect on cholesterol. A study from Finland showed a six-fold (600 percent) decrease in the risk of heart attack and stroke in Pill users over non-Pill users (Darney 1996). This dramatic difference continued for fifteen years after the women had discontinued using the Pill.

Unfortunately, up to 30 percent of perimenopausal women on the Pill experience diminished sexual desire (Leventhal 1997). Taking the Pill reduces the available testosterone in your body, which is the source of sexual desire and sexual fantasies. One solution is to add a small dose of testosterone in a cream or tablet form; it is not necessary to go off the Pill. (Chapter 7 provides a full discussion of testosterone supplementation.)

Injectable Progestins: Norplant and Depo-Provera

Progestins are synthetic progesterones that can be taken in pill form. Natural progesterone, the hormone you make during the second half of your menstrual cycle, can only be taken by injection or absorbed through your skin. Both Norplant and Depo-Provera contain long-acting progestins, which have three mechanisms for preventing pregnancy:

- **Hostile cervical mucus:** The character of the cervical mucus is changed so that sperm cannot penetrate it; in other words, it acts as a barrier.

- **Endometrial change:** The character of the endometrium is altered to make it hostile to sperm.

- **Interrupted ovulation:** There is no egg to fertilize.

Norplant (levonorgestrel implants) delivers the progestin levonorgestrel in six small permeable capsules. These are placed under the skin of the inner side of your upper arm so they don't show. They are effective for five years, after which they need to be removed and replaced if contraception is still desired. The insertion and removal are done in a doctor's office under local anesthetic. Your arm may be black and blue for about a week after the procedure, but discomfort is not a major problem during either insertion or removal. A new version of Norplant is being studied that uses only two pellets, which are larger and easier to remove (Grimes 1997).

Depo-Provera (depo-medroxyprogesterone acetate, or DMPA) is an injection given every three months. It has been the mainstay of contraception in the Third World for the last thirty years and is now used increasingly in the U.S. (Kaunitz 1996; Fraser 1994). In contrast to birth control pills, there is no contraindication to DMPA use in women who smoke, have high blood pressure, or are on medication to prevent blood clotting. Long-term use does lead to decreased bone density (Scholes 1999), however DMPA is a beneficial contraception for women with mild estrogen depletion who are not yet menopausal (Nelson 1996). Estrogen replacement therapy can be added for women who need it to control perimenopausal symptoms and prevent osteoporosis. In addition, DMPA decreases the risk of uterine and ovarian cancer.

When Norplant is removed, the hormone effects are gone immediately; however, Depo-Provera continues to have some effects for up to nine months after it is discontinued. Most women do not have periods while using either of these methods. The majority of women using Norplant or Depo-Provera are very satisfied with these methods of contraception (Fraser 1994; Kaunitz 1996), although side effects can include weight gain, irregular bleeding, headaches, acne, mild depression, and increased PMS. While women using Norplant may also have painful functional ovarian cysts (fluid-filled sacs that produce hormones), women using Depo-Provera do not. Fewer than 15 percent of women experience these side effects. Unlike birth control pills, Depo-Provera and Norplant are not affected by antibiotic usage. (Note: Norplant and birth control pills don't work for you if you are on anticonvulsive medications, but anticonvulsants have no adverse effect on Depo-Provera [Grimes 1996].)

Monthly Injectable Contraceptive

Injectable contraception in the form of Depo-Provera has been widely used throughout the world for over thirty years. Recently, the FDA has approved the use of a monthly injectable combination contraceptive that combines both estradiol cypionate and medroxyprogesterone acetate. The first injection is given within the first five days of your menstrual period and then each subsequent injection is given the same day of the week at four-week intervals. The monthly injectable contraceptive does not have the serious side effects that are sometimes seen with the Pill, such as blood clots and high blood pressure. However, it has slightly higher mild side effects than the Pill does. These include headache, bleeding, and weight gain. Nevertheless, women using this method are extremely happy with it and continue to use it. The pregnancy rate around the world and among the first 780 American women who used it was zero, a much lower rate than is seen with the Pill (Shulman 1999). There are costs associated with monthly visits for your injection which need to be considered.

Emergency Contraception—The Morning-After Pill

If you have had unprotected sex midcycle, about the time you should be ovulating, emergency contraception using the so-called morning-after pill can be effective. It must be started within 72 hours of the time sex occurred. Several methods of emergency contraception are in use, but the one most frequently used until recently is the Yuzpe method. This involves taking two oral contraceptive pills twelve hours apart for a total of four tablets (Grimes 1997). Because of the 50 percent incidence of nausea and vomiting with the Pill, levonorgestrel, a progestin-only medication, is now being used with lower pregnancy rates and minimal side effects. The dosage is two 0.75 milligram pills taken twelve hours apart (Grimes 1998).

Other emergency contraception methods include the use of synthetic estrogens, conjugated estrogens (such as Premarin), insertion of an IUD, and antiprogesterones such as RU-486, the "French abortion pill," which is now available for use in the United States.

TIP! You can call the following toll-free number to find out the correct medication to take for emergency contraception: 800-584-9911, or ask the 800 operator for the emergency contraception hotline number.

What's New

Contraceptive research in the U.S. has slowed to a glacial pace since about the 1970s, largely due to political posturing, liability concerns, and bureaucratic regulation. Other industrialized countries and even Third World countries have benefited much more from new contraceptive devices and techniques than we have (Grimes 1997). In spite of this, several new methods are on the horizon:

- **Polyurethane condoms** which are thinner, stronger and less allergenic than latex condoms (Qureshi 1999).

- **Spermicides** are being developed that are stronger and will inhibit HIV, chlamydia, trichomonas, and other infectious agents from multiplying in the vagina or adhering to vaginal walls. They are being tested in new disposable diaphragms.

- **Biodegradable implants** using cholesterol and other compounds are under investigation (Qureshi 1999).

- **A single-rod implant** containing the progestin desogestrel is being studied and appears to be effective (Qureshi 1999).

- **Vaccines against sperm or fertilized egg,** although attractive ideas, are not working (Frayne 1999). Research is continuing on a vaccine against the hCG hormone, which is necessary to maintain an early pregnancy (Reichman 1996).

Permanent Sterilization

Sterilization remains the most popular form of contraception in the United States (Piccinino 1998). As a woman, you have several options.

Tubal Sterilization

Tubal ligation is a surgical procedure in which the fallopian tubes are closed, thereby preventing the egg from traveling to the uterus. However, it may not be a permanent solution to birth control. Statistics show the failure rate to be 1.8 percent, not 0.1 percent as was thought in the past (Grimes 1997). The failure rates of the IUD, birth control pills, and monthly injectable contraceptives are lower. In some cases, tubal ligation can be intentionally reversed.

Hysterectomy

If you have small fibroids, heavy periods, menstrual cramps, prolapse (sagging uterus), or stress incontinence, you could benefit from a vaginal hysterectomy. A hysterectomy is another form of permanent sterilization. A vaginal hysterectomy (removing the uterus through the vagina) has a shorter recovery period than an abdominal operation. Your ovaries can be left behind so you continue to produce hormones, but you won't bleed anymore, and you can't get pregnant. Also, with your uterus gone, when you reach menopause, you can take estrogen alone instead of the combination therapy recommended for other women.

Summary

Pregnancy during perimenopause stirs a variety of emotions, depending upon where you are in your life plan. You may be worried that pregnancy will be fraught with health difficulties for you and risks for a fetus. You may fear that you cannot become pregnant, although you still want to try. You may have completed your childbearing years and be afraid you might become pregnant again. In this chapter we have explored all these areas of uncertainty. Your health-care provider can help you address concerns specific to your situation. As you have learned, all the answers aren't in yet, but you have a number of options for dealing with a midlife pregnancy.

○ ○ ○ ○

3

PMS Can Change You: Premenstrual Syndrome in Your Transitional Years

Hippocrates (as in the Hippocratic oath) wrote about menstrual disorders for the first time in recorded history. He coined the term hysteria, which he thought was caused by the uterus "wandering" throughout the body, causing trouble wherever it went. Premenstrual tension was described in 1931 (Frank), but the term "premenstrual syndrome" was coined by Dr. Katharina Dalton (Greene 1953). Who cares what it's called! It's real, and it can make you feel as though you aren't in control of your emotions. It's as though you are suddenly outside of yourself, watching in horror as you make really stupid mistakes and comments. The bad news here is that it gets worse during the perimenopausal years (Revlin 1990). The good news is that it goes away once you reach menopause. This chapter will give you a clearer understanding of whether or not you have PMS, what causes it, and how you can treat it.

Diagnosis

Premenstrual syndrome (PMS) is defined as a variable collection of physical and psychological/emotional symptoms recurring on a regular basis in the week or two preceding a menstrual period. It includes symptoms such as mood disturbances, headache, bloating, and weight gain. PMS doesn't affect every woman, but *some* of the symptoms affect 85 to 90 percent of women

(Parker 1994)—and maybe the other 10 to 15 percent just aren't paying attention! In diagnosing PMS, doctors look for the following general conditions:

- **Time of onset:** The symptoms must begin during the two weeks before your menstrual period is due—the luteal phase of your cycle.

- **Duration of symptoms:** The symptoms must resolve within one or two days after the start of your menstrual bleeding.

- **Symptom-free period:** There must be a symptom-free period during the first week after your menstrual period. The first two weeks of your cycle are called the follicular phase.

- **Persistence of symptoms:** Your symptoms must be present over several menstrual cycles, and they must not be accounted for by some other disorder.

- **Severity:** Your PMS symptoms must be severe enough to disrupt your normal lifestyle. Sound familiar? You are not alone. Ten percent of women experience symptoms severe enough to disrupt their lives (Parker 1994).

There are over 150 symptoms ascribed to PMS. The most common of these are insomnia, anger, depression, forgetfulness, sore breasts, weight gain, headaches (including menstrual migraines), tearfulness, acne, and recurrent cold sores. A more complete list can be found in Table 3.1. About 70 percent of PMS sufferers also report one or more positive symptoms, such as increased sex drive, greater creativity, and more energy. (At least there's a ray of light!)

Premenstrual syndrome is now recognized as a valid diagnosis by psychiatrists in the latest edition of the *Diagnostic and Statistical Manual of Mental Disorders*. There has been a move to change the name to premenstrual dysphoric disorder (PDD), although it's probably way too late to make a dent in the well-established public acceptance of the term premenstrual syndrome. To make the specific diagnosis of PDD, you must have one of the following four symptoms as well as four other symptoms, either from this list or from the emotional or behavioral list found in Table 3.1:

- Depressed mood

- Marked anxiety

- Sudden tearfulness, sadness, or increased sensitivity to rejection

- Persistent anger or interpersonal conflicts

Causes of PMS

Whatever you call PMS, hormones from all over the body have been implicated in creating it. They include:

Table 3.1. Common Symptoms of PMS	
Physical	**Emotional or Behavioral**
Breast swelling and tenderness	Anxiety
Fluid retention and weight gain	Depression
Headaches, migraines	Tearfulness
Bloating	Anger
Fatigue	Hostility
Acne, cold sores	Aggression
Heart palpitations	Mood fluctuations
Constipation	Irritability
Dizziness	Forgetfulness
Muscle aches	Poor concentration
Hot flashes	Insomnia
Sleepiness	Food cravings
	Sexual desire up or down
	Poor coping skills
	Panic attacks
	Suicidal attempts
	Feeling overwhelmed or out of control
	Lethargy

Adapted from: American Psychiatric Association. 1996. *Diagnostic and Statistical Manual of Mental Disorders.*

- Ovarian hormones (estrogen and progesterone)

- Pituitary hormones (FSH, LH, and possibly prolactin)

- Endorphins (produced in the midbrain and hypothalamus) and adrenal hormones

- Neurotransmitters

Serotonin, a neurotransmitter in the brain thought to be responsible for chemical depression, is now felt to be the main player in PMS (Barnhart 1995), but your symptoms probably come from a combination of factors.

Hormones

First of all, it really isn't just your raging hormones that are to blame for PMS. It is a combination of your ovarian hormones plus your cortisone, serotonin, endorphins, heredity, and life stresses. Premenstrual syndrome knows no boundaries. It does not correlate with race, culture, marital status, or education, though it seems to be more prevalent in perimenopausal mothers who work outside the home (Ekholm 1994).

Heredity

You've probably heard this one: "PMS has been found to be hereditary—you get it from your kids!" Actually, it may indeed be hereditary. Studies of identical twins (Condon 1993) show a 93 percent chance of their both having PMS. (There is a lesser correlation in fraternal twins.) If your mother had PMS, you are more likely to have it too (Wilson 1991).

Diet

Certain dietary excesses are known to aggravate PMS, including the following:

- **Salt:** Most women experiencing PMS will have increased their salt and carbohydrate intake premenstrually and thereby unwittingly increased their PMS symptoms.

- **Sugar:** A high intake of sweets results in salt retention by your body. The increased presence of salt causes fluid retention and increases premenstrual bloating.

- **Caffeine:** Consumption of large amounts of caffeine, found in coffee, tea, cola, and chocolate, has been reported to worsen the symptoms of PMS (Parker 1994). Caffeine can increase anxiety, tension, depression, and irritability and contribute to insomnia.

Nonhormonal Treatment of PMS

A wide variety of nonhormonal options are available to help you manage the symptoms of PMS.

Diet

In the last section, we pointed out several dietary factors that can contribute to PMS; changing what you eat and drink can make a difference. A diet rich in carbohydrates diminishes mood swings.

Sugars—including fructose and sucrose—are simple carbohydrates. Vegetables, fruits (but not fruit juice, which has no pulp), legumes, rice, pasta, and so on are complex carbohydrates. Both vegetables and fruits have simple sugars within them. When cooked, some vegetables (potatoes and carrots, for example) release their simple sugars.

Serotonin building blocks are found in complex carbohydrates, so the "carbo-cravings" so common in PMS may indicate a natural need to increase serotonin levels. For years, the recommendation for PMS sufferers was to increase proteins and limit simple carbohydrates (donuts, cakes, sweets, and so on). However, there is increasing evidence that meals high in complex carbohydrates and low in protein improve mood symptoms of PMS sufferers, including depression, tension, anger, confusion, fatigue, and lethargy (Barnhart 1995).

You know that as you near your menstrual periods, you crave sweets. The fact is that hypoglycemia, or low blood sugar, does not occur premenstrually any more often than at any other time in your cycle (Barnhart 1995). If you succumb to your sweet craving, the sugar you take aboard causes water retention and results in bloating. What to do about it? At times like this, change your sweet attack signal to a complex carbohydrate attack. You should try to limit sweets and emphasize grains, vegetables, pastas, and fruits. These are all complex carbohydrates that will help your symptoms. Watch out, though: One penalty for a sudden increase in complex carbohydrates, which dramatically increases your fiber intake, is that it can produce a lot of gas.

Fluid retention and bloating are common complaints during the premenstrual period. Many women gain more than five pounds each month. You might think that if you restricted your salt intake, water retention would be reduced. This sounds like it would work, but it doesn't. The solution to fluid retention and bloating, surprisingly enough, is to increase your water intake. Hard to believe it works, but it does. Increased water pulls salt from the tissues, and it is excreted in the urine. The more water you drink, the more salt-laden fluid you excrete.

Vitamins and Minerals

Let's take a look at the effects of several vitamins and minerals on decreasing or eliminating PMS symptoms.

Vitamin B₆

In doses of 100 to 150 milligrams a day throughout the month, vitamin B_6 may help symptoms of PMS. This vitamin is necessary in the synthesis of serotonin and prostaglandins, which play a role in PMS. Prostaglandins are chemicals manufactured throughout the body that exert a hormonelike effect and influence involuntary muscular contraction (including contraction of the uterus), circulation, and inflammation. Vitamin B_6 supplements have been used in the treatment of PMS for years (Wyatt 1999). Complaints of fatigue, irritability, and depression may respond to supplements of this vitamin.

CAUTION! More B₆ is not always better. There have been many reports (Parker 1994) of permanent nerve damage with as little as 200 milligrams a day.

Vitamin E

Vitamin E offers some relief from sore breasts. Indeed, 85 percent of women with PMS-induced sore breasts reported significant relief taking 600 to 800 IU (international units) of Vitamin E daily (Severino 1995). The usual recommended adult dose is 200 to 400 IU. Vitamin E can be toxic at very high levels (3,000 IU). Additional information on vitamin E and its antioxidant benefits is extensively covered in Chapter 9.

Calcium and Magnesium

Calcium and magnesium show modest success in reducing PMS symptoms. (Note: Single mineral therapy with other minerals, such as zinc and copper, has never been shown to diminish the symptoms of PMS.) Both calcium and magnesium are necessary for your nerves to transmit impulses. Several studies have shown calcium to be equal to fluoxetine (Prozac) in reducing PMS symptoms (Thy-Jacobs 1998). The dose is 1,200 milligrams of calcium a day. One small study found 1,080 milligrams of magnesium daily reduced symptoms as well. This is twice the dose recommended for ordinary use (Fachinetti 1991). Both calcium and magnesium can help relieve mental as well as physical symptoms of PMS. Almost all over-the-counter PMS medications contain both of these minerals.

CAUTION! In addition to causing loose stools, using twice the normal dose of magnesium can prevent adequate calcium absorption and increase your risk of osteoporosis in later years (see Chapter 4). For this reason, take the increased magnesium dose only premenstrually, and discontinue it as soon as your period starts.

L-Tryptophan

Taking an oral amino acid called L-tryptophan significantly reduces PMS symptoms, especially irritability (Steinberg 1999). L-tryptophan converts to tryptophan in the body. Tryptophan is an amino acid (protein building block) that is in most common proteins, such as milk. Tryptophan can help alleviate PMS symptoms because it is a precursor for serotonin, a neurotransmitter that promotes relaxation. (That explains why mothers give babies warm milk before bedtime.) High amounts of tryptophan are found in turkey meat and may explain why you get so sleepy after Thanksgiving dinner.

The usual dose of L-tryptophan is six grams per day, beginning at ovulation, and ending with the onset of your period. The good news is that L-tryptophan is an over-the-counter substance that works. The bad news is that it is expensive and may cause drowsiness. The pills found in health food stores contain 50 to 100 milligrams, not grams, and cost $22 for fifty tablets. L-tryptophan in powdered form, available through your pharmacist, may prove to be a less expensive alternative. You might add the powder to the glass of milk you drink with your turkey sandwich.

Exercise

Muscle contractions of your lower legs force extra fluid out of your tissues and into your bloodstream. This is why walking, jogging, bicycle riding, and swimming all help get rid of those puffy feet. Aerobic exercise has been demonstrated to decrease the severity of the negative mood and some of the physical symptoms associated with PMS. Aerobic exercise (walking, jogging, swimming, and biking) is superior to strength training (weight lifting) in reducing premenstrual symptoms (Moline 1993). Research has shown that frequency, such as thirty minutes daily, rather than intensity, is the most important factor in ameliorating your symptoms and increasing your feeling of self-worth. There is, however, no evidence that increased endorphins (morphinelike chemicals made in the brain in response to exercise, pain, and stress) released in vigorous exercise have any effect on PMS. (For more information about exercise, see Chapter 9.)

Evening Primrose Oil

Oil extracted from evening primrose seeds contains vitamin E, prostaglandins, linolenic acid, and several other active substances that are said to have therapeutic effects on a number of conditions. Four trials comparing evening primrose oil with a placebo found the oil reduced premenstrual breast tenderness (Kleijnenn 1994), but found no benefit for the other symptoms of PMS (Khoo 1990).

Behavioral Modification for Mild PMS

Gaining control over your life and its stresses reduces the impact of PMS. Stress control, relaxation techniques, meditation, changes in your diet, and exercise programs have all been shown to help. Prayer is thought to be of benefit, possibly in the same way meditation has been shown to help. Unfortunately, for women with severe PMS, the symptoms themselves shape their lifestyle rather than the other way around—PMS turns out to be the stressor. Still, it's beneficial to have a handle on other stresses in your life. To improve your chances of successfully coping with PMS, the following are some stress management goals that can help:

- Try not to take everything personally.

- Learn to accept that which you are not in a position to control.

- Avoid unnecessary complications; simplify your life.
- Do not procrastinate. (That's a big one!)
- Judge yourself by your own standards to bolster your self-esteem.
- Avoid being judgmental of others.
- Exercise every day.

Do's and don'ts are easy to list, but they are frequently difficult to accomplish, especially when it comes to modifying your behavior. (For a more thorough discussion of stress management, be sure to read Chapter 11.)

Peer-Group Therapy

Peer groups work well for PMS. Using a combination of symptom intervention that includes self-monitoring, personal choice, self-regulation, and environment modification improves most of the psychological symptoms of PMS and increases your self-esteem. Furthermore, the results of this combined approach were equal to those found with the use of medication. Unfortunately, to maintain these results, women must continue long-term treatment (Taylor 1999).

Light Therapy

In one study, women using a "10000 1x cool-white fluorescent light" for thirty minutes every evening during the luteal phase significantly reduced depression and premenstrual tension compared to the placebo group, who used a standard fluorescent light source. These women did not have seasonal affective disorder, just ordinary PMS (Lam 1999).

Sleeping Aids

Insomnia and early awakening are very common complaints in perimenopause. The cause of the insomnia can be a hot flash during the night, or simply feeling warm. (You may not recognize it as a hot flash.) Sleeplessness can also be due to depression, anxiety, life stresses, and physical illness (Danjou 1999). If you do sleep all night, you may still feel tired when you awaken. Regardless of your perception of what is wrong, your symptoms may be due to decreased estrogen. Estrogen supplements can make a big difference, especially if you take them at bedtime (Revlin 1990).

There are also several lifestyle changes you can make to help alleviate this disruptive occurrence:

- **Avoid caffeinated beverages after lunch:** If this doesn't help, stop them altogether. Go off them gradually to avoid withdrawal symptoms.

- **Avoid alcohol within four hours of bedtime:** Although alcohol is a depressant, it has an excitatory phase following the sedative phase. If the four-hour restriction doesn't help, try stopping altogether.

- **Continue to exercise,** but do so in the morning or afternoon. If you exercise within three or four hours of going to bed, you may be too stimulated to get to sleep.

- **Do not eat a heavy meal just before retiring:** Take a light snack if you need food shortly before bedtime.

- **Do something relaxing for the hour or so before going to bed:** In other words, don't pay your bills, study for school, or work.

- **Stop worrying about getting to sleep:** This is the most important item! Just let it happen.

When insomnia isn't helped by behavioral modification and diet changes, you may need to use medication. Sleeping pills are effective for a limited number of days or weeks. After you have taken them for some time, your body adjusts to them, and you simply fall back to your old pattern of sleeplessness. Two new sleeping pills promise some relief from early awakening, however: zaleplon (Sonata) and zolpidem (Ambien). Patients on zaleplon showed no daytime sedative effect and no rebound insomnia when used for four weeks or less. Patients taking zolpiden showed some rebound sleeplessness but had similar daytime alertness as long as the medication was taken at least five hours before awakening (Danjou 1999; Vermeeren 1999; Elie 1999). Small doses of L-tryptophan may also help insomnia. Hops and Kava kava, both over-the-counter herbs, help decrease insomnia as well, and your body does not adjust to them. Kava kava used frequently and in large doses may turn your skin yellow (Hendrix 1998).

TIP! Continuous use of melatonin has been reported to reduce serotonin levels, so you may find your PMS is becoming a lot worse. If so, it is best to avoid using melatonin during the second half of your menstrual cycle. However, taking 10 milligrams of melatonin for five days beginning just before ovulation and continuing for a few days after ovulation, instead of all month long, significantly reduces late luteal-phase PMS symptoms (Kirby 1999).

"Give Me Drugs!"

Many different medications have been used to decrease or eliminate the physical symptoms of PMS, but none of them has proven to be a cure. For example, diuretics reduce fluid retention and a nonsteroidal anti-inflammatory drug (NSAID) like naproxen or ibuprofen will help headaches.

Until recently, the only effective treatments for the psychological symptoms of PMS were medications that altered or halted ovarian activity. While ovarian function is necessary for PMS to flourish, we now know that serotonin in varying levels is the major player. The selective serotonin reuptake inhibitors (SSRIs), such as fluoxetrine (Prozac), paroxetine (Paxil), and sertraline (Zoloft) have been the major breakthrough in the treatment of the psychological symptoms of PMS. The SSRIs will be discussed in a separate section. For now, though, let's take a closer look at some of these other medications.

Diuretics

Most diuretics help reduce bloating, weight gain, fluid retention, and sore breasts. A type of diuretic called spironolactone has become the most popular for the treatment of PMS-related fluid retention (Parker 1994). The dose is 25 milligrams twice a day, taken premenstrually. Although spironolactone is very effective for fluid excess, it has been disappointing in its effect on emotional symptoms. Potassium loss is a worry with spironolactone, as with all diuretics. Prolonged use of spironolactone also can cause cramping and diarrhea, drowsiness, headache, and (rarely) mental confusion. Other diuretics are generally reserved for patients who have no success with spironolactone therapy.

CAUTION! Diuretics sometimes become drugs of abuse, especially in women who are highly concerned about excess weight.

Nonsteroidal Anti-Inflammatory Drugs (NSAIDs)

Some women get menstrual cramps before their period begins. *Nonsteroidal anti-inflammatory drugs* (NSAIDs) help both premenstrual cramps and cramps occurring during the menstrual period. Chemicals called prostaglandins are known to be responsible for menstrual cramps; they make the uterus contract during labor, too. Before prostaglandins were discovered, menstrual cramps were thought to be psychological. The discovery that NSAIDs are antiprostaglandins led to their use to temper the pain many women experience. Ibuprofen and naproxen have become the mainstays for treating menstrual cramps but they are not beneficial for the emotional symptoms of PMS (Mortola 1994). NSAIDs remain the first choice for menstrual cramps.

CAUTION! NSAIDs often cause stomach upset, can lead to ulcers, and, in the elderly and diabetic, may cause kidney problems if used over a prolonged period of time.

Selective Serotonin Reuptake Inhibitors (SSRIs)

How do *selective serotonin reuptake inhibitors* (SSRIs) such as fluoxetrine (Prozac) work? As you learned in Chapter 1, serotonin is a neurotransmitter chemical. When serotonin is outside the neurons (brain cells) that produce it, it has a calming effect on moods. Neurons can reabsorb the serotonin, however, and when they do this in sufficient quantities, the calming effect is diminished or lost. SSRIs keep the neurons from reabsorbing serotonin, which is why SSRIs are so effective in the treatment of premenstrual symptoms (Stone 1990): With more serotonin available, your sense of well-being is enhanced and your mood swings and anger are reduced.

Serotonin levels are decreased in the late luteal phase of women with PMS. This discovery has finally pinned down a chemical cause for severe symptoms of PMS and led the way to a treatment that works. A multicenter Canadian study of fluoxetine was conducted in women with PMS severe enough to impair their daily lives (Steiner 1995). The results showed a 44 to 52 percent improvement in the fluoxetine group compared to 7 percent improvement in the placebo group. The optimal dose was 20 milligrams a day for most patients. Many other studies have shown similar results using other SSRIs (Zoloft, Paxil, Effexor, and Serzone). These drugs become effective much more quickly for women with PMS than for women with other mood or anxiety disorders (Eriksson 1999). Several studies have shown that a woman can take sertraline (Zoloft) or fluoxetine premenstrually *only*, as opposed to continuously (Jermain 1999). Short-term use of these drugs appears to be superior to daily use. Investigators feel this may be due to the development of a tolerance when used daily (Eriksson 1999).

CAUTION! Medications such as fluoxetine appear to be safe for everyone except people with bipolar disorder (what used to be called manic depression). See Chapter 11 for a more complete discussion of this disorder.

The major problems with SSRIs are insomnia or disturbed sleep, sleepiness, shakiness, headache, and lack of orgasm. You can alleviate the sleep disturbance by changing the time you take the medication: If the medication makes you sleepy during the day, take it at night; if it keeps you awake, take it in the morning. Most people find that the side effects decrease over time (Barnhart 1995).

Although SSRIs work wonders for most people, 35 to 67 percent of women and men may have problems with sexual desire or orgasm while taking these medications (Modell 1997). Desire may be lessened and/or orgasms diminished or absent. Since the only good thing about PMS is your increased sex drive, losing it may sound like you've thrown out the baby with the bathwater. Infrequently, sexuality is heightened by these medications (Modell 1997). Luckily, sexual symptoms are less likely to occur at all if you take the medication premenstrually instead of all of the time. Sexual dysfunction is also dose related and sometimes goes away on its own. If not, switching to a different SSRI may help. The addition of bupropion (Wellbutrin) can eliminate sexual side effects (Labbate 1994). Several investigators have given sildenafil (Viagra) to their patients on SSRIs with excellent return of sexual function and desire (Fava 1998; Pallanti 1999). (**Note:** The older antidepressants, tricyclics (not SSRIs) like imipramine (Tofranil) and amitripyline (Elavil), have many more side effects than do SSRIs. These old-timers don't mess with your sex life, but they don't treat PMS either (Freeman 1999).

Tranquilizers such as alprazolam (Xanax), lorazepam (Ativan), and diazepam (Valium), which are not SSRIs, may help some mood changes. Some psychiatrists suggest taking these medications the week before a period is expected, to treat irritability. However, all of them are addicting, and you may get withdrawal symptoms unless you decrease them gradually. By contrast, if you don't like the effects of an SSRI, you can just stop taking it, without fear of withdrawal symptoms.

A new generation of SSRIs is being developed that will not cause significant sexual dysfunction. Citalopram (Celexa) has been used to treat depression without sexual side effects (Pallanti 1999). These new SSRIs will be more site-specific than those currently available. In other words, the new SSRIs will be able to attach to only those receptors in your cells that influence your PMS or depressive symptoms. They will leave your sexuality alone (Leventhal 1997).

Hormone Treatment of PMS

Premenstrual syndrome is almost exclusively the result of normal menstrual cycles. Fluctuations in the hormones without ovulation have been associated with PMS-like symptoms, but those symptoms are rarely as severe as when ovulation takes place (Rubinow 1992). For thirty years, researchers and clinicians alike have thought that variations of estrogen and progesterone were in some way causative of the 150 or so PMS symptoms that plague so many perimenopausal women. Over these years, all sorts of hormonal manipulation has been tried with varied success. With each subsequent generation, a new "cure-all" emerges. Each one claims to eliminate the plethora of annoying to life-altering symptoms we know as PMS. One such recent brouhaha is the use of "natural" progesterone.

Progesterone Therapy—Does It Have an Effect on PMS?

Natural progesterone vaginal suppositories were the main therapy for PMS during the 1980s. The enthusiasm for natural progesterone waned, however, when studies showed that the 80 percent effectiveness of the suppositories was essentially the same as for a placebo (Mortola 1992). In the other 20 percent of women studied, neither the placebo nor the progesterone had any effect (Smith 1993; Epperson 1999). Additionally, no differences in PMS benefits could be demonstrated from using either a low or high dose progesterone suppository (Freeman 1990). Finally, progesterone blood levels were found to be the same in women suffering from PMS and those who were not (Schmidt 1993). Since PMS is not due to an altered progesterone state, women are not benefited by the addition of progesterone.

Progestins and PMS

Progestins are synthetic compounds that act like progesterone but can be taken orally. They don't treat PMS either, and they may make the symptoms worse. Progestins are one of the hormones in birth control pills and are effectively used to control abnormal bleeding. When given to menopausal women to help prevent cancer, they may cause a PMS-like syndrome.

Micronized Natural Progesterone and Creams

Natural progesterone can't be absorbed when taken orally, so scientists have tried to find ways to adapt natural progesterone in the hopes of avoiding the side effects of the progestins while retaining the benefits in treating abnormal bleeding and preventing cancer. This has led to some interesting discoveries. Natural progesterone manufactured from wild Mexican yams and soybeans can be absorbed orally when pulverized into minute particles, a process called micronization.

Several studies of the efficacy of micronized progesterone cream for uses other than PMS are ongoing in Europe and are quite promising. Micronized progesterone can also be absorbed through the skin from a skin patch and is successfully used in combination with estrogen to treat menopausal women.

There are, at last count, twenty-seven different progesterone creams on the market. *Phytoprogesterones*, found naturally in a variety of plants, are a popular treatment for PMS because they are perceived as safer or more effective than synthetic hormones. You cannot absorb those over-the-counter products that contain phytoprogesterones in their raw form because your body lacks the chemical pathways to convert the phytohormones into progesterone. Some contain varying amounts of micronized progesterone as well as phytoprogesterone. Many of the phytohormone creams add a number of other chemicals—chamomile extract, medicinal herbs (black cohosh, burdock root, and ginseng), aloe vera, and vitamin E—to the basic yam extract. Remember, unless they also contain micronized progesterone, none of the phytoprogesterone from the raw yams in the product will even be absorbed; the only chemicals you will absorb are the additives. The manufacturers claim these creams help all sorts of female problems (Lee 1996), but none have been reliably tested against a placebo (Schagen van Leeuwen 1993). Don't be fooled by the claims that these creams will help PMS—they won't (Smith 1993; Epperson 1999).

Estrogen May Help

Many premenopausal women use the estrogen skin patch successfully to alleviate anxiety, migraine headaches, and negative feelings associated with PMS. Some researchers believe that estrogen is not a cure for most PMS, but that it does cure the PMS that has its onset during the premenopausal years—the five years before the onset of menopause (Revlin 1990). They feel that premenopausal PMS is really due to a late luteal phase decline in estrogen levels. If you have never had significant PMS prior to age forty-five to fifty, extra estrogen (by either patch or pill) during the week to ten days before your period is due will usually relieve your symptoms. Unfortunately, your bloating, sore breasts, or menstrual cramps will not be helped and your menstrual flow may get a little heavier.

How do you use the patch? Apply it once you begin to experience PMS symptoms. Place the patch away from your breasts and away from skin creases. The estrogen will begin to work within an hour.

CAUTION! Ten percent of women using the patch get a skin rash sufficient to discontinue its use.

If your PMS symptoms are very predictable, beginning like clockwork, you may get relief from taking oral estrogen, such as low-dose estradiol (Estrace). Take it every day beginning seven to ten days before the expected menstrual period.

Monocyclic birth control pills alleviate many of the symptoms of PMS for the majority of women (Forrest 1979). This is thought to be due to these pills' constant levels of estrogen and progesterone. In contrast, with tricyclic birth control pills, both estrogen and progesterone doses vary throughout the month. Tricyclic birth control pills are less effective in the treatment of PMS.

Some women find their symptoms are worse on the Pill, regardless of whether it is mono or tricyclic; these women have an adverse sensitivity to progesterone (Leventhal 1996).

CAUTION! Migraine headaches may first appear with the use of birth control pills, in which case they must be discontinued.

Prevention of Ovarian Function

Women who don't ovulate don't have PMS. If other treatments for PMS don't work, you may need to block the ovaries from producing hormones, but the cure may be worse than the disease! These treatments will relieve PMS symptoms, but they have other long-term side effects.

GnRH Agonists

GnRH agonists (such as Lupron Depot or Synarel) relieve PMS but cause bone loss. GnRH agonists prevent ovulation by shutting down the pituitary gland and, therefore, the ovary and its hormones. After the initial administration of a GnRH agonist, there is an outpouring of FSH and LH reserves from the pituitary gland, which increases estrogen and progesterone levels. PMS symptoms may get worse for a short period of time. Once the pituitary shuts down, though, PMS shuts down, too. Unfortunately, once a woman's estrogen level drops, she is thrown into a false menopause. With it come the accompanying risks for osteoporosis and heart disease, not to mention hot flashes, memory loss, and vaginal dryness. "Add-back" therapy, using low doses of estrogen with or without progesterone (discussed in Chapter 7), has successfully relieved these symptoms but is not as effective as when the GnRH agonists are used alone (Leather 1999). At about $400 a month, treatment with GnRH agonists is extremely expensive.

Danazol

Danazol is a testosterone derivative that shuts down the pituitary and thereby suppresses ovarian hormones, so PMS symptoms are stopped. In double-blind studies (Dalton 1987), danazol is superior to placebos in reducing overall symptomatology, both physical and mental. However, danazol itself has side effects that can mimic those of PMS, including depression, weight gain, and bloating. Since the drug is derived from testosterone, it may also cause decreased breast size, acne, excess hair growth, and deepening of the voice. (If you use your voice professionally, be especially leery of taking this drug.) Long-term danazol use may accelerate cardiovascular disease. Low-dose danazol used only premenstrually doesn't have these side effects but doesn't relieve any general PMS symptoms either. It does markedly reduce breast tenderness, however (O'Brien 1999). Danazol is an expensive medication, costing about $43 per cycle.

Ovarian Removal

All studies on the surgical treatment of PMS show that a hysterectomy without removal of the ovaries does nothing to improve PMS symptoms. Removal of the ovaries, however, does relieve the symptoms completely. If you are under forty and lose your ovaries, though, you will have great difficulty adjusting your estrogen replacement therapy (Riggs 1986). Inconsistent levels will result in an increase in the risk of osteoporosis and heart disease, even with replacement therapy. Therefore, ovarian removal should be considered only as an absolute last resort.

Depression and PMS

"I don't have any good days; my symptoms just get worse before my period." Does this sound like you? If it does, you may have an underlying depression that is worsened by your PMS. Psychiatrists call this premenstrual magnification (Bailey 1999). Figure 3.1 illustrates the difference between PMS and depression worsened by PMS. As you can see from the graphs, severity of symptoms is the same in the second half of the cycle after ovulation, but the symptoms increase in the first half. There are a number of depressive disorders ranging from major life-altering depression to disorders with only mild emotional effects, but they share similar symptoms. (See Chapter 11 for more complete discussion of types of depression in relation to stress.)

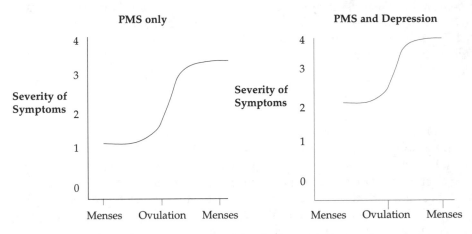

Figure 3.1.   Premenstrual Syndrome with Depression

Menstrual Migraines

Menstrual migraines are severe headaches occurring a few days before your menstrual period is due to start, or the first few days of your bleeding. What is the difference between a migraine headache and the more common tension headache? Table 3.2 illustrates how they differ.

Table 3.2. Characteristics Differentiating Migraines from Tension Headaches		
Characteristics	**Migraine Headaches**	**Tension Headaches**
Location	One or both sides	Both sides
Frequency	Intermittent	Intermittent
Duration	8 hours (2–72 hours)	Variable
Pain	Throbbing (50%)	Often bandlike
Severity	Moderate to severe	Mild to moderate
Associated symptoms	Nausea, vomiting, photophobia	Uncommon
Family history	Often Present	Present

Adapted from: S. D. Silberstein. 1990. "Advance in the Understanding the Pathology of Headaches." *Neurology.* 42 (2):6–10.

Symptoms

A mood change, a food craving, or difficulty concentrating commonly precede a migraine headache. Just before the headache begins, about 15 percent of migraine sufferers experience an "aura." Symptoms during the aura can include a particular smell, flashing lights, or any other unusual occurrence that doesn't makes sense in terms of what is actually going on. Following the aura, a pounding headache begins. Other symptoms include nausea, vomiting, and photophobia (sensitivity to light). If you experience these symptoms, you end up in bed. They may be severe enough to keep you home for a couple of days. The special distinction of menstrual migraines, of course, is that they occur *every month*.

Prevention and Treatment

Let's take a look at some things you can do prevent and treat menstrual migraines.

- **Estrogen:** One of the theories about menstrual migraine is that it results from the change in the estrogen level as it drops just before a period begins. Some women avoid this drop and prevent a migraine with the estrogen skin patch. Patch use begins one week before a period is due. Oral estradiol is superior to other oral estrogens (see Chapter 7) for the treatment of menstrual migraines.

- **NSAIDs:** Some women do well with the antiprostaglandin effects of NSAIDs, which we talked about earlier in this chapter. NSAIDs are taken every six to eight hours for a week before a period is due and into the first two or three days of the menstrual period.

- **Vasoconstrictors:** Two commonly used constrictor drugs are DHE (dihydroergotamine) and sumatriptan succinate. Both are given by injection, though sumatriptan succinate is also available in pill form. The usual treatment is to take one shot by self-administration at the first sign of the headache, and, if needed, to take a second dose one hour later. Only two shots can be used in a twenty-four-hour period. Because sumatriptan succinate can cause a heart spasm, it is first given in a hospital setting.

- **Prevention with Testosterone:** While the vasoconstrictors described above work quite well for migraines, you would probably prefer to prevent the headache than to treat the symptoms. Some success has been found clinically with the use of testosterone pellets injected beneath the skin (Lanka). With this method, the testosterone from the pellet goes directly into the bloodstream. Testosterone is converted into estrogen in a woman's brain (Leventhal 1997). The increased estrogen level in the brain may explain its effectiveness in some patients who have not been helped by other therapies (Lanka). (Note: The new testosterone patch used by men for various reasons contains too high a dose for women. When cut in quarters, the patch may give relief to migraine sufferers and allow them to avoid the discomfort of an injection. Unfortunately, cutting the patch into quarters lessens its adhesiveness. See Chapter 7 for more about testosterone.)

- **Alternative medical therapies:** Alternative medical therapies can be remarkably effective in reducing migraine pain. These techniques can be the answer if you have been plagued by medication side effects or choose to use them instead of more conventional treatments. Biofeedback and acupuncture work quite well for many women. These programs usually require a series of treatments, but they are both good for stress reduction, and stress is a well-known migraine trigger. Hypnotherapy, massage therapy, and osteopathic manipulation can also be effective in moderating migraine pain, especially if you seek treatment at a time when you are vulnerable to an attack (such as premenstrually).

Summary

During perimenopause, PMS increases in severity and duration. Current treatment that works better than a placebo includes diuretics for physical symptoms and SSRIs for emotional ones. Proper diet and exercise also mitigate physical and emotional symptoms. For women who develop PMS for the first time late in their perimenopause, estrogen treatment may be sufficient. The good news is that PMS symptoms will disappear when you reach menopause.

O O O O

4

Serious Changes: Cardiovascular Disease and Osteoporosis

Heart disease and osteoporosis typically first appear during menopause, but you may be sowing the seeds of these diseases during perimenopause. There are steps you can take now to reduce your risks and avoid a harvest of ill health. Perimenopause is your wake-up call. Now is the time to learn about these diseases in order to have a more vibrant and healthy future.

Cardiovascular Disease (CVD)

Alphabet Soup	
CVD	Cardiovascular disease
HDL	High-density lipoprotein
LDH	Low-density lipoprotein

Cardiovascular disease (CVD), which is a disease of the heart and/or vascular system (arteries, veins, and capillaries), is the leading cause of death for women in the United States. To put it in perspective, one in two women will eventually die of heart disease or stroke as compared to one in twenty-five who die because of breast cancer (American Heart Association 1997). Every year, 550,000 people die because of CVD, and 250,000 of them are women (Wenger 1993). Compare that number to 60,000 annual cancer deaths in women over age fifty from all reproductive structures *combined*, including breast, uterus, ovary, cervix, and vagina. For women over fifty, CVD is an enormous personal and public health problem.

You're Not Menopausal—Why Worry?

You don't need to lose sleep over the possibility that you will develop CVD during your transitional years. Keep in mind, however, that estrogen is one of your guardians and that it begins decreasing after your mid-thirties. Men are at far greater risk for CVD than you are during these years, but the gradual decline in estrogen begins to narrow the gap, so you are not immune to heart disease simply because you are still having menstrual periods. Prevention needs to start whenever the risk starts increasing; and for you, that is now.

Risky Business

Until recently, guidelines for preventing heart disease were like the blue jeans of the 1960s. They were based on the anatomy and physiology of men, but they were supposed to fit women too (Harvard Women's Health Watch 1999). When it became clear that the unisex approach was not valid, the American Heart Association and the American College of Cardiology issued new gender-specific guidelines for preventing heart disease in women. See Table 4.1 for a summary of the guidelines. As you can see, many of the risk factors for future heart disease are within your control. Now is the time to get a handle on these factors and take charge of your own personal prevention program to help ensure a better long-term quality of life.

Table 4.1.   Risk Factors for Heart Disease

Estrogen deficiency

Unfavorable lipid profile (cholesterol, HDL, LDL, triglycerides)

Hypertension (high blood pressure)

Cigarette smoking

Sedentary lifestyle

Obesity: 20% more weight than recommended for your age and height

Diabetes

Alcohol abuse

Heavy stress in your life

Family history of coronary heart disease

Estrogen Deficiency—Your Heart Is at Risk

During your perimenopausal years, one of the least evaluated risk factors for CVD is estrogen deficiency. Few women or their physicians think about this until estrogen deficiency symptoms appear or menstrual periods stop. Estrogen deficiency plays a much larger role during the transitional years than many women and health-care providers realize. For example, it is obvious that loss of the ovaries for any reason (such as surgical removal, premature menopause, chemotherapy) will result in a dramatic decline in estrogen. But it is not widely known that many studies have shown a hysterectomy, even with conservation of ovaries, will result in menopause at an earlier age than would normally be expected. This happens as a result of disturbed blood flow to the ovaries from the surgery (Nachtigall 1995). If your uterus has been removed, be especially alert to symptoms of estrogen deficiency. If they appear, talk with your health-care provider about estrogen supplements or low-dose birth control pills.

If you are an overweight smoker with high blood pressure and an unfavorable lipid profile (high cholesterol, low HDL, high LDL, high triglycerides—more on these substances in a moment), you have a lot of CVD risk factors going against you. If estrogen deficiency symptoms are also present, serious consideration should be given to hormone supplementation. There is still time to implement lifestyle changes and start hormone supplements. Don't wait until you need cardiac rehabilitation. Older women who have already developed coronary heart disease may not be able to rely on estrogen to prevent further progression of the disease (Hully 1998).

Mechanism of Estrogen Protection

To understand how estrogen protects you from CVD, we need to explain some basics of how hardening of the arteries (atherosclerosis) develops. The problem is caused by the gradual buildup of plaque on the walls of arteries. Plaque is a lipid (fatlike substance) that results from deposits of excess cholesterol circulating in the bloodstream. It narrows arteries and restricts blood flow, leading to high blood pressure, heart attacks, and strokes. The process of plaque buildup, called atherogenesis, has both lipid and nonlipid components. The lipid component is all about cholesterol, which we explain in a moment. The nonlipid component involves altered functioning of the endothelium (the lining of the arteries).

The endothelium regulates the tone of arteries by releasing compounds that influence whether the vessel is relaxed or constricted. It is easy to see that too much constriction narrows the vessel and reduces blood flow so that more pressure is required to force blood through it. That causes high blood pressure. The endothelium also has surface properties that prevent blood clotting and adhesion of certain blood elements (platelets and white blood cells). This prevents obstruction of the artery. We'll come back to this.

The lipid component of atherogenesis involves cholesterol. Cholesterol is a lipid that is synthesized by your liver. It is also present in animal fat, so the most common external source is from what you eat. Your body utilizes cholesterol for energy and as a precursor for hormones. *Lipoproteins* are the cholesterol carriers in your bloodstream, and estrogen has a potent influence on them. The two most important of these are *high-density lipoprotein* (HDL) and *low-density lipoprotein* (LDL). HDL, the "good guy," carries cholesterol away from the artery walls and other tissues to the liver, where it is broken down and excreted from the body in bile. LDL, the "bad guy," also carries cholesterol in the bloodstream, but it allows the cholesterol to be deposited as plaque on artery walls, causing narrowing of the channel.

With that as a background, let's turn to how estrogen influences atherogenesis. Just as atherogenesis has lipid and nonlipid components, estrogen's heart-protecting effect has both lipid and nonlipid mechanisms (Clarkson 1997).

Estrogen's lipid-related effects include:

- Decreases total cholesterol

- Raises HDL (good) cholesterol 10 to 15 percent

- Lowers LDL (bad) cholesterol 10 to 15 percent

- Decreases lipoprotein(a), another source of atherogenesis

- Raises triglycerides (an unwelcome effect)

- Prevents oxidation of LDL (estrogen is an antioxidant), which keeps LDL from being deposited as plaque

- Inhibits the usual postmenopausal accumulation of central abdominal fat, which is associated with hardening of the arteries. With adequate estrogen, fat tends to accumulate about the hips, and a woman's body shape is typically pearlike. In estrogen deficiency, fat accumulates about the abdomen, and body shape more closely resembles an apple.

Nonlipid protective effects of estrogen include:

- Normalizes regulation of arterial wall constriction and relaxation, preventing high blood pressure. Estrogen deprivation results in inappropriate constriction of artery walls.

- Improves the metabolism of glucose by increasing the body's sensitivity to insulin. Lower levels of circulating insulin result. (Too much insulin is associated with atherogenesis.)

- Increases antiplatelet aggregation factors, which means the risk of blood clots is reduced

- Has a direct strengthening effect on heart muscle (called the inotropic effect), which results in more efficient heart action. This means that more blood is pumped per heartbeat.

The assumption has always been that estrogen's heart protection comes from the favorable effects it has on lipids. However Clarkson's report (1997) showed that 65 to 75 percent of the protection derives from the nonlipid benefits, and only 25 to 35 percent from lipid benefits. So our thinking about estrogen has changed from regarding it as simply a reproductive hormone to the realization that it has diverse effects in many tissues and organs throughout the body. The above discussion details the favorable effects of estrogen on your heart and blood vessels, but this book will show you it brings many more benefits.

Adequate estrogen production is a major reason why you are protected (but not exempted) from cardiovascular disease during your reproductive years; and it explains why your risk for CVD begins to rise when estrogen declines. It also explains why women over fifty with CVD risk factors, and who are on HRT, enjoy a 50 percent decrease in heart attack deaths compared to nonusers of HRT. More than thirty published studies have documented this reduced risk of CVD in estrogen users (Speroff 1994).

Cholesterol-Lowering Drugs (Statins)

The statin (anticholesterol) drugs appear to be as effective as estrogen for prevention of heart disease (Darling 1997; Davidson 1997; Downs 1998). A consensus panel of the American Heart Association and the American College of Cardiology recommends that women with coronary heart disease use statins rather than estrogen replacement therapy as a first-line treatment for lowering abnormal blood lipid levels (Harvard Heart Letter 2000). Examples of such drugs include Colestid, Lipitor, Mevacor, and Zocor.

A Little More about Triglycerides

Triglycerides are a type of fat derived mainly from food. The exact role of triglycerides in causing CVD is not certain, but it is known that high triglycerides combined with low levels of "good" HDL are associated with heart disease, especially in women. High triglycerides in diabetics raise the risk of CVD three-fold in men, but two hundred-fold in women (Bass 1993).

It's Not All Good News

A note of caution was sounded regarding estrogen's protection against coronary heart disease (CHD) with the 1998 publication of the Heart and Estrogen/Progestin Replacement Study (HERS) (Hully 1998). HERS was a large, randomized, placebo-controlled study of postmenopausal women from ages fifty-five to eighty who were known to have CHD. Its purpose was to see if hormone replacement would prevent further coronary heart disease events in women with preexisting coronary disease. To the surprise of most, they found that the HRT group had more heart attacks than the placebo group, but only in the first year. After that, HRT was found to be protective. The increased rate of heart attacks in the first year of HERS was thought to be related to the fact that these older women (average age sixty-six) with significant coronary heart disease were starting HRT for the first time and experienced a temporary increase in blood clotting factors. Most of the heart attacks were in the first four months of hormone use.

The Women's Health Initiative (WHI) announced in April 2000 that a similar effect of estrogen replacement was observed in their fifteen-year ongoing study of estrogen's effect on 27,000 enrolled women. It was also observed that it is a temporary adverse effect that occurs in about one in one thousand women who start HRT. WHI will be completed and the final results published in about 2005.

Two 1999 studies may explain the HERS and WHI results. Each found evidence that estrogen replacement raises the level of C-reactive protein, a substance produced by the liver in response to inflammation (Ridker 1999; Cushman 1999). This suggests that estrogen may cause an initial inflammation in the endothelial lining of arteries, predisposing a woman to coronary artery damage. Until further studies are carried out, a concern exists that in women with proven coronary heart disease, estrogen replacement may not increase longevity.

Slight elevations of C-reactive protein plus monitoring cholesterol profiles are powerful predictors of who may be at risk for a heart attack several years in the future (Ridker 2000). A new highly sensitive blood test for C-reactive protein, called Hs-CRP, is now available (Wilson 1999). If you have risk factors for CHD, this test may help in your decision to change your lifestyle to eliminate those risks.

The Bottom Line for HRT and Heart Disease

HRT use in preventing heart disease is a work in progress. The biological evidence (lipid and nonlipid benefits) that estrogen decreases the risk factors is compelling. Dozens of observational studies of estrogen demonstrate a reduced death rate in HRT users, but this type of study is not proof. The proof as to whether or not HRT actually prevents heart disease will come from prospective interventional studies like WHI. Meanwhile the most important preventive factors remain lifestyle interventions (we'll talk about these in a moment).

HRT may not halt progression of heart disease once it becomes established, but it appears to have a significant role to play in prevention. Women without heart disease who are already on HRT should continue in the short-term. After five to ten or more years' use, estrogen replacement has been associated with a slightly increased risk for breast cancer (discussed in Chapter 6), so caution is prudent regarding long-term use pending the outcome of current studies.

Women who are considering HRT should realize there are considerable benefits, but that the risks are not yet fully understood. Ongoing studies will help in determining for which women the benefits outweigh the risks.

The take-home message for you as a healthy perimenopausal woman is, therefore: If you plan to use HRT, start it when your estrogen deficiency symptoms begin and before you develop coronary heart disease. Naturally, it would be better still to do everything you can to avoid getting CHD in the first place. Read on for more on how you can do this.

Hypertension—It's Hard on Your Heart

High blood pressure (140/90 or above) occurs because of increased resistance to blood flow due to atherosclerosis. The heart has to pump harder to get blood through these vessels. Over time, the heart is damaged by this constant extra effort. A low-fat diet, regular exercise, adequate estrogen, and, where appropriate, blood pressure medications are all important in controlling blood pressure and minimizing heart damage.

Smoking—Bad News for Your Heart

Nicotine is a vasoconstrictor. It causes blood vessels to squeeze down, and more pressure is needed to force blood through them. Your heart must work harder. Inhaled tobacco smoke also damages the lungs, which reduces the amount of oxygen that gets into the bloodstream. This forces the heart to speed up blood circulation in order to deliver the oxygen your body's tissues need. Tobacco use also has a toxic effect on your ovaries, leading to an earlier menopause and the risk of CVD from diminished estrogen.

If you smoke, your chances of dying from a heart attack are four times higher than if you do not. Even if you don't smoke, living with a smoker gives you twice the risk of a heart attack death (Kawachi 1997). Lung cancer is also strongly associated with smoking and is the number one fatal cancer in women. Breast cancer makes all the headlines, but lung cancer is much more deadly. Heart disease or lung cancer will ultimately cause the death of 35 percent of smokers. There is some good news, though. The American Heart Association states that if you quit now, in ten years your risk of a heart disease death will diminish to the same risk level as for people who never smoked. As you read this book, you will notice numerous other references to the dangers that smoking poses for you. Your heart is only one of the beneficiaries of your being a nonsmoker.

A Sedentary Lifestyle Is Not Good for Your Heart

Your heart does not tolerate low or nonexistent levels of exercise. Cardiologists and fitness experts throughout the world advise that cardiac fitness is essential to good health, and you can achieve it with only moderate activity.

A total of three hours per week of brisk walking or thirty minutes of aerobic exercise on most days will keep your heart fit for the long term. It's a lot easier to do it now than later, when it is called cardiac rehabilitation. The formula for achieving and maintaining cardiac fitness is examined in Chapter 9.

Obesity—Your Heart Hates It

If you are more than 20 percent over your ideal weight, you have crossed the line: It's not just an issue of physical appearance anymore; it's a health risk. The most accepted method of determining ideal weight is the Body Mass Index (BMI). You can calculate your own BMI by multiplying your weight in pounds by 700, and dividing by the square of your height in inches. (See Chapter 10 for more about BMI.) A BMI of 27 or over puts you at risk for future heart disease and other weight-related health problems. If you become overweight, your heart must work harder in every activity your body performs just to carry those extra pounds around. In addition, the extra body fat you accumulate will likely have resulted from a diet that is too high in fat. This raises your cholesterol level and puts you at greater risk for CVD. A healthy diet is not merely an option for you in your transitional years, it's a must. Slimming down for the long haul involves a permanent fitness program that stresses both a healthful diet and exercise. (Chapter 9 takes a close look at this topic.) A healthy heart will make the next half of your life a lot more livable for you.

Eat a Heart-Healthy Diet

To benefit your heart, base your diet on fruits, vegetables, whole grains, and nonfat or low-fat dairy products. A high fiber intake of 25 to 30 grams per day (from fruits, veggies, and especially whole grains) is associated with a reduced risk for heart disease. Eat only small portions of skinless poultry or lean red meat. Fat should supply less than 30 percent of your total daily calories, so keep animal fats to a minimum. Replace saturated fats from animal foods with monounsaturated fat from plant foods (e.g. olive oil or canola oil instead of butter). Consume no more than 300 milligrams of cholesterol daily. Include fish in your diet about two or three times each week. (Chapters 9 and 10 discuss healthy diet extensively.)

A 1998 report from the Nurses' Health Study found that women who consumed 400 micrograms of folic acid plus 3 milligrams of vitamin B_6 reduced their risk of heart attack by 50 percent (Rimm 1998). Foods rich in folic acid, also called folates, include green leafy vegetables, legumes (beans, peas), citrus fruits, poultry, liver, and whole-grain cereals. Good sources of B_6 include bananas, poultry, liver, seafood, and low-fat dairy products.

Stress and Your Heart

Social and psychological influences in life can add up to enormous stress for some women. Over the long haul, prolonged and frequent jolts from your stress hormones can result in an adverse effect on your cardiovascular system. (See Chapter 11 for more on stress management.)

CVD Summary

Few achievements in the health field can surpass the decline in deaths from cardiovascular disease in the United States. Death rates from all forms of heart disease peaked in the 1950s. For coronary artery disease, the major form of heart disease, death rates peaked in the 1960s and have declined 60 percent since then. Death rates from stroke have declined 70 percent (Wellness Letter 1999). Millions of lives have been extended in the past few decades as a result of this progress. Whether the decline in death rates will continue is questionable, given the rising rate of obesity in both adults and children in our country, and the growing tendency for Americans to pay less attention to high blood pressure.

Osteoporosis

Osteoporosis means porous bones. It is a condition that results from loss of bone mineral density (BMD) and bone protein; this loss causes weakened bones that fracture easily. Some researchers think it is a disease process and not a component of normal aging (Hammond 1998). Osteoporosis is mistakenly regarded as a problem of very old women. While it is true that the devastating effects on quality of life are primarily in postmenopausal women, osteoporosis has its beginnings in a woman's mid-thirties. In fact, you may even have set yourself up for osteoporosis in your teens and twenties. Osteoporosis is largely preventable, but to avoid it, you need to be able to recognize whether you are at risk. This section of the chapter takes a look at who gets osteoporosis, what happens and why, how to prevent it, how to diagnose it, and how it is treated. There are many factors intimately involved in maintaining bone density, such as weight-bearing exercise, adequate calcium and vitamin D intake, and elimination of risk factors, but estrogen is the single most important ingredient in preventing osteoporotic fractures.

Who Gets Osteoporosis

Nearly 30 million Americans are at risk for osteoporosis, and 80 percent of them are women. Americans suffer 1.5 million osteoporotic fractures per year. The National Osteoporosis Foundation estimates that half of all women over age fifty will suffer an osteoporotic fracture sometime during their lives. See Table 4.2 for the magnitude of the osteoporosis problem. Postmenopausal women sustain 250,000 hip fractures every year. This is the most common osteoporosis complication, with an average cost of up to $35,000 per patient (Ray 1997). As many as 20 percent of hip fracture sufferers are dead within one to four months from surgical complications and the heart and lung effects of the inactivity that results from fractures. Half of the survivors are never able to live independently again because of their inability to walk normally. Osteoporosis is a major factor in the rapidly rising number of women who require nursing home care. Indeed, 75 percent of nursing home residents over age sixty-five are women.

Osteoporosis is also implicated in tooth loss from diminished bone support of teeth, although the most important factor in tooth loss is periodontal (gum) disease. Approximately 32 percent of American women over age sixty-five have no teeth. The Harvard Nurses' Health Study and other researchers report that HRT favorably influences tooth retention (Paganini-Hill 1995).

The annual cost of medical care for osteoporosis is $13.8 billion (Ray 1997), and the human toll is appalling. This is an epidemic that can escalate to major proportions when the 38 million women of the baby boomer generation become postmenopausal. In spite of the fact that the vast majority of people at risk are women, a survey of women aged forty-five to seventy-five revealed that 75 percent have never inquired of their health-care provider about osteoporosis (National Osteoporosis Foundation 1998). The numbers quoted above should be dramatically improved when your generation becomes sufficiently informed and motivated to take charge of this threat to your health and your quality of life.

Table 4.2.   Magnitude of the Osteoporosis Problem in the U.S.

- Affects over 28 million women

- 250,000 hip fractures/year in women

- 1.5 million total fractures a year

- 33% of white women will fracture their hips

- 25% of white women will fracture their spines

- 25% of Africa-American women will fracture their hips

- Annual cost estimated at $13.8 billion

Sources: Melton 1997; Ray 1997; Cooper 1992

Nuts and Bolts of Osteoporosis

Bone is a living, dynamic tissue. It is made up of protein collagen fibers, which are infiltrated with crystals of calcium phosphate. Bone tissue is constantly being added and removed, just like skin. This process is referred to as *bone remodeling*. Normally, bone removal and bone formation are in balance, and a sturdy skeleton is maintained. Osteoporosis results when bone formation falls behind bone removal. Loss of estrogen is a primary cause of this imbalance, and here's why. The cells that form bone are called osteoblasts. The removers are osteoclasts. And guess what? Estrogen receptors are known to exist on osteoblasts. This makes the presence of estrogen molecules plugged into those receptors a necessary condition for maintenance of healthy bones. Bone loss therefore begins when estrogen declines and the osteoblasts are not getting their job done.

As you already know, the onset of estrogen decline occurs in your mid-thirties. You do not become ravaged by bone loss at this age. Osteoporosis is very slow and subtle, offering no particular symptoms to alert you to its presence. As a matter of fact, one of the reasons osteoporosis has been such a problem for women in the generations prior to yours is that its effects were often not recognized until about age seventy. A woman would do something as mundane as step off a curb and fracture her hip. Fortunately, enough is now known about the causes and prevention of osteoporosis that you are not dependent upon a personal tragedy to alert you to your risk. You can learn whether you are at risk and take steps to avoid osteoporosis.

Estrogen Replacement and Osteoporosis

Estrogen replacement therapy (ERT) should be started within five years of menopause to get maximum benefit from its use. Women who use estrogen have a 71 percent reduction in nonvertebral fractures. An 80 percent reduction in vertebral fractures occurs when estrogen is supplemented with calcium (Cauley 1995). Once started, ERT should continue long-term because rapid bone loss ensues when ERT is discontinued (Speroff 1999). For women who must not, or choose not to use estrogen, other alternatives exist, such as bisphosphonates (we discuss these later in this chapter). Many risk factors increase a woman's chances for developing osteoporosis, and you can favorably alter many of them; we'll discuss how in a minute. But maximum protection from fractures later in life requires estrogen to be part of the equation. Hormone replacement is covered extensively in Chapter 7.

The Role of Progesterone and Progestins

Promoters of food supplements and "natural" hormonal products have been making a lot of noise in recent years about the use of natural progesterone cream for prevention of osteoporosis. Bottom line: While it's true that natural progesterone and its synthetic forms, progestins, can help reduce the rate of bone loss, estrogen is much better at it. Because progesterone and progestins act as mild antiestrogens, there was concern in the early 1980s that combining the two would inhibit estrogen's demonstrated beneficial effects. Fortunately, that turned out not to be true, and HRT that utilizes both hormones is known to be quite beneficial in preventing it.

Natural progesterone can be produced from soybeans, peanuts, and wild Mexican yams. The only FDA-approved natural progesterone is Prometrium, which is derived from peanuts. A cream form of natural progesterone has been used in Europe for many years, and prescription use is now on the upswing in the United States. A randomized, double-blind, placebo-controlled trial has shown the cream is *not* effective in preventing osteoporosis (Leonetti 1999). In spite of this, some claims imply that natural progesterone cream is adequate on its own for osteoporosis prevention, quite apart from other, proven methods.

The Role of Testosterone and Estrogen

A small study using both testosterone and estrogen demonstrated *increased* bone formation, as compared to estrogen's ability to stop bone loss (Raisz 1996). For such a regimen to be accepted, it must be shown that the necessary dose of testosterone will not lower HDL, which would increase the risk of CVD. Clearly, more study is needed.

Let's Talk Calcium

Calcium is your body's most important mineral. As vital as calcium is to bone integrity, it is also necessary to proper functioning of your muscles, brain, heart muscle, blood-clotting mechanism, and many other bodily needs. Wide fluctuations of calcium levels are not tolerated for long, so an elaborate hormonal system exists to regulate calcium in your bloodstream. The system utilizes: calcitonin, a hormone from the thyroid that stimulates bone production; reproductive hormones (estrogen, progesterone, and testosterone); corticosteroids from the adrenal glands; parathyroid hormone; and vitamin D. If your calcium intake is insufficient to maintain a normal blood level, the regulators get it from their handy calcium storage depot—your bones. In the next few paragraphs you will learn how to keep your calcium regulators happy and your bones strong.

The average American woman's diet is deficient in calcium, containing little more than 200 to 500 milligrams of calcium per day. In 1997 the National Academy of Sciences changed their recommended daily calcium intake for adults from 800 millgrams per day to 1,000 milligrams for premenopausal women and 1,200 milligrams for women (and men) over age fifty-one. In later years, the greater calcium supplements are needed because the intestine becomes less efficient in absorbing calcium. In addition, with declining estrogen, calcium utilization is impaired, so supplements are definitely important from perimenopause on. The safe upper limit is 2,500 milligrams per day (Institute of Medicine 1997).

Look over Table 4.3, which lists the calcium content of various foods. You will see that some of them are high in calcium but also high in fat and/or high in calories. With study and selection, you can achieve a diet with sufficient calcium.

Table 4.3.   Calcium Content in Various Foods

Food		Serving	Calcium	Calories	Fat Gms
Milk					
	Whole	1 cup	288 mg	150	8.1
	Skim	1 cup	296 mg	89	4.7
Cheese					
	Cheddar	1 oz	204 mg	112	9.1
	Swiss	1 oz	260 mg	95	7.1
	Cottage, 2% fat	4 oz	78 mg	100	2.2
Yogurt					
	Whole milk	1 cup	274 mg	141	7.7
	Plain, low-fat	1 cup	414 mg	143	3.4
Ice cream, 10% fat					
	Hard (vanilla)	1 cup	176 mg	270	14.1
	Soft serve (vanilla)	1 cup	236 mg	375	25.6
Ice milk	Hard, 4% fat (vanilla)	1 cup	176 mg	185	4.6
	Soft serve, 3% fat (vanilla)	1 cup	274 mg	225	8.6
Tofu					
	Firm curd	4 oz	6–100 mg	150	8
	Medium curd	4 oz	4–90 mg	90	6
Vegetables					
	Spinach, fresh, cooked, drained	1 cup	150 mg	40	0
	Broccoli, fresh, cooked, drained	1 cup	136 mg	40	0

Continued on the following page.

					Table 4.3. continued
Food		**Serving**	**Calcium**	**Calories**	**Fat Gms**
Vegetables (cont.)					
	Lima beans, fresh, cooked	½ cup	81 mg	120	0
	Collards, fresh, cooked, drained	1 cup	357 mg	65	0
	Turnip greens, fresh, cooked	1 cup	252 mg	30	0
Seafood					
	Shrimp, canned, drained	3½ oz	115 mg	100	0.8
	Salmon, canned, with bones	3½ oz	183 mg	210	14
	Oysters, raw, 18 medium size	3½ oz	258 mg	160	2.0
	Sardines, canned, with bones	3½ oz	425 mg	311	24.4
Nuts and Seeds					
	Almonds, shelled, about 12 nuts	1 oz	45 mg	170	15
	Sunflower seeds, hulled	1 oz	35 mg	159	14

Adapted from: Osteoporosis Foundation table (1992)

What Are Your Chances for Osteoporosis . . . and Your Daughter's?

Ages eleven through sixteen are the most critical years for bone accumulation; that is when bone growth is most rapid (Theistz 1992). A National Institutes of Health study panel reported in 2000 that only 10 percent of girls and 25 percent of boys between ages nine and seventeen get enough calcium. Bone mineral density (BMD) peaks in the late twenties to early thirties. Bone mass is constantly accumulating until that time if you are eating a healthy diet, getting regular exercise, and have plenty of estrogen. In other words, a window of opportunity to build a sturdy skeleton exists between the ages of about eleven and thirty. To accomplish healthy bone growth and bone mass accumulation during those years, girls and young adult women require four ingredients:

- 1,300 milligrams of calcium daily during the teen years, then 1,000 milligrams daily to age fifty (1,200 milligrams daily after fifty). A glass of milk or a plain nonfat yogurt has about 300 mg.

- 400 IU of vitamin D daily. A glass of milk has about 100 IU.

- Regular exercise

- Adequate estrogen

Risk Factors for Osteoporosis

Many additional risk factors exist that you need to know about in order to avert osteoporosis. Some of these factors are not within your control to change, but many of them are.

- **Race:** Caucasian and Asian women are more at risk than African-Americans because African-American women produce higher levels of calcitonin.

- **Family history of osteoporosis:** This is a strong indicator that you may be at risk, especially if a first-degree relative (mother, sister) has had an osteoporotic fracture.

- **Estrogen deprivation:** Delayed onset of menstrual periods, no full-term pregnancies, absence of ovaries, and early menopause are all conditions that decrease lifetime exposure to estrogen and the beneficial effects of estrogen on bone mineral density.

- **Skeletal size:** Small-boned women are more at risk. Having less bone mass makes a difference because your body uses the same amount of calcium each day, whether you have large or small bones. If your intake of calcium is inadequate, your body gets it from your skeleton.

- **Low body weight:** Underweight women are more likely to have osteoporosis. A weak form of estrogen called *estrone* is made from the conversion of body fat. Your body composition should be about 22 percent fat to avert diminished estrone. A "fashion model" body is definitely under 20 percent.

- **Sedentary lifestyle:** Weight-bearing exercise prevents bones from becoming weak. If calcium supplements and vitamin D are combined with exercise, bone density is increased even further (Prince 1995).

- **Low calcium intake:** If you had a low calcium intake in your past or if it is low now, you are at risk. During your transition, you need about 1,000 milligrams of calcium daily. If your diet doesn't give you that much, use a supplement. (Postmenopausal women need 1,200 milligrams unless they are on HRT, in which case 1,000 milligrams is enough.)

- **Cigarette smoking:** This is a triple whammy. First, nicotine interferes with your ability to absorb calcium. Second, tobacco smoke has a toxic effect on the ovaries (Windham 1999), leading to earlier menopause and major estrogen depletion. Third, smoking changes the metabolism of estrogens in the liver, reducing the level of active hormone available to your body. Smoking increases the risk of hip fracture 40 to 45 percent (Speroff 1999). Half a pack a day is all it takes.

- **Alcohol:** Alcohol interferes with calcium absorption from the intestine by toxic alterations to vitamin D. The risk level is exceeded by more than two alcoholic beverages per day. On the other hand, moderate consumption of five drinks per week is associated with increased estrogen and calcitonin levels, resulting in greater bone density in the spine (no change was noted in the hip) (Feskanich 1999).

- **Caffeine:** More than two caffeine beverages, such as coffee or cola drinks, is enough to increase risk. The risk can be blunted with adequate dietary calcium.

- **Phosphate-containing carbonated sodas:** These can be a problem. Too much phosphorus stimulates the parathyroid gland to become more active in removing calcium from your bones. Red meats and processed foods often contain phosphates as well. Moderation is advisable.

- **Absence of menstrual periods:** If you haven't had a menstrual period for an extended time (except during pregnancy), low estrogen levels result. Anorexia, bulimia, excessive exercise, and prolonged severe stress can cause your periods to stop.

- **Fad dieting:** If you are on a metabolically imbalanced high-protein/low-carbohydrate diet now or have been in the past, your risk for osteoporosis is increased (Wellness Letter 2000). The Atkins Diet is an example. High-protein/low-fiber diets interfere with calcium absorption by speeding up the transit time of food through the intestine. There is less time to absorb calcium. In addition, when protein consumption exceeds the recommended daily intake by 50 percent, calcium is lost in the urine. (Chapter 9 discusses protein needs.)

- **Hyperthyroidism or hyperparathyroidism:** These conditions both result in calcium loss at the expense of your bones.

- **Long-term corticosteroid use:** Corticosteroid (such as cortisone and prednisone) use in a long-term regimen can deplete bone mass by 30 percent in as little as six months. Screening for BMD is important in this situation and treatment should be instituted if BMD declines.

- **Depression of long duration:** This puts you at higher risk for osteoporosis at any age. Dr. Philip Gold, chief of neuroendocrinology at the National Institute of Mental Health, showed that women with depression had 10 to 15 percent lower bone density in their hips than normal for their age. The average woman in his study was age forty-one, but with a bone density level equivalent to that seen in seventy-year-old women. The cause was felt to be elevated levels of the stress hormone cortisol. This finding was confirmed in a separate 1996 study by Michelson.

Two Minerals and a Vitamin You Should Know About

Magnesium has a function similar to calcium in maintaining the proper contracting ability of muscles and transmission of nerve impulses. However, excess magnesium adversely affects bone density by inhibiting utilization of calcium. Ordinarily your intake of magnesium should never be more than half that of calcium. If you estimate the calcium in your daily diet to be 500 milligrams daily, magnesium should be no more than 250 milligrams. If you are taking a 500 milligrams calcium supplement for a total of 1,000 milligrams daily, magnesium can be 500 milligrams. Ironically, high doses of magnesium in the range of 1,000 milligrams are beneficial for PMS. If you are treating PMS with this level of magnesium, it should be as short a course of therapy as possible. Magnesium food sources include nuts, green leafy vegetables, legumes, and seafood.

Phosphorus is a major component of bone, but an excessive intake leads to bone loss. The parathyroid gland is a major regulator of calcium, and high levels of phosphorus cause the parathyroid to remove calcium from bones. As mentioned above, carbonated sodas, red meat, and processed foods are loaded with phosphates.

Vitamin D receptors exist in the intestinal tract and enhance the absorption of calcium. About 400 IU per day of vitamin D are needed to maintain optimum calcium absorption. The safe upper limit for vitamin D is 2,000 IU per day (Institute of Medicine 1997). Exposure to sunlight is another source of vitamin D, and people who have little sun exposure may need 800 IU.

"Tell Me If I've Got It"—Diagnosis

The early stages of osteoporosis are free of symptoms, so this is a blind alley for diagnosis. Routine X-ray is nearly useless because it does not disclose osteoporosis until bone mass loss approaches 30 percent. By that time it is usually too late to completely replace lost bone. The most reliable test is dual-energy X-ray absorptiometry (DEXA). It can detect as little as a 1-percent loss. This is a low-dosage X-ray technique that takes about three to five minutes to measure bone density. DEXA evaluates your spine, wrists, and hips, which are the most common sites for fractures. At present, DEXA is the gold standard for evaluating bone density.

Computed tomography (CT scan) has also been used for diagnosis, but it is more expensive, uses more X-ray irradiation, and does not evaluate the hip very well.

Ultrasound has a role to play as a screening technique. Quantitative ultrasound scans of the heel and kneecap have been shown to correlate well with DEXA results in evaluating bone density and predicting fracture risk. The advantage of ultrasound is that it does not utilize X-ray and is less expensive than DEXA.

The National Osteoporosis Foundation does not recommend a DEXA screening until age fifty-five. If you know you are at high risk for osteoporosis, however, you should start an aggressive prevention program immediately. In addition to changing the risk factors that are changeable, you should consider estrogen supplements during perimenopause if you have deficiency symptoms. The low-dose birth control pill works well for this, and you can take it right up to menopause. In fact, it serves not only as prevention, but as treatment as well.

Treating Osteoporosis

Until the 1990s, "treatment" for osteoporosis consisted of little more than an aggressive prevention program, as we discussed above. Few of you will require treatment during your transition, but let's take a look at some of the breakthroughs that have been made in treatment, in case you need it further down the line. Prevention of osteoporosis has been called the *only* game in town; but now that various treatments are available, prevention can be thought of as the *best* game in town.

Bisphosphonates are a nonhormonal class of drugs that have been shown to be beneficial in replacement of lost bone mineral density (BMD). They inhibit bone removal. The second generation of these drugs (alendronate and pamidronate) increases BMD and strength if taken with calcium and vitamin D. Spinal and hip fractures are reduced 50 percent (Hosking 1998; Black 1996). Alendronate is marketed as Fosamax. Although alendronate increases BMD, it only reduces fractures in those women proven to have osteoporosis, so it should not be used to prevent osteoporosis, only to treat it (Cummings 1998). Treatment with alendronate over four years produces a higher BMD than estrogen replacement therapy. It has now been shown that combining alendronate with estrogen works better than either used alone (Lindsay 1999). Therefore, in women with osteoporosis established via a DEXA scan, both of these helpful therapies can be used. A new bisphosphonate called resendronate became available in 2000, and additional similar drugs are likely to appear in the future.

Raloxifene (Evista) is a relatively new type of estrogenlike drug that is FDA-approved for treatment of osteoporosis. It is one of the "designer estrogens" called a *selective estrogen receptor modulator* (SERM). Raloxifene has been designed by cellular biologists so that it will attach to estrogen receptors on bone, but will not attach to breast receptors or endometrial (uterine lining) receptors. Raloxifene does result in increased BMD, but estrogen is 30 percent more effective (FDA 1997). Raloxifene reduces the risk of vertebral fractures, but not hip fractures (Ettinger 1999). Theoretically, it should reduce uterine cancer risk, and this was confirmed in recent studies showing no increase in endometrial thickness (hyperplasia) in up to three years of use (Cohen 2000). Endometrial hyperplasia is a precursor of cancer. The risk for breast cancer is 76 percent lower in raloxifene users (Ettinger 1999). (More on this in Chapter 6).

Another form of treatment is use of calcitonin, a hormone that reduces bone loss and causes a small increase in bone mass. It is synthesized from salmon and is available in an injectable form and a nasal spray, marketed as Miacalcin. Daily use combined with adequate calcium will increase bone density in vertebrae, but there is no significant benefit to hips or wrists, which are common fracture sites. Vertebral fractures were reduced 36 percent in one study (Silverman 1998). Another study showed that calcitonin was not effective in the first four years after menopause, but was helpful for those women who were more than ten years postmenopausal (Campodarve 1994). In advanced osteoporosis, salmon-calcitonin may be of considerable help in chronic pain from vertebral crush fractures.

Estrogen and testosterone taken together have been shown to increase bone density, but as we mentioned earlier, this form of treatment requires more research before it can be widely advocated.

The birth control pill (BCP) suppresses bone turnover more effectively than HRT (Taechakraichana 2000). This study confirmed previously held beliefs that using the BCP during perimenopause and the early years of postmenopause is beneficial in terms of osteoporosis prevention as well as lowering risk factors for coronary heart disease.

Sodium fluoride may be a new method in the wings for treating osteoporosis. Dr. Charles Pak, director of the Center for Mineral Metabolism Research at Texas Southwestern Medical Center, has studied this method. He reports that a slow-release form of sodium fluoride, when accompanied with calcium citrate, can build new bone and prevent spinal fractures. In the past, fluoride was shown to build bone, but it did not reduce the fracture rate. This slow-release method also builds bone but, apparently, stronger bone (Eastman 1997). The FDA has reviewed this method, but has not approved it.

Vertebroplasty is a new treatment for painful vertebral compression fractures. It involves injecting a surgical cement into the collapsed vertebra to strengthen it and alleviate pain.

Phytoestrogens may have a positive role to play in prevention and treatment of osteoporosis in postmenopausal women. Phytoestrogens are plant compounds structurally resembling estradiol. They are found in many fruits, vegetables, and grains, but especially in leguminous seeds (soybeans, chickpeas, lentils, beans). The three main classes of phytoestrogens are isoflavonoids, coumestans, and resorcyclic acid lactones. Of these, isoflavonoids have the most potent hormonelike activity. Like estrogen, isoflavone molecules can attach to receptor sites in bone, heart, and bladder tissue, where their estrogenlike activity can occur. But during the reproductive years, isoflavones behave as antiestrogens. It is not until estrogen deficiency is occurring that isoflavones begin to act as weak estrogens (Blair 1996). Bottom line: If you have risk factors for osteoporosis, dietary supplements of fourteen servings of soy protein per week can help prevent it. Such an intake provides an average of 16 to 20 grams daily of soy protein, plus 32 to 40 grams of isoflavones. If you already have osteoporosis, twenty-one servings of soy protein per week are recommended (Nisly 1999).

For those who can't consume sufficient dietary isoflavones, concentrates of isoflavones are available as food supplements. A precaution in the use of concentrates is that they may inhibit the effect of any estrogen preparations you may be taking, so their concomitant use is discouraged. Promensil is an isoflavone concentrate currently marketed as a food supplement.

A synthetic isoflavone derivative called ipriflavone (IP) has been used in Europe for many years. One of its metabolites (or products when it's metabolized) is daidzen, which has been shown to inhibit bone resorption and possibly stimulate bone formation (Civitelli 1997). Adverse drug reactions, consisting of gastrointestinal complaints and allergic reactions, have been reported in up to 14 percent of those studied (Agnusdei 1997). Ipriflavone is available in the United States as a food supplement.

Isoflavone concentrates and ipriflavone have been shown to be not as effective as HRT, raloxifene, or alendronate in either prevention or treatment of osteoporosis. For this reason, the recommendation for their use is limited to women at risk for or with diagnosed osteoporosis, who cannot tolerate or decline to use HRT, raloxifene, or alendronate, and who are unable to increase their dietary consumption of isoflavones to a beneficial level (Nisly 1999).

On the horizon, Amgen, a large American biotechnology company, has discovered a protein it calls osteoprotogerin, which regulates bone mineral density. A search is underway for a drug to treat osteoporosis utilizing this new discovery. Another avenue researchers are exploring is how to promote bone formation. All treatment methods currently in use target prevention of bone resorption. One new possibility is the use of parathyroid hormone (PTH) to directly stimulate new bone formation. One study reported a 45 percent increase in spinal BMD over two years (Lane 2000). PTH has been approved by the FDA, so its future is secure, but no preparation is likely to be on the market until 2001 or later (Lukkin 2000).

As you can see from all of the above, osteoporosis is the subject of intense interest and scientific research. This bodes well for the huge numbers of your generation who are entering the phase of life when osteoporosis becomes more than a theoretical consideration of some future problem.

Summary

This is the time in your life to assess your personal risk for the future development of cardiovascular disease. If you can identify certain CVD risk factors that apply to you, give them the serious consideration they deserve. Most of the risks listed earlier in Table 4.1, are amenable to change if you become proactive in managing them.

Osteoporosis must be avoided if you are to enjoy a full life after you become menopausal. If you and the rest of your boomer cohorts live en masse into your eighties as predicted, osteoporosis is one of the major threats to your maintaining the ability to live independently. Now, before you have to experience it, is the time to take the steps necessary to avert this devastating incursion on the second half of your life. The bottom line is that while calcium, vitamin D, cessation of smoking, moderation of alcohol use, limitation of caffeine and phosphorus intake, and weight-bearing exercise are all important to maintaining bone density, estrogen is the underlying necessity for prevention of fractures. Be alert to the signs and symptoms that your estrogen levels may be declining. If they are, consider starting an estrogen supplement, and jump all over a prevention program now.

Discuss your concerns about cardiovascular disease and osteoporosis with your doctor, and establish a plan for altering the risks in your favor. With your commitment and the support of an informed health professional, you can implement changes now that will improve your chances for a better quality of life in the best half of it.

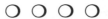

5

The Great Imitator: Thyroid Change Can Fool You

In transitional women, thyroid disease can mimic many of the symptoms you have been learning to associate with estrogen decline. Fatigue, sweating, disturbed concentration, short-term memory loss, depressed mood, irritability, and diminished sexual desire all may result from thyroid disease of one type or another. It's best that you know about this, because abnormal thyroid function is commonly missed by health-care professionals. For transitional women, thyroid symptoms more frequently trigger a suspicion of ovarian hormone decline. If female hormones are prescribed for these symptoms and they fail to improve, testing for a thyroid abnormality should be the next step. This chapter describes the signs and symptoms that can alert you to a thyroid problem and concludes with diagnosis and treatment.

The Thyroid Foundation of America says that by age fifty, 10 percent of women will suffer from hypothyroidism, which means the thyroid gland is underactive. As many as half don't even know they have a failing gland. Hyperthyroidism, which means an overproduction of thyroid hormones, is much less common. If all types of thyroid disorders are included, the frequency is up to twenty times more in women than in men. The incidence in women peaks during the forties and continues well into old age. For these reasons, it's important to know that your perimenopausal symptoms may not be entirely a result of estrogen decline.

What Should You Look For?

Thyroid disease can imitate many illnesses, including major depression, heart disease, arthritis, and even cancer. In addition, the symptoms of an overactive or underactive gland can simulate many of the complaints commonly seen with estrogen decline in perimenopausal women. Some have called thyroid disorders "the great imitator," and with good cause. We compiled Tables 5.1 and 5.2 to illustrate the similarities between abnormal thyroid function and perimenopausal changes.

Table 5.1. Comparison of Complaints Common to Hypothyroidism and Estrogen Deficiency

Complaint	Hypothyroidism	Estrogen Deficiency
Fatigue, sluggishness, no energy	Persistent	May wax and wane
Depression	Very persistent	May wax and wane
Menstrual change	Irregular to absent	Same
PMS Symptoms	Aggravated or initiated	Same
Decreased sexual desire	Common	Same
Difficulty becoming pregnant	Common	Same
Short-term memory loss	Common	Same
Diminished concentration	Common	Same
Loss of hair	Common	Late forties and beyond
Brittle hair	Common	Maybe
Dry skin	Common	Same

These tables show why thyroid disease can be easily overlooked in perimenopausal women. It is important not to miss this diagnosis, however, because thyroid disease is easily treated and resolved. If you do have thyroid disease but you or your doctor are misled into an investigation of diminished sex hormone levels, a trial of estrogen supplements will not improve your symptoms. If your FSH and estradiol blood levels are checked, they will be normal. At this point, don't throw up your hands in despair at failing to find the cause of your symptoms. The next step in diagnosis is thyroid testing.

Table 5.3 is a listing of additional hypothyroidism and hyperthyroidism symptoms that are not comparable to transitional changes. If you have some combination of these noncomparable changes plus estrogen deficiency–like

Table 5.2. Comparison of Complaints Common to Hyperthyroidism and Estrogen Deficiency

Complaint	Hyperthyroidism	Estrogen Deficiency
Increased sweating	Common	Hot flashes are similar
Scanty menstrual periods	Common	Common
Irritability and moodiness	Common	Common
Heat intolerance	Common	Common
Trouble sleeping	Common	Common
Pounding of heart	Common	Common

symptoms, a thoughtful evaluation of them may suggest thyroid disease and lead to thyroid testing and an earlier diagnosis; but your doctor must be a skillful listener. The appropriate tests are discussed later in this chapter. First, let's take a look at how your thyroid gland works.

Table 5.3. Additional Thyroid Symptoms

Hypothyroid	Hyperthyroid
Weight gain and difficulty in losing it	Nervous energy, inability to sit still
Dry, scaly skin and scalp	Rapid resting pulse rate
Brittle hair and nails	Unexplained weight loss
Cold intolerance, inability to get warm	Increased appetite
Sleeping more than usual	Buttoned collars fit too tightly
Slow heart rate	Eyes bulge slightly
Sluggish tendon reflexes, knee jerk	Frequent diarrhea
Puffiness of face, ankles	Frequent indigestion
Tingling in wrists and hands	Swollen ankles
Aching muscles and cramps	
Multiple joint aches	

How Your Thyroid Gland Works

Alphabet Soup	
SHTH	Subclinical hypothyroidism (SHTH)
T3	Triiodothyronine
T4	Thyroxine
TSH	Thyroid stimulating hormone
TSI	Thyroid stimulating immunoglobulin

Your thyroid weighs about one ounce, but it is a powerhouse. It is butterfly shaped and straddles the trachea (windpipe) at the base of your neck. Its function is to regulate the body's metabolism, which means it has major control of chemical and physical changes throughout your body. It influences growth and development of every body tissue and organ, and it regulates how much oxygen cells consume and how much energy is expended. The thyroid accomplishes its regulatory function by manufacturing and releasing its hormones into the bloodstream, which carries them to every tissue and organ—even your fingernails!

Your thyroid produces two hormones: triiodothyronine (T3), which is the biologically active hormone, and thyroxine (T4). Once T4 is released into your bloodstream, it is converted into T3. Your pituitary gland monitors and controls the amount of thyroid hormone in the bloodstream. The pituitary works with your thyroid in much the same way it does in regulating the production of estrogen and progesterone by the ovaries (see Chapter 1). The pituitary releases a hormone called thyroid stimulating hormone (TSH), which is carried in the bloodstream to your thyroid and directs it to deliver just the right amount of T3. When T3 is too low, an increase in TSH causes your thyroid to replenish the supply; when T3 is too high, TSH is lowered. If your thyroid cannot produce enough T3 to satisfy the pituitary, more TSH is sent to it, and then more, and maybe still more. This forms the basis for thyroid testing. A high TSH blood level confirms an underactive gland, and hypothyroidism. The reverse situation is seen in hyperthyroidism. A newer, more sensitive test called sTSH is now being used in hyperthyroidism when very low TSH levels are found (Klee 1994).

Hypothyroidism—Underdoing It

Ninety percent of hypothyroidism occurs in women. (It hardly seems fair, does it?) The gender difference is not well understood as yet, but it is reasonable to assume that a disparity this large must be related to a feature that women have and men do not—estrogen! Hypothyroidism seems to be associated with women who are overweight and have an early onset of menstrual periods, a large number of full-term pregnancies, and a late menopause. In women between the ages of forty and sixty, 3 percent will develop clinically demonstrable hypothyroidism, and another 10 percent will develop a subclinical form of it, which means that the thyroid hormone is a little low, but not enough to produce the usual signs and symptoms.

The cause of hypothyroidism for 90 percent of women who have it is the development of antibodies that attack the thyroid and its hormones (Dyan 1996). This is called an autoimmune reaction, and the condition has been named Hashimoto's Disease. If you have a reaction like this, your thyroid gland becomes inflamed, and tissue damage renders it unable to produce enough thyroid hormone. Your pituitary then generates more TSH, causing the thyroid to work harder. This works for a while, but at the expense of the thyroid cells multiplying and becoming larger. (An enlarged gland is called a goiter.) Ultimately, your thyroid can't keep up with hormone demands. Your pituitary's TSH is whipping a tired horse, and thyroid hormone eventually drops low enough to cause the classic symptoms of hypothyroidism shown in Tables 5.1 and 5.3.

Hyperthyroidism—Overdoing It

Hyperthyroidism is most commonly seen in the thirties and forties. It affects about 2 percent of women. There are several forms of this disease, the most common being Graves' disease. Graves' disease is caused by a rogue antibody called thyroid stimulating hormone receptor antibody (TSHR-Ab). When TSHR-Ab plugs into thyroid receptor sites ordinarily occupied by TSH, it causes the thyroid to produce more hormone than normal (Franklin 1998). This condition speeds up heart rate, steals sleep, causes a fine hand tremor to develop, increases appetite, and causes eyes to protrude slightly. Blinking the eyes becomes less frequent, and the skin is warm and moist most of the time. Menstrual periods may stop, which triggers concerns of pregnancy at first, and then of premature menopause when pregnancy test is negative. Women who already have coronary artery disease may develop angina or have a heart attack. If you have Grave's disease, you may act fidgety and feel as though you're about four inches off the ground all the time.

Your doctor can confirm a diagnosis of hyperthyroidism by hearing your story, doing a physical examination, and ordering lab tests. The tests will reveal a high level of TSHR-Ab, and the sTSH level will be low.

The Ovary/Thyroid Connection

The ovaries and thyroid interact with each other in terms of hormone production. Estrogen and progesterone receptors exist in the thyroid, and T3 receptors are in the ovaries. Not surprisingly, then, a diminished female hormone effect may cause your thyroid to function sluggishly. Your perimenopausal symptoms from lessened estrogen may then be exaggerated by the additional symptoms of hypothyroidism. A confusing array of symptoms may be present. If you are on HRT but find that relief has not occurred for such things as a depressed mood, short-term memory loss, or difficulty in concentration, a thyroid check may be in order. If both glands are malfunctioning, supplementing both hormones can be magic.

The other side of the coin is this: Thyroid disease can cause a malfunction of the ovaries. Hypothyroidism or hyperthyroidism can be the root cause of several significant health problems for women:

- **Menstrual irregularity:** Hypothyroidism prevents ovulation, resulting in a thickened endometrium. As a result, your cycles become prolonged and heavy. Hyperthyroidism prevents the development of your endometrium, resulting in shortened cycles initially, followed by scanty flow and then cessation of bleeding altogether. It is a good idea for transitional women with menstrual irregularities to insist on a thyroid check before agreeing to a D&C or other surgical treatment, such as a hysterectomy, for uncontrolled bleeding

- **Loss of sexual desire:** One of the less frequently recognized causes of loss of sexual desire is an overactive or underactive thyroid. Nearly 90 percent of hypothyroid and 50 percent of hyperthyroid women have loss of sexual desire (Eskin 1995). The causes vary all the way from vaginal dryness to depressed mood to overpowering fatigue. Happily, when thyroid disease is identified and treated, the problem usually disappears.

- **Infertility:** Infertility is a common accompaniment of hypothyroidism. Ovulation fails to occur because of inadequate levels of thyroid hormone. This situation is easily treatable, which is why a thyroid check should be part of every infertility investigation.

- **Postpartum blues:** As many as 40 to 60 percent of women suffer from postpartum blues. For most, it is mild and self-limiting. However, estimates are that about 10 percent of the afflicted women are actually suffering from an inflammatory condition called thyroiditis (Hayslip 1988). This is an autoimmune problem caused by antibodies that attack the thyroid, causing an inflammatory reaction. Thyroid-related postpartum blues generally occur six to twelve weeks after delivery, unlike typical postpartum blues, which start within a few days.

The bottom line for you is the importance of being aware of thyroid disease as a possible cause of your symptoms. Once your suspicion is aroused, a trip to the doctor should be next on your agenda.

What Your Doctor Will Do—Diagnosis

The symptoms and signs may not be obvious at first. As their severity increases, however, the initial subtleties become easily recognizable changes. Your doctor must take a number of factors into account in determining your diagnosis, including your own report of what has been happening, a physical exam, and testing.

Your Story

Whether you perceive your body's altered status as featherlike or sledgehammerlike, it's important to report these changes to your doctor, who will then take a medical history. It is unlikely that your history alone will nail down a diagnosis, but a skillful listener will be able to eliminate all but a few culprits.

Your Body

Physical examination plays an important diagnostic role in distinguishing whether it is a hypothyroid or hyperthyroid problem. Table 5.4 lists some key observations.

The physical signs of hypothyroidism are usually late in appearing. This means that in the early stages of an underactive thyroid gland, physical examination may not be particularly revealing of your condition.

Table 5.4. Physical Symptoms in Hypothyroidism and Hyperthyroidism		
Physical Examination of	**Symptom in Hypothyroidism**	**Symptom in Hyperthyroidism**
Resting pulse	Too slow	Too fast
Blood pressure	Lowered	Raised
Reflexes (knee jerk)	Slow and sluggish	Brisk and intense
Eyes	Slow lid movement	Eyes may bulge slightly; infrequent blinking
Thyroid gland	May be enlarged	May be enlarged

Your Lab Results

Both thyroid hormones, T3 and T4, can be measured with blood tests, but the pituitary hormone (TSH) blood test is a more sensitive indicator of thyroid function. For this reason, most doctors skip the T3 and T4 tests. If you have an underactive gland, your pituitary attempts to spark it up with more TSH. If your thyroid is overactive, the pituitary cuts back on TSH stimulation.

Small lumps, or nodules, are common in the thyroid. A small percentage of them can be detected by physical exam, but with an ultrasound scan, about one-third of women can be shown to have one or more small nodules. They are usually harmless, but it is important to have them evaluated; they have been associated with hypothyroidism, hyperthyroidism, and cancer. Several methods exist for evaluating lumps, as well as for testing a diffusely enlarged thyroid without lumps. These include ultrasound, needle biopsy, and radioactive iodine uptake with a thyroid scan.

Treatment of Hypothyroidism

The best treatment for hypothyroidism is simple hormone replacement, and that is a happy thought because there is no cure. Thyroxine, or T4, is your native hormone, and this is what you will be taking. Thyroxine is a safe, inexpensive, and reliable treatment. The correct daily dose will require some adjustment from time to time until you hit upon the right one for your particular needs. Monitoring your TSH level is a reliable method to assess the effectiveness of your dose. The correct thyroxine intake will gradually bring your TSH back down to normal.

A controversy exists as to whether subclinical hypothyroidism (SHTH) should be treated—it is, after all, a symptomless condition. The problem is that up to 25 percent of SHTH eventually progresses to full-blown hypothyroidism (Danese 1996). In addition, some evidence exists showing that women with SHTH are more at risk for coronary artery disease and subsequent heart attacks because of unfavorable lipid profiles. A cardiac contraction abnormality called atrial fibrillation is associated with SHTH and there is an increased possibility that osteoporosis may occur. Since treatment with thyroxine is simple, safe, and inexpensive, a good case can be made for utilizing it.

Some advice and precautions about thyroxine use:

- Aluminum-containing antacids (Gelusil, Amphogel, Tempo, Maalox Plus in tablets, and Mylanta liquid) adversely affect thyroxine absorption.

- Iron adversely affects absorption. Take thyroxine and iron at different times of the day.

- Take only the amount prescribed as necessary to keep your TSH level normal. Overdose causes bone resorption and puts you at greater risk for osteoporosis; it also causes symptoms of hyperthyroidism, such as sleepless nights, nervousness, pounding heart, and diarrhea and can even damage your heart muscle.

- To maintain even levels, take thyroxine the same time every day in the morning on an empty stomach and wait one hour before eating or drinking anything else.

- Get a TSH blood test once a year after your thyroxine dose is stabilized to stay on top of maintaining the right dose.

- If you become pregnant, be certain your obstetrician is aware that you are taking thyroid hormone replacement. Your requirements for thyroxine supplements will often fall in the first trimester but rise in the third trimester. Therefore, your TSH should be checked several times during pregnancy. The correct dose must be maintained to protect your baby.

Treatment of Hyperthyroidism

Prior to starting treatment for hyperthyroidism, a beta-blocker medication is usually prescribed. This type of drug strengthens the heart muscle and lowers blood pressure. Hyperthyroidism can seriously damage the heart muscle, so this is an important first step. Two commonly used beta-blockers are propranolol and atenolol.

Three methods are currently in use to manage an overactive thyroid:

- Antithyroid medication: This is usually the first line of treatment. Drugs in this category prevent your thyroid from making all that extra hormone. The two most commonly prescribed are propylthiouracil (PTU) and methimazole. They are taken in tablet form once daily for six months to a year. Over several months of treatment, you will gradually revert to normal from the "weird looking, fidgety, nervous wreck" you used to be.

- Radioactive Iodine Therapy (RAI): If drug treatment fails, RAI may be the next best form of controlling your runaway gland. RAI is taken orally. Your thyroid selects the radioactive iodine from the bloodstream and concentrates it in the overactive cells, which are then destroyed. The net result is that your thyroid can't produce as much hormone as it had been doing, and things settle down. And no, you won't glow in the night, because the radioactivity disappears from your body in a few days. About 50 percent of people treated with RAI become hypothyroid and require thyroid hormone supplements (Franklin 1998).

CAUTION! RAI therapy must be avoided if you are pregnant because it can have an adverse effect on a developing fetus. Bernard Eskin reports (1995) that the ovaries may absorb some of the RAI, so he recommends avoidance of this therapy if you are planning a pregnancy in subsequent years.

- Surgical removal: Sometimes, surgical removal of all or part of your thyroid is necessary. If you have only a single overactive nodule, simple removal of that nodule may be all you need. Most of the time, the entire gland is too active, and a total, or near total, thyroidectomy is necessary.

Any of the treatment methods we just described for an overactive thyroid can result in an underactive gland, so it is important for you to have annual thyroid evaluations.

Summary

Thyroid problems are often subtle and easily overlooked. This is especially true for perimenopausal women. You or your doctor may be misled by symptoms that are more commonly attributed to decline in female hormone production. It is worthwhile to have a TSH blood test every five years after age forty. This ensures that abnormal functioning of your thyroid will be picked up early. An underactive thyroid is the most likely thyroid dysfunction, and its treatment is almost always simple, inexpensive, and safe. Vigilance and awareness are your best friends in identifying thyroid problems.

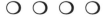

6

Frightening Changes—Cancer

Cancer risks are not high for you in your transitional years. Why, then, discuss them in this book? First of all, your chances are not zero either, as you no doubt know, so a discussion of these potential threats is appropriate to arming you with information about your health after age thirty-five. And, as you'll learn in this chapter, there are steps you can take during the transitional years to reduce your chances of getting cancer. This chapter covers the four most common female cancers: breast, uterine, cervical, and ovarian. In addition, because they are also common (in both women and men), we take a look at lung and colon cancer. You will also learn what cancer is, what your risks are for getting it, how it is diagnosed, the all-important prevention methods available to you, and current treatments.

What Changes?

In cancer, cells change. Each of your several trillion cells has genes that control all aspects of cell life. The genes determine what chemicals are manufactured, when the cell reproduces itself, and how long each cell lives. As time passes, genes may be changed by the aging process and by the effects of outside agents you consume or to which you are exposed, such as pesticides, preservatives, tobacco smoke, alcohol, fat, various foods, and other environmental carcinogens (cancer-causing agents). These genetic changes are called mutations. After a mutation has taken place, the altered gene operates the cell in a different fashion. Most of the time, the change is relatively inconsequential, but sometimes the mutation produces a cancer-causing gene (an oncogene). All subsequent generations of that cell possess the oncogene and have the potential to become cancer cells if the oncogene is activated by one of the outside influences mentioned above. Some people are born with oncogenes they inherit from their parents that lie dormant unless or until activated later in life. Cells also have tumor suppressor genes that control how a cell grows. If the tumor suppressor gene is damaged, it can no longer control the growth rate, and the cell takes off on its own to produce a cancerous growth. Cells can also become cancerous if they are no longer able to respond to the tumor-suppressor signals.

Once the oncogene is active, the cell it controls no longer behaves in a normal way. It becomes a rogue cell, producing an anarchy of uncontrolled growth and invasion of neighboring cells, tissues, and organs. Cancer cells cannot perform the same functions as normal cells, and the body suffers as these functions are lost. If the cancerous tissues are not removed or their growth halted, the body in which they exist will not survive.

A revolution is taking place in genetics. Scientists worldwide are making huge gains in methods of identifying oncogenes and neutralizing them with gene therapy. Research is now under way that will enable physicians to identify the genetic makeup of each cancer sufferer's tumor. Armed with that information, the selection of treatment options will be much more accurate. Right now, treating cancer is largely a high-risk guessing game. Most chemotherapy drugs work only about 20 to 30 percent of the time, and figuring out which one to use is an art as opposed to a refined science. Scientists are also working on several methods of starving cancer cells without harming healthy cells. It appears that the future is promising, but we must still stay vigilant in terms of prevention, early diagnosis, and treatment methods, our knowledge of all of which is steadily improving.

The risk of your developing a cancer is not dependent upon a sole factor, such as the presence or absence of an oncogene. Other factors include the state of your nutrition, the competence of your immune system to combat abnormal cells, your genetic makeup, and uncounted external hazards to which you may be exposed. Cancer development is the sum of diverse circumstances and conditions that are brought to focus on regulating cellular growth. Some of your risk for cancer is based on a shuffle of the genetic deck, and some of it is luck. The good news is that some of it is under your direct control.

Breast Cancer

Alphabet Soup	
BSE	Breast self-exam
HDI	High-definition imaging
MRI	Magnetic resonance imaging
PET	Positron emission tomography

Breast cancer is a hot-button issue if there ever was one. It is the second most common cause of cancer death in women (lung cancer is first). Breasts are an important feature of femininity, so it is not surprising that the thought of breast cancer should cause such concern and fear in women. You should know as much as you can about breast cancer because you may need to make some important decisions during perimenopause that hinge on accurate information.

First, Some Numbers

Currently, 182,000 American women develop breast cancer annually, and this results in 46,000 deaths each year. Breast cancer constitutes 29.7 percent of cancer in women. The risk of getting breast cancer has doubled since 1940. This increased risk may be explained in part by a longer life expectancy and a greater likelihood of diagnosis. The actual incidence of diagnosed breast cancer plateaued in 1987 and has been declining since 1990. The five-year survival rate for cancer that has not spread beyond the breast tissue (about 60 percent of breast cancers) has risen from 72 percent in the 1940s to 97 percent in 1997. If the cancer has spread to regional lymph nodes in the armpit, the five-year survival drops to 71 percent; and it drops to 18 percent if there are distant metastases (American Cancer Society 1997).

The rate of breast cancer has increased by over 50 percent, from 1 in 12 in 1940 to the current figure of 1 in 8. This statistic, however, is misleading; it applies only to women who are currently age twenty and will live to age eighty-five. You have a better chance of understanding your own risk for breast cancer by looking at Table 6.1. The odds of getting breast cancer increase as you age, the majority occurring after menopause. By age forty they are 1 in 217, for example, but by age sixty-five, they are 1 in 17. This means that if you are cancer-free at forty, your chances by age sixty-five are more than twelve times higher (217÷17 = 12.7). Many women (and their physicians) actually believe that one in eight American women now living will develop breast cancer. It simply is not true. The one in eight figure mentioned above is true only if you are a twenty-year-old woman who will live to age eighty-five. But you are forty, not twenty, and your lifetime risk to age eighty-five is much lower if you are now cancer-free, because you have already survived nearly half your life without breast cancer.

What Are Your Risks?

A number of conditions and situations influence the risk of developing breast cancer. You have the ability to control some of the risk factors; others are just the cards you have been dealt.

Age

Breast cancer increases in frequency with age. Nearly 80 percent occurs after age fifty, 15 percent occurs in women under age fifty, and 6.5 percent under age forty. A woman at age seventy has about seven times the risk as a woman at age forty-five. So growing older is the single most important risk factor. Indeed, 85 percent of women who develop breast cancer do not have

Table 6.1. Odds of Developing Breast Cancer by Age	
By age 25	1 in 19,608
By age 30	1 in 2,525
By age 35	1 in 622
By age 40	1 in 217
By age 45	1 in 93
By age 50	1 in 50
By age 55	1 in 33
By age 60	1 in 24
By age 65	1 in 17
By age 70	1 in 14
By age 75	1 in 11
By age 80	1 in 10
By age 85	1 in 9
Lifetime	1 in 8

Source: 1987–88 data, SEER Program of the National Cancer Institute and the American Cancer Society.

any identifiable risk factor other than age (Speroff 1998). Therefore every woman must be considered at risk.

Family History

If your mother or sister (called first-degree relatives) has had breast cancer before age fifty, your risk is double that of someone without that history. If the cancer occurred after fifty, your risk is less high, but still 1.4 times more than usual. If two or more relatives (mother, sister, aunt, grandmother) have had breast cancer, especially before menopause, you are also at higher risk. This is called familial breast cancer, and it may be inherited (Colditz 1993).

Two genes (called BRCA1 and BRCA2) have been identified that can predispose their carriers to breast cancer. There may be others. When these genes are normal, they have a protein that functions as a tumor suppressor. It is estimated that mutation of these genes (into oncogenes) accounts for 3 to 5 percent of all breast cancer (Newman 1998; Malone 1998). The mutated gene has abnormal or nonfunctional tumor suppressor protein and may fail to prevent normal cells from overgrowing. When the mutated gene is activated by other influences, the breast cells these genes control are no longer prevented from unrestrained growth, and a cancer starts. More than one hundred mutations of BRCA1 are now known, and it is possible to identify them with DNA testing. Although it may be an overestimation, studies have shown that a woman with a mutated BRCA1 gene has an 87 percent lifetime risk of early-onset (before menopause) familial breast cancer and a 40 to 65 percent increased risk for ovarian cancer (Hoskins 1995). Each of her children of either sex has a 50 percent chance of inheriting BRCA1 from her. Her male children who inherit a mutated BRCA1 gene have a threefold-increased risk for prostate cancer and a fourfold-increased risk for colon cancer. Estimates are that only a tiny number (0.04 to 0.2%) of American women may be carriers of a mutated BRCA1 gene (Krainer 1997).

Carriers of a mutated BRCA2 gene have a similar lifetime risk for early-onset familial breast cancer as BRCA1, but a lower risk for ovarian cancer. (Male carriers of BRCA2 have an increased risk of breast, pancreatic, and prostate cancer.) Among women of Ashkenazi Jewish descent, the prevalence of BRCA1 and BRCA2 is about 2 percent (Struewing 1997).

What all this means is that assessing your risk for familial breast cancer must include evaluation of both the maternal and paternal sides of your family. DNA testing for these genes is possible through genetics departments at medical centers, but it is very complex and expensive. A drawback is that it does not predict with accuracy which carriers of mutated genes will actually develop a cancer. At present, DNA screening is not recommended except for families with the following characteristics:

- Early onset of breast cancer within the family (before menopause)

- One or more relatives with ovarian cancer

- Three or more relatives with breast cancer

- Ashkenazi ancestry and one family member with breast or ovarian cancer

Smoking

And you thought the cancer risk of smoking was to the lungs. That's still true, of course, but the complex toxins in tobacco smoke are apparently causing cancerous changes in breast cells also, because smokers have more breast cancer than nonsmokers (Bennicke 1995). Just another good reason to be a nonsmoker.

Estrogen and Reproductive Experience

Life situations that result in prolonged and uninterrupted cyclic estrogen exposure, seem to predispose women to breast cancer. Table 6.2 lists these factors. Use of birth control pills, however, do not increase your risk of breast cancer (Darney 2000).

Hormone replacement therapy is a complex issue in regard to breast cancer and is thoroughly discussed in Chapter 7

Table 6.2.   Reproductive Risk Factors and Breast Cancer

Factor	Result
Early onset of menstrual periods (before age 12)	More lifetime years of monthly estrogen cycles and monthly changes in the breasts
Late menopause (after age 54)	More lifetime years of estrogen cycles
Having a first baby after age 30 or having no pregnancies	More uninterrupted years of estrogen cycles
Prolonged infertility from lack of ovulation	If ovulation is not occurring, progesterone's antiestrogen protection is lost
Obesity (more than 20 percent above ideal weight)	Excess estrogen results from conversion of fat to estrogen
Prolonged perimenopause with absence of ovulation	Causes unopposed estrogen exposure
The woman's birth weight	A birth weight over 4,000 grams (8 lbs., 8 oz.) seems related to high estrogen exposure during fetal life (Michels 1996)
History of several pregnancies	Multiple pregnancies are protective, apparently because they interrupt the monthly breast changes caused by the normal hormonal cycle

Dietary Factors and Obesity

It is well known that the incidence of breast cancer is increased in countries where affluence, unfavorable diets, and lack of exercise are common. In most of these scenarios, too much circulating insulin is seen (hyperinsulinemia), as well as resistance to the glucose-lowering effect of insulin (insulin resistance). Hyperinsulinemia is found more often in women with breast cancer (Bruning 1992).

Japanese women, whose diet traditionally includes only 10 to 20 percent of calories from fat and animal protein, have 75 percent less breast cancer than American women. However, when Japanese women convert to a typical Western diet, their rate of breast cancer increases, in one or more generations, to that of American women (Ziegler 1996). The typical American diet (if such a thing truly exists) averages 30 to 40 percent of calories from animal fat and another 12 percent from protein.

Soy consumption causes a reduction in the circulating levels of estrogen by increasing the level of sex hormone binding globulin (SHBG) (Lu 1996). SHBG binds to estrogen molecules and essentially takes them out of play. When soy intake is high, there is less breast, endometrial, and prostate cancer. Speculation is that the isoflavones in soy, which resemble estrogen molecules, occupy estrogen receptor sites and displace natural estrogen. No one knows this for certain, however, since scientific data are rather limited on links between soy and breast cancer. It may be that soy intake is associated with other factors in lifestyle and diet that are themselves protective. Nevertheless the aggressive food supplement industry is trumpeting soy protein as if a clear protective benefit against breast cancer and breast cancer recurrence has been established.

As for dietary fat and breast cancer, the trend in thinking has been that fat is not a causative factor. A major ongoing prospective study called the Women's Health Initiative is looking at this relationship and should provide more definitive answers by about 2005 (Seltzer 1996).

It may turn out that the role of dietary fat is that a high fat diet is high in calories and is therefore associated with obesity. Excess body weight influences the risk of breast cancer differently in premenopausal and postmenopausal women. Before menopause, overweight women have a lower risk than women of normal weight. After menopause, excess weight is associated with a slightly increased risk (Potischman 1996). This is explained by the fact that postmenopausal women have less SHBG. Estrogen can be manufactured in fat; so in obesity, estrogen levels are higher and a low level of SHBG allows more unbound, free estrogen to be in circulation.

Well-done red meat increases the risk of breast cancer. High cooking temperatures produce substances called heterocyclic amines, which are mutagens, or chemicals that cause DNA changes in breast cells. The Iowa Women's Health Study found a 4.6 times higher risk for breast cancer in women who consumed well-done red meat as compared to those who ate it rare or medium-cooked (Zheng 1998). No correlation was found in the degree of cooking with chicken and fish.

Data from the Nurses' Health Study revealed that breast cancer risk was reduced in women who consumed more than moderate amounts of alcohol if they had an adequate intake of folates. Folates occur naturally in green leafy vegetables (think foliage), but the predominant source in most American diets is from breakfast cereals fortified with folic acid and from standard multivitamins (Zhang 1999).

Alcohol

Many studies have shown that having more than two alcoholic drinks per day increases the risk of breast cancer by about 30 to 40 percent. A 1998 study found a linear relationship between alcohol consumption and breast cancer—meaning the greater the consumption the greater the risk (Smith-Warner 1998). This report on 322,647 women found a 9 percent increased risk with 0.75 to 1 drink per day, and a 41 percent increase with 2 to 5 drinks per day. It is thought by many that alcohol has an adverse influence on the liver's metabolism of estrogen, which results in less SHBG binding and more circulating estrogen than nondrinkers. With lower SHBG levels in postmenopausal women, there is greater risk for breast cancer from alcohol consumption than before menopause. So, depending on your age, abstinence may be the best policy, with moderation definitely in second place.

Exercise

The effects of exercise in reducing breast cancer have been studied for premenopausal women to date; but postmenopausal exercise research is under way. The Harvard Nurses' Health Study found that breast cancer risk was reduced by 18 percent if women exercised about seven hours per week (Rockhill 1999). The risk was even lower if regular exercise had been part of a woman's lifestyle dating back to her teens and twenties. Be sure to share this information with your daughters, and consider joining them if you are not already an exercise devotee. (Exercise is covered in Chapter 9.)

Birth Control Pill

It is widely known that long-term Pill users have a decreased incidence of uterine and ovarian cancer, and that the protection lasts twenty years after they stop taking the Pill. Long-term Pill use has no influence on breast cancer. It neither increases nor decreases the risk (Darney 2000). In women who were previous Pill users and who later in life developed breast cancer, the type of cancer was more localized, with less metastatic spread (Collaborative Group 1996). Pill use does not increase the cancer risk in women with family histories of breast cancer, nor in women who have benign breast conditions, except in women who are carriers of a mutated form of genes BRCA1 or BRCA2. In addition, there is no evidence that Pill use prior to the onset of breast cancer has any effect on the prognosis (Holmberg 1994).

New Method for Individual Risk Assessment

Your doctor can determine your individual risk for breast cancer with the Breast Cancer Risk Assessment Tool. This is a computer program developed by the National Cancer Institute (NCI) and the National Surgical Adjuvant Breast and Bowel Project. You provide answers regarding your personal history of breast abnormalities, current age, age at first menstrual period, age at first live birth, the breast cancer history of close relatives, whether you have ever had a breast biopsy, and your race. These data are fed into the program and it estimates your risk of developing breast cancer for two time periods: over the next five years and for your lifetime. The assessment tool is free to your doctor from the NCI at 800-4-CANCER or online at www.nci.nih.gov.

Screening for Breast Cancer

The traditional screening methods for breast cancer have been breast self-examination (BSE) and physician exams; and since the 1980s, mammograms have become a regular part of the mix. Other more sophisticated, and sometimes more expensive, methods are also emerging.

Breast Self-Examination (BSE)

Breast self-examination is an important element of breast cancer detection; it is for anyone who has breasts and for as long as she has them. It's important to know what to look for when examining your breasts. Check with your health-care provider or the American Cancer Society (800-ACS-2345 or www.cancer.org) for information and videos on the correct technique for looking at and feeling your breasts. After a few exams you will have become acquainted with your breasts, becoming the single most qualified expert on what they feel like. The advantage for you is that with this internal database established, you become acutely aware if there is a change.

Change is what you are looking for. The natural lumpiness in some breasts can be noted to undergo subtle changes as hormones fluctuate during the cycle. But cancer is not subtle, and it doesn't change as your hormone levels change; so a hard lump that is distinctly different than the usual consistency of your breast and one that persists through two cycles, deserves further evaluation. It is difficult, but possible, to detect lumps much smaller than one half inch (1.3 centimeters) in size; but the more expert you become, the better your chances of recognizing a small one. The earlier you find it, the better.

The best time to do a BSE is just after your period, because there is less congestion and less tenderness in your breasts. You can examine your breasts firmly without its being painful, and with lessened glandular swelling, you are more likely to recognize a new lump. If your periods have stopped, just select a regular date you are likely to remember, like the first or last day of each month.

Keep in mind, though, that self-examinations, and those by a health provider, can detect only relatively large breast lumps. This means that by the time you or your doctor can feel a cancerous lump, it may have been present for a considerable period of time—possibly more than two years. Regular mammograms, on the other hand, can detect lumps that are too small to feel by BSE, and they are being relied on more than BSE to detect new lumps. However, it is not yet time to abandon BSE. Mammograms miss about 10 percent of breast tumors because some of them do not contain calcium, an important identifying sign of cancer.

Physician Breast Examination

A thorough annual breast exam should be part of any physical exam and gynecological checkup. Your doctor's exam should be regarded as part of your backup system. Although you are the established expert on what your breasts feel like, an experienced physician has felt many more abnormal lumps than you have. If you are concerned about a difference you have noticed, this is the person whose opinion you should solicit. Once you know that what you are feeling is not suspicious, you can be less concerned. If, on the other hand, you both agree that something suspicious is present, an investigation will begin. The next exam will likely be a mammogram.

Mammography

Since 1987 there has been a continuing decline in the death rate from breast cancer (Tarone 1996). This is attributed to earlier diagnosis as the result of screening mammography and to improved treatment with tamoxifen (discussed below). Mammograms can detect tumors as small as 5 millimeters, or about the size of a large pea. This is about one-half the size found by the average woman's self-exam. Since early detection is a major key to surviving breast cancer, it is obvious that mammography plays an important role.

A sixteen-year English study confirmed the role of mammography in reducing breast cancer mortality. It compared women who did breast self-examination after special training, to women who had regular mammograms plus physician breast exams. The breast cancer mortality was 27 percent lower in the group having mammograms and clinical exams (Moss 1999).

Mammography is done with an X-ray machine that passes radiation through your breasts after they have been compressed to a flatter shape. This can be uncomfortable, so be sure to avoid getting it done in the latter half of your cycle, when your breasts may be naturally tender. The X-ray film shows the general architecture of the breasts and any abnormal densities within them. Cancer densities are different in character than others, and they usually have certain clustered calcium flecks that can be recognized by a radiologist.

A 1999 law requires you and your physician to be notified of mammogram results in writing within thirty days. If evidence of cancer is found, you must be notified within five days. Be sure that you have your mammogram in an FDA-certified facility. To find one, call the National Cancer Institute at 800-4-CANCER, or check their Web site: (www.nci.nih.gov) or the FDA web site at (www.fda.gov/cdrh/mammography/certified.html).

TIP! Be sure to avoid using body powder before a mammogram; the powder granules may be misleading on the X-ray film, masking calcium flecks in a tumor.

About one in ten screening mammograms discloses an abnormality. In this situation an additional magnification view may be necessary. An ultrasound exam may also be done to get a better look at a suspected cyst. One or two in ten of these follow-up exams may lead to a recommendation for a biopsy of the suspicious area, 75 percent of which are found to be noncancerous (Harvard Women's Health Watch 2000. Breast Imaging).

A big question is how often and at what age you should have a mammogram. The long-term survival studies of breast cancer showed that women in their forties who have had mammogram screening survive their breast cancer better than women who did not have mammograms (ACOG 1997). Add to that the American Cancer Society statistics showing about 19 percent more breast cancers in women aged forty to forty-nine than in women aged fifty to fifty-nine, and the need for mammogram screening in the forties becomes obvious (American Cancer Society 1998). However, mammograms in women under age fifty produce a higher percentage of false positive readings. This results in four times as many biopsies as in women over fifty. The reason is that younger breasts are more dense, and this results in more suspicious shadows on the X-ray film. Recent studies found that women on HRT have greater breast density than nonusers, which results in more false positive mammograms, as well as more false negative results (Greendale 1999; Kavanagh 2000).

Mammograms of younger breasts may lead to unnecessary biopsies, but early detection of cancer by means of a mammogram may pay off by saving your life. New evidence has shown that cancer grows more rapidly in younger breasts, and annual mammograms are indeed justified in women under fifty (Antman 1999). Two separate studies showed that mammograms reduce breast cancer deaths of women in their forties by 44 percent and 35 percent (ACOG 1997). The American Cancer Society recommends annual mammograms starting at age forty, and the National Cancer Institute recommends mammograms every one to two years after forty.

To what age should women have mammograms? A study from Sweden found no reduction in breast cancer mortality after age seventy in women who had annual mammograms. Screening all women to age sevevnty-nine saves 0.3 days of life per woman (Kerlikowske 1999). These authors suggested that since low bone mineral density (BMD) in elderly women is associated with a lower incidence of breast cancer, checking BMD and deferring mammogram screening in those with low BMD would be more cost-effective than annual mammograms.

TIP! Augmentation breast implants may somewhat diminish the effectiveness of mammography. (Scar tissue around the implant may hinder the breasts from being compressed adequately.) Most X-ray facilities have special techniques for dealing with this, so ask them about it when you make your appointment.

Ultrasound

Ultrasound is a useful backup tool for mammography. Sound waves pass through structures if they are composed mostly of water, but they are bounced back if they strike something solid. This creates an image on a monitor that can then be interpreted and evaluated. Ultrasound is not a good primary screening tool for breast cancer because it will not pick up lumps smaller than 1 to 2 centimeters. In addition, ultrasound cannot distinguish the tiny calcium flecks that are so important in recognizing early cancer. Its main usefulness is in distinguishing between breast masses that are cystic (fluid filled) and those that are solid. Mammograms do not make this distinction. If a lump is cystic, it may not be necessary to do more than drain the cyst with a tiny needle. A solid mass is more ominous and usually requires biopsy or removal. Ultrasound saves a lot of biopsies.

Thermography

Cancer gives off more heat than normal tissue. Thermography, a radiation-free technique detects increased heat, but has failed to be useful because many benign masses also give off increased heat, leading to an unacceptable number of false negative and false positive results. Thermography using computers to analyze the images may identify cancerous masses better, and may eventually be resurrected as an adjunct to mammography.

New Developments in Breast Cancer Screening

In 1996, the FDA approved an advanced high-definition ultrasound machine designed to distinguish between benign and malignant breast lumps. Conventional ultrasound produces a rather grainy image, but a process called high-definition imaging (HDI) is much more distinct. In several other countries where HDI has been used for some time, studies showed that it is 99 percent accurate in predicting that a breast lump is noncancerous, but it is only 60 percent correct when it predicts cancer. This means a 40 percent false positive cancer prediction; but it has the potential to reduce by 40 percent the 700,000 breast biopsies that are done each year. This can represent a huge advantage in reducing the pain, inconvenience, and expense of diagnosing or ruling out cancer by biopsy.

Another new technique uses digitized computer technology in mammography. This will eliminate problems with denser breasts using standard mammography.

Magnetic resonance imaging (MRI) is another option. It is expensive and can be a daunting procedure—the patient must lie still in a narrow tube during the test. The newer, horseshoe-shaped open MRI tube alleviates this claustrophobic effect. MRI offers these advantages in breast screening:

- It can aid in deciding whether a breast lump is benign or malignant, possibly avoiding an unnecessary biopsy.

- It can detect whether a cancerous lesion is the sole tumor or or whether there are multiple locations.

- It utilizes no radiation.

- It can detect a leaking silicone breast implant.

A disadvantage is that MRI will detect breast lesions that are noncancerous and yet still lead to needless biopsies. It is not a practical tool for primary screening at this time, so it is being used as a mammography backup. Let's hope future innovations can make MRI a practical tool for primary screening.

Another scanning process, called positron emission tomography (PET), measures the uptake of a radioactive sugar by a cancerous breast tumor. Because cancer cells have a high metabolic rate, they need more sugar for energy, and they concentrate the radioactive sugar more than normal cells. This creates a "hot spot" on the scan. The cost is quite high, so PET is not a first-line-of-defense screening device. The National Cancer Institute has funded a study to see whether PET can identify cancer cells in lymph nodes. If it can reliably do this, it will save painful lymph gland surgery in women with proven breast cancer, if the glands can be shown to be free of cancer cells. A similar scanning procedure, called scintimammography (SMM), involves injection of a radioactive compound that is taken up selectively by malignant cells. PET and SMM cannot accurately detect masses smaller than 1 centimeter.

A new scanning technique called breast biofield examination (BBE) is now available. BBE detects disruption in the normal external-to-internal electrical differences in cells. Cancer cells have a different electrical profile than normal cells. BBE is 98 percent accurate in detecting cancer cells. This gives it an advantage over mammography in evaluating younger women with denser breasts.

Traditional surgical biopsy can often be avoided by sampling a suspicious lump with a tiny needle which removes cells by suctioning them into the needle. It is called fine needle aspiration cytology (FNAC). The aspirated cells are then examined microscopically. If no abnormalities are found, nothing further may need to be done. If the lump is a cyst, the fluid inside is removed by FNAC and the cyst collapses. When suspicious cells are noted on FNAC, a larger needle may be used to take a core sample of the lump; this provides a larger tissue sample. If suspicion of cancer persists, standard surgical biopsy of the lump may then be needed. FNAC is part of a triple approach to diagnosis, involving breast examination, mammography, and FNAC. Failure to detect a malignancy with at least one of these diagnostic tests is unlikely (Vetto 1995).

As mentioned earlier in this chapter, it is now possible to identify the mutated forms of BRCA1 and BRCA2 genes that raise the risk for breast cancer to over 80 percent. The DNA screening technique for identifying these genes is available in research centers, but it is labor-intensive and quite expensive. The question arises as to who should be screened. Shattuck-Eidens (1995) and Hoskins (1995) believe that a strong family history of breast and/or ovarian cancer before menopause justifies screening a woman. They also believe genetic screening by DNA analysis reveals you have the mutated form of the gene, your family should also be screened.

Difficult questions arise as to how the information from such DNA tests should be handled. If you are cancer-free and discover you carry the mutated gene, you must take many things into consideration: Should you have both breasts and your ovaries removed? What should you do about getting married? Does your fiancé have a right to know you may face a serious health threat at some future time? Should you plan a family? Does your employer have a right to know? How will this affect your health insurability? Must future disease potential be disclosed if it becomes known? You can see where this is leading. A mountain of genetic information is about to descend upon us in the next few years, and we are not well prepared to handle it medically, morally, ethically, or legally. Science is beginning to outdistance the wisdom necessary to utilize its discoveries. There are no easy answers to these questions. However, the American Society of Clinical Oncology (ASCO) is working to keep on top of these issues. Guidelines were issued in May 1996 to help physicians advise their patients regarding breast cancer prevention, recognition of risk factors, early detection, counseling about familial cancer, and utilization of genetic screening (Gershenson 1996).

Treatment of Breast Cancer

In the last decade, 150,000 women per year were diagnosed with breast cancer. Of these, 70 percent will die of a disease other than breast cancer. This is a reflection of earlier diagnosis and therefore more effective treatment.

Current surgical treatment of breast cancer with lumpectomy manages to prevent over two-thirds of complete breast removals (mastectomies). Surgical reconstruction of a new breast is available if your breast must be removed. Treatment of breast cancer is too broad an issue to be covered completely here. A great many options are available with regard to management. This means, of course, that if you are diagnosed with breast cancer, you have many decisions to make. Your best decisions will come from a base of good information about treatment. You can gather information from breast surgeons, plastic surgeons, radiation therapists, and oncologists (cancer specialists), as well as from a broad choice of literature and on the Internet. Check for a local support group in your area. Enlist the support of your family and close friends. It isn't easy to make important decisions when you are under the stress of contemplating survival issues; a compassionate partner, friend, physician, or counselor can be of immense help.

Tamoxifen Treatment for Prevention of Breast Cancer Recurrence

Tamoxifen (Nolvadex), a complex drug with both estrogenic and antiestrogenic properties, is used as a follow-up treatment in women who have been treated for breast cancer. It is molecularly similar enough to estrogen that it can occupy estrogen receptor sites on breast cells and thus prevent estrogen from stimulating cancer growth in any residual cancerous cells or in the other breast. For this reason, tamoxifen is called a selective estrogen receptor modulator (SERM). For the first five years of use, it lowers the cancer recurrence rate dramatically and reduces the mortality rate by 26 percent. In a trial of healthy women to prevent breast cancer, tamoxifen reduced the incidence by half (Wellness Letter 1999). This drug also helps prevent osteoporosis, and has a positive effect on cholesterol and lipoproteins. What a great drug, right? That was the good news.

The bad news is that when tamoxifen occupies the estrogen receptor sites on the cells of uterine endometrial glands, it may stimulate the glands to overgrow and cause hyperplasia (an increase in cell growth). This can lead to endometrial cancer. This risk is higher with increased duration of tamoxifen use, as well as in women with prior estrogen replacement, and in women who are overweight (Bernstein 1999). In May 2000, the government listed tamoxifen as a carcinogen.

So what is a body to do? The best course for tamoxifen users is to be alert to abnormal uterine bleeding. If hyperplasia is proven by endometrial biopsy (an office procedure), a course of progesterone therapy will usually reverse it. If it is not reversed and you wish to continue tamoxifen, your doctor may recommend a hysterectomy. Tamoxifen also increases the risk for other potentially serious problems, including deep vein thrombosis (blood clots in major veins) and pulmonary embolism (blood clot in the lung). Less threatening side effects include an earlier menopause, cataracts, and vaginal discharge. So a benefit versus risk assessment must be used here, but for most breast cancer survivors, the benefits outweigh the risks by more than thirty times.

New Gene-Based Drugs for Advanced Breast Cancer

Cellular biologists continue to produce new drugs for more effective management of advanced breast cancer. About 30 percent of breast cancers have a very active gene called HER2. If HER2 is identified in a breast cancer, it can be treated with a drug called trastuzumab (Herceptin), which inhibits the activity of a protein produced by HER2. When trastuzumab is combined with chemotherapy, a 50 percent shrinkage in tumor size occurs. That compares favorably with chemotherapy alone which shrinks the tumor only about one-third. Paclitaxel (Taxol) is another drug that enhances chemotherapy with a 26 percent smaller death rate than with chemotherapy alone. The hope is that these innovative medications, and others sure to come, will keep advanced breast cancer under control, and make it a manageable chronic disease as opposed to a potentially fatal illness.

Breast Cancer Prevention

Tamoxifen was approved by the FDA in 1998 for use in preventing breast cancer in women who are at particularly high risk for it. The National Cancer Institute reported, from the Breast Cancer Prevention Trial, that tamoxifen reduces the risk of breast cancer by 49 percent (Fisher 1998). Because of the side effects mentioned earlier in this chapter, women who opt for preventive tamoxifen must be carefully screened.

Raloxifene is one of the "designer estrogens," meaning it was designed by cellular biologists so that it will attach only to certain estrogen receptor sites. This type of drug is known as a selective estrogen receptor modulator (SERM). Raloxifene attaches to bone receptors and is therefore useful for preventing osteoporosis. It was designed not to attach to breast or endometrial receptors, which reduces the risk of cancer in these tissues. Investigators in the Multiple Outcomes of Raloxifene Evaluation (MORE) found a 76 percent decreased breast cancer risk in postmenopausal women who are at normal risk (Cummings 1999). It still isn't known if raloxifene is better than tamoxifen, but the Study of Tamoxifen and Raloxifene (STAR), which began in 1999, will enroll 23,000 women and hopes to determine this.

Preventive mastectomy involves total removal of both breasts to avoid cancer. It seems like a radical step, but in a woman with a mother and/or sister who has died of breast cancer, and who has a mutated BRCA1 or BRCA2 gene with a 50 to 80 percent chance of breast cancer, preventative mastectomy can be a serious consideration. Some women who choose this option do so after they have completed their childbearing. Unfortunately, such surgery is not foolproof, because it is not possible to surgically remove every last breast cell. Nevertheless, preventive mastectomy is more than 90 percent effective in preventing cancer and reduces the risk of fatal breast cancer by 81 percent (Hartmann 1999).

Summary of Breast Cancer

Breast cancer is a frightening prospect. It may not be an everyday worry for you as a transitional woman, but it is important to assess your personal risk factors for breast cancer and let this information help you chart your life course. Prevention techniques, in those areas you can control, are important. In addition, new discoveries about breast cancer continue to be made that promise to enhance the available methods of prevention, early diagnosis, and treatment.

Endometrial Cancer

Cancer of the endometrium (uterine lining) is the most common genital cancer in women over forty-five (ACOG 1993). It is primarily a disease of postmenopausal women. Approximately 33,000 cases are diagnosed each year, and almost 6,000 deaths result. The annual risk rate is 1 per 1,000 women. Endometrial cancer ranks as the fourth most common female cancer of any type. (Lung, breast, and colon cancer are the first three, in that order.) In recent years, the frequency of this cancer's death rate has been diminishing. Speculation is that the decrease is due to better recognition of the disease in its early stages, as well as to the practice of adding progestin to the regimen of women who use estrogen replacement.

Hormones and Endometrial Cancer

In 1975, two studies reported that the frequency of endometrial cancer was increased in women on hormone replacement therapy (HRT) who used estrogen with no added progestin. Further research by numerous investigators confirmed the increase in endometrial cancer, indicating that this estrogen-only HRT causes an increased cancer risk of five to eight times the normal range (Gershenson 1997). More important, the research also showed that if progestin was added to the HRT, the increased risk was reversed to the same level as in those women who took no hormones at all.

The protective mechanism of progestin is based on the effect that your natural, native progesterone (what your body produces) has on endometrial cells. Estrogen causes growth of endometrial cells, and progesterone inhibits and limits the extent of the growth. Progesterone is an antiestrogen It reduces the number of available estrogen receptors on the cells and induces enzymes in the cells to convert estrogen from estradiol, its most potent form, to estrone, the least potent. These mechanisms protect the endometrium by reducing the degree of estrogen stimulation and, in turn, the risk of abnormal growth. Later in the cycle, both hormones decrease, and the endometrium is shed in a menstrual period. In HRT using both hormones, the endometrium-protecting effect of progestin works in the same fashion.

The net effect of too much estrogen stimulation, whether from unopposed estrogen replacement or from life events, is that the endometrial glands become enlarged, and the endometrium thickens (called hyperplasia). Over time, the excess stimulation results in distorted glands, called atypical hyperplasia, which is a precancerous condition.

Are You at Risk?

The risk factors for endometrial cancer are increased by estrogen stimulation without the modulating effect of progesterone. The following are known risk factors.

Absence of Ovulation

Most of the progesterone you produce occurs after ovulation. A variety of situations can result in failure to ovulate, called anovulation, and underproduction of progesterone. This can occur during the perimenopausal transition; if you are having irregular menstrual cycles, there may be prolonged periods of anovulation. This can lead to hyperplasia and abnormal bleeding. Be sure to get a consultation for any change in your bleeding pattern.

Failure to ovulate can also occur as a result of infertility from a hormonal cause. Another condition, polycystic ovary syndrome, can result from abnormal estrogen production, an increase in male hormone, and irregular or absent ovulation. Women with this condition are also at increased risk for endometrial cancer.

Obesity

Fat acts as a catalyst to convert ovarian testosterone and adrenal male hormones to estrone, the weak form of estrogen. This estrogen source is constant, rather than cyclic like the estradiol produced in your ovaries. After years of extra stimulation from estrone, an endometrial cancer can finally result. The more overweight a woman is, and the longer that condition exists, the greater the risk. Obesity is associated with an almost four times greater risk (Shoff 1998).

Diabetes and High Blood Pressure

Many diabetics are overweight and at risk from extra estrone produced by fat. Even diabetics of normal weight, however, are at a twofold increased risk because diabetes itself is an independent risk factor; diabetes plus obesity is a double whammy and the increased risk is threefold (Shoff 1998). Many diabetics are hypertensive from hardening of the arteries. If high blood pressure is also added to the mix, endometrial cancer is even more likely.

Screening and Diagnosis

How does your doctor detect endometrial cancer? Abnormal bleeding is the single most important clue. When this occurs, ultrasound and tissue sampling are the primary means of evaluating it.

Ultrasound as a Diagnostic Adjunct

When the endometrium becomes thickened by hyperplasia, an ultrasound can measure this thickness. (The procedure involves inserting a specially designed probe into the vagina.) It is only reliable in postmenopausal women, however, because premenopausal women normally have a thickened endometrium. Saline can be instilled into the uterus at the same time, which may help differentiate between hyperplasia and other causes of abnormal bleeding.

Tissue Sampling

When abnormal vaginal bleeding suggests that endometrial tissue must be evaluated, tissue sampling is the next step. Several methods are available to accomplish this:

- **Dilation and curettage (D&C):** This was the traditional method of obtaining tissue samples until the last decade or so. It involves dilating the canal of the cervix (the opening of the uterus) sufficiently to introduce instruments for removing a sample of the uterine lining. It is a blind procedure—the tissue being removed cannot be seen. As you might surmise, a D&C has built-in inaccuracies. This procedure is covered in detail in Chapter 14.

- **Endometrial biopsy:** This is a simplified version of the D&C. A tiny tube, called a canula, is inserted through the canal of the cervix into the uterine cavity. Dilation of the cervix is not required because the canula is about the same diameter as the cervical canal. This is an office procedure, and it takes only seconds to obtain a tissue sample. The disadvantage is that, like a D&C, it's blind, and it hurts like a menstrual cramp for a few seconds.

- **Hysteroscopy:** This is done under anesthesia in conjunction with a D&C. A hollow metal tube with an eyepiece and internal fiber-optic lighting is inserted into the uterine cavity, offering a view of the entire endometrial surface. Abnormalities can be pinpointed and accurately biopsied.

Prevention of Endometrial Cancer

What can you do to prevent endometrial cancer? Let's take a look at the options.

Be Alert to Your Bleeding Pattern

Abnormal bleeding is a convenient (yes, we really mean that) marker for endometrial disease. Hyperplasias and cancers bleed easily and early. Knowing this can get you under care promptly and increase your chances for a complete cure. If hyperplasia is present, it can usually be reversed with progesterone therapy (see the next section), and a potential cancer can be avoided. Early treatment of endometrial cancer approaches a 100 percent cure rate.

CAUTION! Do not, repeat *not*, ignore an abnormal pattern of vaginal bleeding.

Hormones

Proper and timely administration of progesterone can reduce your risk for endometrial cancer. Absence of progesterone puts you at risk. The less you are exposed to unopposed estrogen stimulation during your lifetime, the less your likelihood of this cancer. The low-dose birth control pill, which uses small doses of estrogen and synthetic progesterone, can provide what you need. Any time you are anovulatory for a period of many months or years, the Pill can help. This can occur in the early teens, when anovulation is common, and in the perimenopausal years as well.

Studies show that for women on the Pill, the endometrial cancer risk is lower by more than half compared to those who never used it. If Pill use continues for ten years or more, the risk reduction is 80 percent, and the protection continues at a 30 percent reduction for about twenty years after the Pill is discontinued (Reichman 1996). The take-home message is that if you have risk factors for endometrial cancer such as diabetes, obesity, and anovulation, taking the Pill in your forties protects your endometrium into your fifties and sixties.

Other forms of progesterone are available for you if you cannot or must not take estrogen.

Treatment of Endometrial Cancer

A hysterectomy is usually required to treat endometrial cancer because lymph glands in the pelvis must be removed. When endometrial cancer is diagnosed early, the cure rate is 95 to 98 percent. In more advanced stages, postoperative radiation and chemotherapy may be needed.

Summary of Endometrial Cancer

Endometrial cancer death is mostly preventable. Recognition of your risk factors and becoming proactive in altering them favorably is crucial to avoiding this disease. All that is necessary is to get a consultation if you have abnormal vaginal bleeding, be aware of the risk factors you may have, and have the diagnostic studies your doctor suggests. If you catch it early on, you can almost certainly be cured.

Lung Cancer

Lung cancer is numero uno. Every year there are more than 72,000 new cases, and since 1987, more women have died of it each year than of any other malignancy. Breast cancer causes 46,000 deaths annually, but the American Cancer Society says that lung cancer kills 59,000 women each and every year, and the numbers are continuing to rise. It is much less curable than breast cancer, with an overall five-year survival rate of only 13 percent. Even if lung cancer is caught early, the five-year survival rate with intense treatment is still only 37 percent. Lung cancer symptoms are usually a late-in-the-disease event. Screening with routine chest X-rays has little positive value in early detection. A new type of imaging, called spiral CT scan, is better than a chest X-ray in identifying early lung cancer, but up to 75 percent of abnormalities are false positives. This leads to many unnecessary follow-up tests, including surgical lung biopsies. It may not make front-page news, but the current means of diagnosis and treatment of lung cancer are clearly inadequate.

Risk Factors

In a word, smoking. The "smoking gun" that links tobacco use to lung cancer—an ingredient of tobacco tar called benzo(a)pyrene—has been identified. The experts agree that cigarette smoking accounts for 85 percent of lung cancer cases. The converse is therefore obvious: that you can eliminate 85 percent of your risk for the most common cancer you face by being a non-smoker. Your odds improve still more if you have always been a nonsmoker and you were never exposed to secondary tobacco smoke.

The fact is, secondhand tobacco smoke causes 3,000 to 4,000 lung cancer deaths annually in nonsmokers (Harvard Women's Health Watch 2000. Tobacco Smoke). Nonsmoking women who live with smokers have a one and a half times increased risk for any kind of cancer. If you were raised by smokers, your lung cancer risk is already 17 percent higher than if you were not. Ex-smokers still have double the risk of nonsmokers, even after many years of having quit. Still, that's better than the thirty-five-fold increased risk of long-term smokers.

What other factors play a part in lung cancer? One of them is fat. The National Cancer Institute found in a study of nonsmokers that a high saturated fat intake increases the risk of lung cancer by six times. Other diseases, such as chronic bronchitis, tuberculosis, asthma, and emphysema, add to the risk as well. Environmental pollutants are also a factor. Be sure your house is free of asbestos and radon gas, two well-established carcinogens. Atmospheric smog has not been linked to lung cancer, but it seems to have an additive effect if you are a smoker.

Lung cancer is a discouraging disease because there are no early symptomatic markers, there is no effective screening tool, and treatment does not result in a favorable survival rate. The best we've got is prevention: Don't smoke, and don't hang out with smokers. Keep in mind, too, that one of the best services you can do for your children is to set an example by being a nonsmoker.

Colon and Rectal Cancer

Colon and rectal (colorectal) cancer is the number three cancer killer of women. Actually, it's about the same in both genders. About 75,000 women are diagnosed with colorectal cancer yearly, and 28,000 deaths are recorded. Your lifetime chances of getting a colon cancer are about 6 percent, but with early detection and effective treatment, your lifetime chances of dying from it are only about 3 percent. The chances of getting colorectal cancer are eleven and a half times greater after age fifty than during your perimenopausal years. Why talk about it now? Because there are some changes you can make now that will decrease your risk later on.

What Are the Risk Factors?

Would you guess that factors influencing the risk of cancer in the digestive tract would turn out to include food? You'd be right. Dietary components can be both positive and negative factors. Let's take a look at some of them:

- **Animal fat:** This is the primary risk in your diet, and red meat consumption is the major culprit. The Harvard Nurses' Health Study followed 90,000 women for six years and found two and a half times more colorectal cancer in red meat eaters than in women who ate mostly fish or skinless chicken. That's pretty strong evidence. Dairy products appeared to have no influence on the incidence of colorectal cancer. If animal fat consumption is reduced to 20 percent of total daily calories, colon cancer is reduced by two-thirds and rectal cancer by one-third (Reichman 1996).

- **Fiber:** There is some controversy on the issue of dietary fiber and colon cancer. One study found a lack of fiber in your diet predisposes you to colorectal cancer. If you have a high fiber intake (25 to 30 grams a day), your risk for colorectal cancer is reduced by over 40 percent (Willett 1994). The average American diet has only 10 to 15 grams a day. However, more recent report from the Nurses' Health Study found dietary fiber did not decrease the risk of colorectal cancer, but it did decrease diverticulosis, hemorrhoids, and constipation (Fuchs 1999). (See Chapter 9 for more on fiber.)

- **Heredity:** Heredity also influences this cancer. Your risk is increased 1.7-fold if a first-degree relative has had colorectal cancer under age fifty-five, and 2.7-fold or higher if two or more have had it. When colorectal cancer is a familial trend, there is a greater likelihood that women will develop it in their thirties and forties than after fifty. (Note: A genetically induced condition called inherited polyposis syndrome causes 1 percent of colorectal cancer. The gene has been identified, so if this is in your family, get a consultation from a gastroenterologist or intestinal tract specialist.

- **Colon polyps:** If you have had polyps identified in your colon, your risk of colon cancer is higher, even if the polyps were removed. You can get more of them, so periodic colonoscopy, explained in the next section, is important for you.

Screening—No Fun at All

Screening for colorectal cancer should begin in average-risk people at age fifty. There's nothing elegant about any of the screening methods for colorectal cancer. They all involve poking around a rather sensitive area of your body and doing perfectly revolting things like stool examinations. Keep in mind, though, that this one is the number three cancer killer for you. Let's take a look at the advantages offered by screening for colorectal cancer.

Digital Rectal Examination

A digital rectal examination is a necessary and important component of your annual pelvic exam. It is awkward and uncomfortable, but so is the rest of a pelvic exam, so why not put up with a few seconds more of that for an important check? Polyps, tumors, hemorrhoids, rectoceles (bulging of the rectum into the vagina), and abnormalities on the back of the uterus, as well as ovarian problems, can all be detected by a rectal-vaginal exam. If your annual exam does not include a rectal, ask for it to be done.

Fecal Occult Blood Test

The fecal occult blood test (FOBT) checks for invisible traces of blood in your stool. Bleeding anywhere in the gastrointestinal tract, from the mouth to the anus, can produce a positive FOBT. The test has been useful in detecting colorectal tumors (and for polyps over 1 centimeter in size). You can do the three-day FOBT in the privacy of your home or take stool samples to the laboratory. Several things can trigger a false positive test, so for seven days before you collect three consecutive stool specimens, you must avoid red meats, raw fruits (especially melons), raw vegetables (especially radishes, turnips, and horseradish), aspirin, nonsteroidal anti-inflammatory agents (like ibuprofen), and vitamin C. The dietary restrictions must continue during the three days of stool sample collection. Vaginal bleeding can contaminate a stool specimen, so be certain to avoid collection during your menstrual period. The American Cancer Society suggests that occult blood testing be done annually on women (and men) over age fifty (Winawer 1997).

Colonoscopy and Sigmoidoscopy

A positive FOBT requires a more thorough investigation. One study of over 21,000 people showed that the mortality from colorectal cancer was reduced by one-third in people with positive tests, if colonoscopy (which we explain in a moment) was done and the responsible polyps removed (Mandel 1993).

However, the value of fecal occult blood screening is being questioned by some. It is cumbersome and inconvenient, so strict compliance is difficult for most people. Newer thinking, backed by newer technology, is resulting in less use of this time-honored screening test. Colon cancer experts now feel that integrating family history of colorectal cancer with examination through the use of two techniques, flexible sigmoidoscopy and colonoscopy, are better screening methods. Colonoscopy is an examination of the entire interior length of the colon with a flexible fiber-optic tube. Flexible sigmoidoscopy is similar, but only about one-third of the colon is examined. An alternative recommendation is this: If you have first- or second-degree relatives (that is, parents and siblings or aunts, and uncles, and grandparents) who have had colon cancer under age fifty-five, you should have a colonoscopy at age forty or at an age ten years younger than the relative was at the time of diagnosis (Winawer 1997). If everything is normal, your colonoscopy should be repeated every five years, but it should be every three years if adenomatous (glandular) polyps are found and removed. If there is no colorectal disease in your family, a colonoscopy every ten years should be done starting at age fifty. At this point in time, colonoscopy is not available in all communities. In this situation, the three-day test for fecal occult blood should be done annually starting at age fifty.

Another screening procedure for colorectal cancer is the double contrast barium enema. Barium shows up on X-ray, so filling the colon with it outlines the walls of the rectum and entire colon. Barium enemas disclose about three-quarters of tumors or polyps larger than 1 centimeter. Colonoscopy and trained colonoscopists may be in short supply in some areas, so a barium enema may be the first test done when the occult blood test is positive. If a tumor or polyps are found, the next step is direct visualization and biopsy with sigmoidoscopy or colonoscopy.

In one study, the most years of life saved by screening was with a combination of barium enema and flexible sigmoidoscopy every five years. The fewest years saved was with flexible sigmoidoscopy alone every five years (Winawer 1997). However, any screening strategy is more effective than no screening.

Prevention

We've already looked at diet and screening methods as the two most important preventive methods for colorectal cancer. There are a few more you should know about:

- **Beta-carotenes:** Beta-carotenes play a role in preventing colorectal cancer. These are food pigments that are converted to vitamin A. You will find them in green and yellow vegetables such as carrots, squash, sweet potatoes, pumpkin, spinach, broccoli, and cantaloupe. Those who consume a diet rich in these foods have less colorectal cancer than those who eat little of them.

- **Exercise:** As a preventive measure for colorectal cancer, exercise may surprise you, but consider this: Exercise increases the production of prostaglandins, which stimulate involuntary muscle activity. (See Chapter 3 for more about prostaglandins.) The theory is that prostaglandins decrease the chance of colorectal cancer by speeding up the propulsion of food wastes, thereby reducing the amount of time the colon walls are in contact with any carcinogens that were consumed. Exercise has long been observed to reduce colorectal cancer by half.

- **Aspirin and other nonsteroidal anti-inflammatory drugs (NSAIDs):** These inhibit a type of prostaglandin (PGE2) that is overproduced by colorectal cancers. It is this form of prostaglandin that enables the cancer to promote its own growth into surrounding tissues. The Harvard Nurses' Health Study found that long-term (twenty years) use of four to six aspirin tablets a week reduced the colorectal cancer risk by 50 percent (Calle 1997). NSAIDs such as sulindac are also beneficial by suppressing the expression of cyclooxygenase-2 (COX-2), a substance found in colorectal cancers that has been demonstrated to play a causative role in the cancer (Sheehan 1999).

- **Estrogen:** A review of eighteen published studies on colorectal cancer showed that postmenopausal hormone use was associated with an overall 20 percent reduction in colon cancer and a 19 percent reduction in rectal cancer. For women who took estrogen long-term, the colorectal cancer reduction was 34 percent. Protection was substantially lost within a few years of discontinuation of estrogen, and by five years a benefit was no longer apparent (Grodstein 1999). Speculation on the biological mechanism for estrogen's protection is that estrogen causes a decrease in bile acids, which are associated with promotion of colorectal cancer. It is also known that beta estrogen receptor sites are located in the entire intestinal tract, so a direct inhibitory effect may be occurring. On the other hand, one study found colorectal cancer was unaffected by estrogen use (Jacobs 1999). Long-term ongoing clinical trials will clear up the confusion, but we feel the safest bet at the present is to use HRT.

- **Multivitamins:** The folate in multivitamin preparations is felt to be responsible for a significant reduction in colon cancer. It is estimated that 88 percent of the population has a dietary intake of folate less than the 400 micrograms per day available in standard multivitamins. Folate facilitates a chemical change called methylation, which is essential to normal DNA formation. Hypomethylation of DNA is one of the earliest events in the development of colon cancer. Therefore a daily multivitamin is recommended (Giovannucci 1998).

- **Green tea:** A Shanghai study of 931 women and men found that women who were regular green tea drinkers had an overall risk reduction for colorectal and pancreatic cancer (Ji 1997).

Summary of Colorectal Cancer

Your risk for colon and rectal cancer is much higher than for any of the female genital cancers. As the third most common malignancy you face as a woman, it deserves your attention. This may sound like an old song in this chapter, but let's sing it again: This disease is largely avoidable if you know your personal risks, include the recommended preventive measures in your life, and take advantage of available screening methods. Just as for other malignancies, you must become informed and proactive to be in control of this type of cancer.

Cervical Cancer

Alphabet Soup	
ASCUS	Atypical squamous cells of undetermined significance
HPV	Human papilloma virus
HGSIL	High-grade squamous intraepithelial lesion
LEEP	Loop electrosurgical excision procedure
LGSIL	Low-grade squamous intraepithelial lesion
STD	Sexually transmitted disease

Since 1950, cervical cancer deaths have been reduced by more than 70 percent. Something to crow about, right? No, not yet. If routine screening were available to all women (and unfortunately, it is not) and women took advantage of that screening (and they don't always do so, for a number of reasons), deaths from cervical cancer might be reduced up to 90 percent. Every year 13,500 women still develop invasive cervical cancer, and 4,400 die mostly needless deaths. Cervical cancer is a young woman's disease. About 75 percent of cases are at an age less than sixty-five, and most are premenopausal (ACOG 1993).

Cervical cancer is quite slow to develop. It is estimated that in 95 percent of women with a high-grade cervical lesion (the most severe noncancerous cellular abnormality), it takes eight to twelve years from the time it appears to the development of invasive cancer. In 5 percent, however, a much faster progression, of six to twenty-four months, may occur (Celentano 1989).

What Puts You at Risk?

In a word, sex. And no, this doesn't mean you have to stop it. In recent years, sexually transmitted diseases (STDs) have been linked to cervical cancer. This has given additional meaning to the term "safe sex." Several factors are known to play a role.

Human Papilloma Virus (HPV)—the Main Player

Like other cancers, the causes of cervical cancer are not yet completely understood. But it is known that the human papilloma virus (HPV) is present in more than 95 percent of all cervical cancers worldwide. The virus has more than seventy-five known strains, twenty-four of which are known to infect the genitals of both sexes. As additional types of this virus are discovered, its presence in cervical cancer approaches 100 percent (Paavonen 1999). Researchers have shown that any of thirteen specific strains of HPV, called oncogenic HPV, are necessary to the development of cervical cancer.

Oncogenic HPV strains in themselves are not completely sufficient to cause cancer. Other factors, which we'll look at in a moment, can also influence your risk.

The health risk of HPV is not a serious one—except in women! If you are infected, the risk of threatening cellular abnormalities in the cervix increases by as much as 25 percent. The risk is especially high for the thirteen oncogenic strains of HPV (Braly 1997). Most women who have been infected with HPV do not develop cervical cancer or precancerous changes in the cervix unless they have one of the cancer-causing strains. HPV is also linked to vaginal and vulvar cancer. A new test, called Digene Capture II HPV, has been approved by the FDA to identify this virus (Wellness Letter 2000). Since the new test is more expensive than the Pap test, and no one yet knows how accurate it will be, the best use for now is in those women who have an abnormal Pap rather than for mass screening in every woman who is sexually active.

A mutually monogamous relationship appears to be the best protection from HPV. If your Pap smear shows evidence of an HPV-induced cellular abnormality, a colposcopic exam (an exam with a binocular magnifying instrument) with appropriate biopsies may need to be done, and treatment initiated. The colposcopic exam should also include your vagina, vulva, perineum (area between vagina and anus), and the anus. Regular follow-up Pap screening is a must.

Other Risk Factors

Now let's look at a few other factors that influence risk:

- **Multiple Partners:** The most significant risk factor for your developing cervical cancer is whether or not you have had multiple sex partners. The more you have had, especially if a barrier contraceptive method was not used, the greater is the likelihood that you will have acquired HPV. The second most important determinant is whether your partner(s) have also had multiple sex partners.

- **Unprotected sex at an early age:** The earlier you started having sex unprotected by condoms, the more at risk you are for cervical cancer, simply because HPV will have been in your cervix a greater number of years. Even the very common chlamydia vaginal infections are associated with a 2.3- to 6.6-fold increase in cervical cancer (Paavonen 1999). Multiple partners and unprotected sex add to the risk for teens, just as for anybody else.

- **Herpes virus:** Herpes is a virus that is readily transmitted sexually. It causes very painful skin ulcerations on the vulva (a woman's outer genitals), as you well know if you have been infected. Herpes can be a life threat to a newborn infant; but in adults it rarely is a serious problem. Nevertheless, women who carry the virus are known to have a higher incidence of abnormal Pap smears. Herpes virus can lead to precancerous abnormalities.

- **Cigarettes:** Cigarette smoking is recognized as a cofactor for cervical cancer. It doubles your risk. Nicotine has been found in the vaginal secretions of smokers at concentrations forty times higher than the bloodstream (Notelovitz 1993). If you smoke, it is just as important for you to have regular Pap smears as it would be under any of the situations already mentioned.

- **Genetic susceptibility:** A 1995 Japanese study report by Nawa indicated that heredity may also be a factor.

Screening—the Pap Smear

The Pap smear is easy, painless, and affordable; insurance covers it. It is done during a pelvic exam. A speculum is placed in your vagina so your cervix can be seen, and then some cells are collected and placed on a slide for analysis. Getting a Pap smear doesn't take long, and it might save you from getting a cancer.

A microscopic examination checks for specific changes in the cervical cells that are the precursors of cancer cells. These changes occur well in advance of cancer, and this is the advantage the Pap smear gives you. It can take eight to twelve years for cervical cells to be transformed from normal to cancerous. When precancerous cells are found, they can be easily and completely removed, preventing the development of a cancer.

A new method of evaluating cervical cells in liquid, called ThinPrep, is available. It can also test for HPV and other sexually transmitted diseases, which in itself is a big step forward. With this method, more cells are available to study. Studies of the liquid method indicate it is 65 percent more accurate in determining not only the presence of abnormal cells, but also the likelihood of whether abnormal cells will go on to become a cancer (Linder 1997). In addition, compared to the standard dry slide technique, there are far fewer cellular abnormalities that are deemed to be of an "undetermined significance."

When Should You Get a Pap Smear, How Often, and for How Long?

The National Cancer Institute, American Cancer Society, and American College of Obstetricians and Gynecologists currently recommend an initial Pap smear by age eighteen (or at any younger age for those who are sexually active). Then, after three consecutive normal smears have been taken annually, a Pap every three years is considered adequate for protection (ACOG 1993). But evidence from studies in Canada, Denmark, Norway, and the United States shows that lower levels of cervical cancer are seen when the screening interval is every two years. The cancer rate is up to four times higher if the test is done every three years. The above recommendations are for those in a stable relationship. If you change sexual partners, yearly Pap smears are advised for the next three years.

It is known that some HPV infections can cause a severe cellular abnormality in the cervix, called high-grade squamous intraepithelial lesion (HGSIL), which in about 5 percent of instances can progress to an invasive cancer within six to twenty-four months (Koutsky 1992). This is why Pap screening must begin as soon as sex begins. It was formerly thought that these abnormalities went through a multiyear process of progressive worsening from low-grade to high-grade precancerous lesions, but this is not the case. In fact, it is possible to have a low-grade squamous intraepithelial lesion (LGSIL) coexisting with HGSIL. On the other hand, LGSIL is not typically a precursor of cancer and it usually does not even progress to HGSIL. LGSIL often disappears without treatment. But a Pap is necessary to tell what may be happening in your cervix.

There is a variation in opinion as to the age at which Pap screening can be discontinued. For women who have had a high-grade cellular abnormality or cervical cancer, Pap testing should continue indefinitely, even if the uterus has been removed. (It is possible to develop a vaginal cancer after the cervix has been removed if high-grade cervical disease was present.) Aside from that situation, an emerging policy in some large clinics is to stop screening in the late sixties to early seventies if there have been three normal Pap tests at intervals of at least one year over the prior ten years. However, gynecologic oncologist Walter Kinney (1997) feels Pap screening should continue indefinitely for most women. He notes that 25 percent of cervical cancers and 40 percent of deaths from cervical cancer are in women who are over age sixty-five, and many women by this age have had multiple sex partners and/or partners with multiple other partners, which puts them at risk. He recommends, for this reason, that Pap smears be done throughout a woman's lifetime.

Evaluating Your Abnormal Pap

Pap screening is your entrée to diagnosis. The American College of Obstetricians and Gynecologists states that the conventional Pap test is still the most effective way to diagnose cervical abnormalities (ACOG 1999). If it is abnormal, the next step will depend upon what the Pap report says. Generally it sorts itself out into one of two recommendations. For a high-grade abnormality (HGSIL), cervical biopsies using a colposcope are needed. Low-grade abnormalities (LGSIL) are not regarded as serious and immediate risks. One option with LGSIL is to do a colposcopy. A second choice is to simply repeat the Pap three times at six-month intervals. If all three repeats are normal, routine screening intervals are resumed. If a second abnormal Pap shows up, a colposcopy and biopsies must be done. ASCUS reports (atypical squamous cells of undetermined significance) are handled the same way as LGSIL.

In a recent meta-analysis (all prior studies reviewed) conducted by the Agency for Health Care Policy and Research (AHCPR), the false negative rate for the conventional Pap test was found to be nearly 50 percent (AHCPR 1999). Because of this, three additional testing options are being advocated to enhance its effectiveness as a screening tool. A major problem with these technologies is their expense. They are not cost-effective for annual mass screening, so they are being advocated as a part of screening about every three to four years (Brown 1999):

1. Both liquid-based cellular collection (ThinPrep) and computerized analysis (AutoPap, PAPNET) decrease the rate of false negative readings (Guidos 1999; Parham 1999).

2. Human papillomavirus DNA testing (Digene Hybrid Capture II HPV) for the oncogenic (cancer-causing) types of the virus will increase the reliability of a normal reading. One study showed that DNA testing for HPV in all ASCUS cases is 89 percent sensitive in picking up high-grade abnormalities that had been missed. Then if all such positives were referred for colposcopy, the overall sensitivity increases to 97 percent (Manos 1999).

3. Direct visual inspection (DVI) of the cervix with low power magnification (speculoscopy) after application of acetic acid (vinegar) highlights any abnormal areas. DVI allows more accurate direction of cellular collection for Pap testing and/or biopsies of the cervix if necessary (Sankaranarayanan 1998). Enhanced visualization of the cervical abnormalities is also being accomplished by application of chemical luminescent materials (Suneja 1998).

Given the current problems with the negative predictability of the Pap test, it is fortunate that 95 percent of cervical cancers develop slowly. If you are getting regular Pap screening, the likelihood of a developing cancer being missed on every Pap smear is small.

Treatment of Precancerous Cervical Abnormalities

The principle involved in treatment of precancerous cervical lesions is to destroy or remove the abnormal cells so that they can be replaced with normal cells. This can be accomplished in several ways:

- **Cryocautery:** This is a method of freezing the targeted tissue with specially designed probes. Extreme cold kills cells just like extreme heat. This method is usually restricted to low-grade lesions that are not very large or extensive. It is an inexpensive office procedure that does not require anesthesia.

- **Surgical removal:** Surgery involves cutting out the abnormal tissue. The tissue is removed intact for microscopic examination to be certain all the abnormality is contained within its borders and to check for involvement that might not have been revealed by smaller biopsy samples. One type of procedure, called LEEP (loop electrosurgical excision procedure), uses electric current to remove the tissue. It can be performed in a doctor's office. Another procedure, surgical conization of the cervix, is performed as a hospital procedure. It is performed when the abnormal tissue has extended into the canal of the cervix or there is a suspicion of more advanced disease, such as an invasive cancer.

After treatment for high-grade cellular abnormalities, it is very important to have Pap screening at increased intervals. Recurrence or progression of cervical disease is most commonly detected in the first years following treatment, even if treatment was a hysterectomy (Gemmell 1990). Therefore, rescreening is recommended at six, twelve, and twenty-four months. If everything stays normal, an interval of every two years is then appropriate.

Summary of Cervical Cancer

Cervical cancer can and should be prevented. The simple Pap test has a pretty good fifty-year track record in reducing the deaths from this disease by 70 percent, but it is still not good enough. Modern techniques and diagnostic tools are very effective in preventing invasive cancer of the cervix, but getting a Pap is the first step.

Ovarian Cancer

Of all gynecologic cancers, ovarian cancer is the most difficult to diagnose, and the most unlikely to be cured, and therefore the most deadly. Luckily, it is also the least common. In every 100,000 women, fifteen will develop ovarian cancer each year. Your lifetime risk for getting this cancer is 1.4 percent (one in seventy); but if you are unlucky enough to develop ovarian cancer, your chances of surviving five years are just 40 percent. The death toll is 14,000 women each year (ACOG 1993). This terrible track record stems from the fact that there are no early symptoms for ovarian cancer and that no effective screening methods are yet available. As a result, about 70 percent of women are already far advanced in the disease when the diagnosis is finally established. Unless you have a strong family history of ovarian cancer, the likelihood of getting this cancer during your perimenopausal years is quite small. Most of it occurs in the sixties and then diminishes in advanced age.

Prevention of Ovarian Cancer

The total number of times a woman ovulates influences her risk of ovarian cancer. The more ovulations, the greater the risk. Four or more full-term pregnancies halves the risk and six months of breast-feeding moderately reduces the risk (Harvard Women's Health Watch 2000. Ovarian Cancer).

It has been known for many years that women who take oral contraceptives can cut their risk for ovarian cancer by half. The longer you use the Pill, the greater risk reduction you'll have—up to 60 percent after six years of use. As a result, Pill use is now recommended for women at high risk for ovarian cancer.

A hysterectomy reduces the risk 30 percent. A tubal ligation may lower the risk up to 70 percent (Harvard Women's Health Watch 2000. Ovarian Cancer).

Other factors weakly associated with ovarian cancer are smoking, a high-fat diet, and use of talcum powder in the genital area. Cornstarch-based powders are okay. After traveling through the vagina, uterus, and fallopian tubes, talcum particles can reach the ovaries, where an inflammatory process is initiated and a cancer may ultimately be started.

Screening Tests for Ovarian Cancer

The search for an ovarian cancer biomarker (screening test) has been ongoing for many frustrating and fruitless years. Annual pelvic exams, pelvic ultrasound scans of the ovaries, and the once highly touted CA-125 blood test have all failed to detect ovarian cancer at an early stage—the only time it counts. That's the bad news. There is some better news, however. A 1998 study reported on a potential biomarker for ovarian and other gynecologic cancers. It is a chemical called lysophosphatidic acid (LPA). It was found to be significantly elevated in the blood of forty-seven out of forty-eight women with ovarian cancer, and it was elevated in nine out of ten who had Stage I ovarian cancer (there is a 90 percent survival rate in Stage I) (Xu 1998). The initial study was far too small to have scientific credibility and general acceptance, so a larger study of 1,000 women is underway at the M. D. Anderson Cancer Center in Texas. LPA blood tests represent a potentially stunning advance on the near horizon in our screening ability for ovarian cancer.

For additional discussion of ovarian cancer, see Chapter 14, where it is discussed in the section regarding ovarian removal with a hysterectomy.

Summary

It isn't pleasant to read about this type of disease. Still, if you made it through this chapter, you have improved your fund of information about a disease process that frightens most of us.

Let's review the most important issues surrounding cancer:

- Cancer is not a high-risk disease for you as a perimenopausal woman, but you must not ignore it as a possibility.

- Many of the risk factors for these cancers can be altered in your favor, but you need to start changing them now, while you are young and there is plenty of time.

- Most, but not all, cancers have effective screening techniques that are readily available.

- Certain body signs and symptoms can tip you off that you may be entering a cancer danger zone. Knowing them can save your life.

As a young woman, you may feel distanced from the diseases discussed in this chapter. For the most part, if they occur at all, they are still well down the road. We hope cancer is not a part of your future and that this chapter assists you in avoiding it.

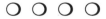

Section II

Changing the Odds

7

You Can Change Your Hormones: The Case for Hormone Replacement Therapy (HRT)

This chapter is about some steps you can take to manage hormone deficiency. It covers the use of estrogen, progesterone, and androgens (male hormones)—their appropriateness, risks and side effects, their dosage, and regimens for effective use. (Chapter 8 takes a look at alternatives to hormone replacement therapy.)

One of the most difficult decisions you will have to make is whether to take hormones as you approach menopause. You hear "take 'em" and "don't take 'em" advice with equal fervor from divided camps. For the past several years an information war has been in progress regarding the issue of hormone replacement therapy (HRT). You and your physician have been in the crossfire of a battle that has produced conflicting reports about the safety and effectiveness of replacing deficient hormones. To no one's surprise, the media have had a field day with the negative reports, and the fear generated has turned many women away from using hormones.

Not even half of estrogen-deficient women take hormones (Keating 1999). This may be partly a result of the information war's conflicting reports and the confusion they cause in the general public, and partly because of unacceptable side effects associated with HRT.

You may have read that hormone use prevents cardiovascular disease and osteoporosis reduces the devastation of Alzheimer's disease, increases blood flow in the brain, and improves long-term memory. Everyone agrees that estrogen alleviates the symptoms of hormone decline. You have also read that there is an increased risk for breast cancer in women taking hormones. So how do you decide what to do?

Basic Science of Estrogen

It is generally believed that women live longer than men because of the cardiovascular protection estrogen provides. Scientific investigations of estrogen have become the most exciting and rewarding of the concerns involving women's health. New concepts about estrogen's effect on the body are being revealed that clarify the benefits and risks of estrogen replacement.

We have come to realize that estrogen's effects are extraordinarily complex. In the past, the concept that estrogen could have effects on a wide array of target organs was never a serious consideration because it was known that an estrogen receptor was required in the cell nucleus of any responding tissue. The presence or absence of this receptor was considered the primary determinant of whether or not a cell could respond to estrogen. And estrogen receptors could not be identified in more than a few organs. Recently, however, cellular biologists discovered a second kind of estrogen receptor, which has demonstrated a dramatic potential for widespread estrogen action.

The original estrogen receptor is now known as ERα, estrogen receptor alpha. The new one is, of course, ERβ or beta. Any particular type of estrogen (there are several) may have a different cellular effect depending upon which type of receptor to which it becomes attached. For example, tamoxifen is an estrogenlike drug used to prevent breast cancer recurrence. When it attaches to breast cell alpha-receptors, it has an estrogen antagonist effect and suppresses cellular growth. But when tamoxifen attaches to beta-receptors in bone, it acts like an estrogen agonist and promotes improvement in bone mineral density. So tamoxifen shows tissue selectivity, and is therefore characterized as a selective estrogen receptor modulator (SERM). Raloxifene, discussed later in the chapter, is also a SERM since it activates receptors in bone but not in the breast. This demonstrates that estrogen exerts different activities in different tissues. In addition, different types of estrogen acting through the same type of receptor can induce different biological activity. This means that all estrogens can no longer be considered interchangeable. Estrogen types are covered later in the chapter.

Hormone Replacement Therapy (HRT) with Estrogen

With the emergence of all this new knowledge about estrogen's expanded effects, we are realizing that estrogen has greater benefits for perimenopausal and postmenopausal women than have been previously recognized. It certainly suggests that the decision for or against estrogen use should be considered from a broad perspective, including both short-term and long-term benefits. Several hormones can be used in HRT, including estrogen, progesterone, and testosterone (male hormone). They are usually used in combination, but we will talk about each of them separately. Let's first look at the use of estrogen.

Benefits of Estrogen Use

Estrogen use offers a number of benefits:

- **Control of symptoms:** Hot flashes, sleep disruption, long-term memory loss, impaired concentration, moodiness, vaginal dryness, diminished sexual sensitivity, and all the other disturbances of perimenopause and postmenopause are not life threatening, but they can threaten the quality of your life. Replacing estrogen reliably and quickly controls estrogen deficiency symptoms.

- **Cardiovascular protection:** The risk of death from coronary heart disease for women over age fifty is 31 percent. Compare that to the mortality from breast cancer (2.8 percent) and from a hip fracture (2.8 percent) (Cummings 1989). Almost three dozen studies in the past quarter-century have uniformly shown the extraordinary benefit estrogen has on the heart. The death rate from heart attacks is reduced by 50 percent if estrogen deficiency is corrected (Judd 1996). Many of the HRT studies have evaluated a reduction in risk factors over the short term, meaning less than five years of use. But there is evidence that long-term use is also beneficial (Grodstein 1996). Indeed, in a report of women using HRT an average of seventeen years, estrogen users had a significantly lower risk of death from any cause, although most of the reduction was in heart and vascular disease (Grodstein 1997). Estrogen has beneficial effects on all aspects of your cardiovascular system. As we've discussed in Chapter 4, about 25 percent of its CVD benefit is in lowering cholesterol, improving lipoprotein ratios of good HDL to bad LDL, and reducing plaque formation in arteries. About 75 percent of the protection is from prevention of plaque adhesion to the walls of arteries, lower blood pressure, strengthened heart muscle, and improved cardioprotective function of the endothelium (lining of arteries).

    The Harvard Nurses' Health Study of 87,000 women found hormone users who had high risk factors for CVD had a 49 percent reduction in CVD deaths, but in low-risk women it was 11 percent (Grodstein 1997). This suggests, of course, that if you are in good health and you stay that way, estrogen replacement may not be as important to you for prevention of CVD. Grodstein also noted that the reduced risk of CVD mortality was lost by the fifth year after discontinuation of estrogen.

A common criticism of past studies showing CVD protection from HRT use has been "selection" bias or "healthy user" bias. By this, the critics mean that women who enter such studies are more likely to be better educated, of a higher socioeconomic status, in better health, with a better diet, regular exercises, motivated to take estrogen, and more. But a large prospective study in Finland of estrogen therapy in postmenopausal women found the same dramatic reduction in CVD deaths as other studies and the effect of estrogen was the same regardless of socioeconomic status (Sourander 1998).

- **Osteoporosis prevention:** Adequate calcium, weight-bearing exercise, vitamin D, a healthful diet, and avoidance of alcohol and tobacco are beneficial in preventing osteoporosis, but they can't get it done as well without estrogen. Bone density can be improved by these other methods, but bone strength sufficient to lessen the fracture rate doesn't occur without estrogen (Cauley 1995).

- **Better brain function:** Memory and other thought processes depend on adequate estrogen levels. Estrogen receptors in your brain cells receive estrogen molecules, which then improve the transmission of impulses from one neuron (nerve cell) to the next. In addition, estrogen use increases the actual number of functioning nerve cells. The more neurons you have, the larger the network of functioning nerve cells, and the better your brain functions. Estrogen supplements in elderly women have been shown to decrease the incidence of Alzheimer's disease (AD) by 29 percent (Yaffe 1998), but in women who already have AD, estrogen does not slow the progression (Mulnard 2000). Using single photon emission computed tomography (SPECT), it has been demonstrated that estrogen-deficient women have reduced blood circulation to the brain, particularly to the areas responsible for memory. During hot flashes, such women have even further decreases in cerebral circulation. In fact, these women had temporary vascular changes during a hot flash typically seen in women with mild to moderate Alzheimer's disease (Greene 1998). Hormone replacement normalized cerebral blood flow. This suggests that hot flashes over time could contribute to neurodegenerative changes. Women have brain glucose needs 19 percent higher than men and are more susceptible to diminished circulation (Baxter 1987). This may explain the higher incidence of Alzheimer's disease in estrogen-deficient women than in men.

- **Preventing and healing of vaginal dryness and thinning (atrophy):** Estrogen can not only prevent these problems, it can clear them up if you already have them. Advanced atrophy, with thinning of the vaginal walls, loss of their elasticity, and painful sex, is unlikely to happen to you during perimenopause, but it's important to stay alert to estrogen deficiency symptoms.

- **Preventing of prolapse of pelvic organs:** Loss of elasticity in the supporting structures of your uterus, bladder, and rectum may allow them to sag so far out of position that they protrude through your vagina. Childbearing and aging both play major roles, but loss of estrogen is a facilitator (Cutler 1992).

- **Preventing of urinary incontinence:** As in prolapse, loss of elasticity and atrophy can cause stress urinary incontinence, but estrogen depletion contributes to both. Estrogen replacement does not restore lost tone or cure incontinence (Jackson 1999), but use of estrogen replacement may help prevent this problem.

- **Cancer prevention:** Prevention? Yes; evidence is accumulating that estrogen significantly reduces the incidence of colorectal cancer, your number-three cancer risk (Grodstein 1999).

- **Better skin:** Estrogen is necessary to maintaining normal collagen and elastin in skin. These two connective tissues are responsible for keeping your skin smooth and pliable. When estrogen declines, you start losing both collagen and elastin. If skin thickness diminishes from loss of collagen and skin elasticity declines from loss of elastin, guess what you get? Wrinkles. Estrogen is not a fountain of youth for skin, but it helps.

- **Macular degeneration:** Age-related macular degeneration (AMD), the leading cause of legal blindness in the United States, may be reduced by HRT (Eye-Disease Case-Control Study Group 1992). About 17 percent of the population between ages forty-three and eighty-six years have this type of AMD. After age seventy-five, about 35 percent of people have it. The cause of AMD is poorly understood, although smokers have a two- to threefold increased risk. A Dutch study linked AMD to loss of estrogen from early menopause, finding a 90 percent increased risk compared to women whose menopause was at the usual age (Vingerling 1995). One study found a 1 to 4 percent reduction in AMD per year of HRT use depending upon the severity level of AMD (Klein 1994).

If you add all this up, you can see that estrogen can have short-term and long-term benefits. Short-term improvements include control of estrogen deficiency symptoms. Long-term, estrogen has beneficial effects on your heart, blood vessels, bones, brain, vagina, bladder, colon, skin, eyes, and cancer prevention. Before you back the truck up to your pharmacy for a load of estrogen, though, be sure to read the next section.

Estrogen Risks

Alphabet Soup
CE   Conjugated estrogen

If all the good news about estrogen were the complete story, the decision to use HRT would be a snap. Like most medical regimens, though (and like life in general, for that matter), the good news must be tempered by downside risks. To be effective and to avoid side effects and risks, estrogen must be used in appropriate situations and in appropriate doses. Both you and your doctor need to know your personal health risk factors and the role estrogen may play in influencing them.

Estrogen risks are at the top of the list for most women when the subject of HRT comes up. A commonly expressed fear is, "They say it causes cancer." Of course you don't want a malignancy, so let's address that issue first.

Endometrial Cancer Risk with Estrogen Replacement

If a woman takes unopposed estrogen (estrogen without the addition of progesterone), her risk of endometrial cancer goes up five to eight times compared to nonusers. The magnitude of the increased risk depends on the dose and duration of use. One study found that as little as six months of unopposed estrogen use increases the risk of endometrial cancer fourfold, and the increased risk lasts for several years (Grady 1995). Even with the addition of progesterone after unopposed estrogen use, the risk is lowered only to twofold. Combining estrogen with progesterone for more than twelve days per cycle results in a cancer risk at the same level as for women not on HRT (Pike 1997). If you are obese or have diabetes or hypertension, you still have an increased risk for developing endometrial cancer.

Breast Cancer Risk with Estrogen Replacement

Researchers studying estrogen today think that in the few instances where an increased association of estrogen replacement and breast cancer exists, it is related to the total length of time breast cells are exposed to estrogen molecules (Zhang 1997). Numerous studies put this risk at about 5 percent. This is based on the observation that there is a slightly greater association of breast cancer with native (produced by the body) estradiol replacement than with conjugated estrogen (CE) derived from synthetic and animal sources.

The evidence to date strongly suggests that estrogen may speed up the growth of an existing cancer. It may not start the fire, but it can fan the flames. What most women fear, though, is that estrogen will cause cancer if they use it for replacement or supplementation.

In 1997, a worldwide reanalysis of all observational studies on the relationship of hormone use and breast cancer was published (Collaborative Group 1997). The authors estimated that HRT use for four years would result in one more case of breast cancer than expected per 1,000 users, and HRT use of thirteen years would result in one more case than expected per 100 users. This is less than that associated with obesity or daily alcohol consumption (Speroff 1999). The worldwide study also found that women who develop breast cancer while taking HRT have a reduced risk of dying from it. This is because of: (1) better surveillance of women on HRT, resulting in earlier detection; and (2) acceleration of tumor growth by estrogen, so that tumors are discovered earlier, at a less virulent and aggressive stage.

The implications of these studies are that a reappraisal must be made of whether lifetime use of hormones should be advocated. It certainly suggests that the decision for or against hormone replacement must be individualized. For many women, the benefits of hormone use may not compensate for the fear of acquiring breast cancer. For women with low risk factors for heart disease and osteoporosis but at high risk for breast cancer (see Chapter 6 for risk factors), the benefits of hormone replacement may not outweigh the perceived risks. One exception to hormone use and risk factors for breast cancer is that hormone users with a family history of breast cancer are not at any more risk for breast cancer than nonusers (Grodstein 1997).

All observational studies fail to show statistically significant evidence that breast cancer is associated with short-term use (less than five years), and many have failed to develop evidence that long-term HRT use increases the risk (Speroff 1999). Some epidemiologists (researchers who study large-population disease trends) say there is actually some reassurance in the fact that breast cancer studies disagree. They point out that if there were a close relationship between breast cancer and estrogen use, the studies would all be in agreement. These scientists reason that if there is a cause-and-effect relationship, it is in a specific subset of women that is too small for current methods of epidemiological investigation to reveal. However, the 1999 Iowa Women's Health Study of 37,105 women did report on a small subset of women on HRT who had a greater risk of developing a nonaggressive (less dangerous) type of breast cancer (Gapstur 1999). Four rare cancer types were identified as linked to estrogen use. These four have a favorable prognosis with treatment, and constitute only 5 percent of all breast cancers. The researchers also found that HRT was not associated with the four most common types of breast cancer. Experts have questioned the scientific validity of this study's methods of evaluating data (Berga 1999), so the argument rages on.

There is no question that women on HRT who are unlucky enough to get breast cancer may have the cancer's growth accelerated by taking estrogen. But, other than the questionable Iowa study, there is very little credible evidence that HRT actually causes breast cancer. So the bottom line in any woman's decision on whether or not to take HRT must be based on a balancing of the risks with the expected benefits.

The birth control pill (BCP) has been widely used for over forty years. Studies from all over the world have failed to show any association of BCP use with breast cancer (Darney 2000). This is in spite of the fact that the estrogen dosage in BCPs is about 75 percent higher than the dose in HRT. Even in women with a family history of breast cancer, BCP use has not resulted in higher rates of breast cancer. This is also true for HRT users (Sellers 1997). The exception to this is a higher rate in women who carry the mutated form of the genes BRCA1 and BRCA2. If estrogen causes breast cancer, we should be seeing a huge increase in the disease in view of the 150 million BCP users since 1960, but we are not. Like breast cancer that occurs in HRT users, breast cancer in BCP users shows up at an earlier stage, treatment is more successful, and death rates are lower.

There is one more reassuring point about estrogen and breast cancer. Look over Figure 7.1. It demonstrates the incidence of female cancer in women who are *not* taking estrogen. Figure 7.1 shows that the incidence of endometrial cancer (which, it has been established, can be caused by estrogen use) decreases after menopause, but the incidence of breast cancer increases. If estrogen is a factor in causing breast cancer, it would make sense for its incidence to decrease after menopause, when estrogen production is lost, but

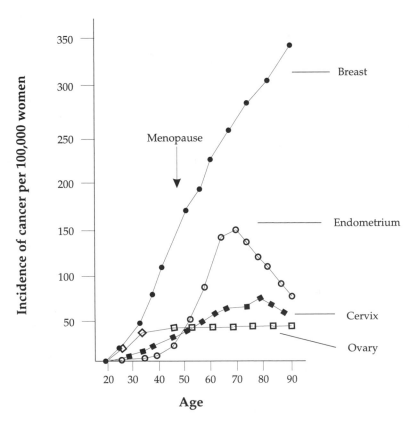

Adapted from: Grombell et al. 1983

Figure 7.1.   Female Cancer Rates in Nonhormone Users

it does not. This strongly suggests that estrogen is not a major risk factor. An additional point this diagram demonstrates is that breast cancer is not a disease of young women; nearly 80 percent of it is in postmenopausal women. Thus, the two most significant risk factors for breast cancer are: being a woman, and aging.

Widely publicized articles containing negative information about estrogen have resulted in uncounted numbers of women discontinuing their estrogen and have discouraged others from starting it. The definitive answers will come from the Women's Health Initiative (WHI), a fifteen-year prospective study of 63,000 women that started in 1993, sponsored by the National Institutes of Health. WHI is the largest clinical study of women's health ever undertaken. One of the issues WHI is examining is the relationship of estrogen use to breast cancer. Their results will not be known until about 2005 to 2007. Meanwhile, your best bet is the credible sources of information available from current studies, the preponderance of which show that estrogen does not cause breast cancer.

Gallstone Risk with Estrogen

Formation of cholesterol stones in the gallbladder is a small risk associated with estrogen use. Estrogen enhances the level of "good" HDL (high-density lipoproteins), which brings cholesterol to the liver. The cholesterol is then concentrated in the gallbladder and excreted in bile. (Bile is an intestinal aid in the digestion of fat; it passes out of the body in bowel movements.) If cholesterol concentrations are high while bile is being stored in the gallbladder, stones can be formed. Small ones are passed into the intestine with liquid bile, but larger stones remain in the gallbladder. Pain and vomiting after eating fatty foods results.

Increased risk factors for cholesterol gallstones occur with high levels of estrogen in the bloodstream, caused by pregnancy, high-dose HRT, and obesity. The higher the level, the greater the risk. Other factors related to stone formation include a high-fat diet and a sedentary lifestyle.

Risk of Blood Clots

HRT has been linked to a small increased risk for deep vein thromboembolism. This occurs when a blood clot in a deep vein, usually in a leg, breaks off and travels in the bloodstream to the lungs, causing a pulmonary embolism. It can create a life-threatening emergency. In women who have had deep vein blood clots in the past, using HRT dramatically increases the risk for thromboembolism, so HRT should not be used.

Estrogen Side Effects

Side effects of estrogen range from breast tenderness and enlargement to headaches, nausea, and irregular bleeding. They are not serious health threats, but they certainly influence quality of life. For the most part, side effects appear soon after a woman starts estrogen replacement. They tend to diminish or disappear as the body becomes accustomed to the new estrogen level. This is similar to the way a woman gets used to the huge estrogen increases during pregnancy.

If you are experiencing side effects, it may be necessary to change the dose of estrogen, the type you are taking, the route of administration, the schedule of taking it, or all of the above. For example, women with headaches and nausea problems do better on the skin patch or a continuous oral regimen using native estradiol. Bloating and PMS-like symptoms are improved with a continuous schedule, rather than a cyclic regimen. More than half a dozen types of estrogen are available, so switching can be the answer. In other words, hormone replacement must be individualized for you. A "one size fits all" mind-set simply does not work. The bottom line is this: Don't give up on this important health benefit because of side effects. A caring physician who is knowledgeable about hormone replacement and perimenopausal changes can help you.

Types of Estrogen

There are several types of estrogen available in a variety of forms from a number of pharmaceutical companies. They sort themselves into three categories: native (human) estrogen, animal-derived estrogen, and plant-derived estrogen. We'll take a look at each of them here.

Human Estrogens

The amount of each of the human estrogens present in your body at any given time is determined by a variety of life situations, including age, pregnancy, diet, amount of body fat, lifestyle habits that can affect your ovaries, and your genetic makeup. There are three types:

- **17-beta estradiol:** For simplicity, we will refer to this type as estradiol. It is the predominant form of estrogen in your body from puberty through menopause. Produced in the ovaries, it is the biologically active form of estrogen that acts at the cell receptor sites throughout your body. It influences over 400 of your body's functions. This is the form of estrogen that starts declining after age thirty-five and finally reaches very low levels after menopause. It affects your heart, blood vessels, bones, brain, skin, hair, vagina, bladder, and other organs. It would seem the logical choice for hormone replacement, but conjugated estrogen, described in the next section, has been the predominant choice for decades in the United States. The commercial brands of estradiol are molecularly the same as what your ovaries produce, but they are derived from plants and micronized (broken down to fine particles) for better absorption. They are available as tablets, a vaginal cream, a vaginally inserted ring, and skin patches. Estradiol is commercially available in the tablet form as Estrace.

- **Estrone:** This is the predominant estrogen after menopause, following the decline in estradiol. Estrone is produced by the ovaries and by conversion of body fat. It is also made in the liver, which converts estradiol to estrone. Since estrone can be converted back into estradiol, estrone serves as a reservoir the body can use for its primary form of estrogen. After menopause, body fat continues as a source of estrone, so it wins the estrogen race by default. Estrone is a weaker form of estrogen than estradiol, so it takes a higher dose to be effective in hormone replacement. Postmenopausal obese women, when compared to slender women, are less likely to develop osteoporosis but more likely to develop endometrial cancer, breast cancer, and gallbladder disease; researchers speculate that excess estrone may be the source of the increased risk. Estrone is commercially available as Ogen and Ortho-Est.

- **Estriol:** This is biologically the weakest estrogen. It is not present in measurable amounts normally, but it is produced in large amounts during pregnancy. Estriol has been tried for estrogen deficiency, but it has not been shown to be as protective as estradiol for the heart, bones, brain, and other organs. Some symptom relief occurs, but it has little beneficial effect on moods, memory, and fragmented sleep. Estriol is not commercially available, nor is it FDA-approved for use as hormone replacement.

Conjugated Estrogens

Conjugated estrogens (collectively known as CE) are derived from pregnant mares' urine (thus the brand name Premarin), so they are also called conjugated equine estrogens. A plant source of CE (sold in the U.S. as Cenestin) is also available. Conjugated estrogens are actually a group of several estrogens rather than a single hormone. Some of these estrogens have a greater ability to attach to estrogen receptor sites than estradiol, so they may in effect displace human estradiol. Some women, especially the elderly, show improved memory with CE—even women with Alzheimer's disease (Henderson 1995). CE is not uniform in its effects on various tissues. Some symptoms may be relieved and others not. Conjugated estrogens stay in the body for two to three months after the last dose, compared to less than twenty-four hours for estradiol, so an adverse effect may be prolonged. On the other hand, research has shown that conjugated estrogens are less frequently associated with breast cancer than estradiol (Cutler 1992). This may be related to their prolonged duration of effect. If CE is occupying the breast tissue receptor sites, estradiol is prevented from doing so. Conjugated estrogens also are more potent than native estradiol in improving lipoproteins by raising HDL (high-density lipoprotein) and lowering LDL (low-density lipoprotein). If this form of estrogen doesn't work for you, don't despair. Other forms of estrogen and other routes of administration are available.

Synthetic Estrogens

The term synthetic refers to manufactured estrogens that are chemically different from your native hormone. By contrast, Estrace, for example, is a manufactured form of 17-beta estradiol, which your body produces; it is molecularly the same as your native hormone and therefore is considered a "natural" hormone. Three representative examples of synthetics are:

- **Ethinyl estradiol:** This synthetic estrogen is most commonly found in birth control pills. It is much more potent than native estradiol and provides more estrogen than is needed for hormone replacement, so it is little used for that purpose in the United States.

- **Estradiol valerate:** About 100 times more potent than native estradiol, so it is rarely used in the U.S.

- **Estrone:** In its brand-name forms (Ogen and Ortho-Est) this is a semisynthetic called estropipate, because piperazine is added to pure estrone to enhance absorption into the body.

Plant-Derived Estrogens (Phytoestrogens)

Certain plants have isoflavones referred to as phytoestrogens. These are compounds that act as precursor molecules from which estradiol is manufactured inside your body. They are found in a variety of plants including soybeans, wild Mexican yams, flaxseed, fruits, nuts, berries, teas, red clover, ginseng, dong quai, and black cohosh.

These last four are herbs widely used to treat symptoms of estrogen decline, such as hot flashes and mood swings. However, ginseng, dong quai, and black cohosh have not been shown to be potent enough to prevent osteoporosis and cardiovascular disease. Dong quai, a traditional Chinese herb, and black cohosh, used by Native Americans, are vasoconstrictors, which means that they cause the blood vessels in the skin to constrict. When you have a hot flash, the blood vessels in your skin dilate. Both dong quai and black cohosh prevent this from happening.

Isoflavones in soy, Mexican yams, flaxseed, and red clover are primarily antioxidants. Among other benefits to the cardiovascular system, antioxidants are known to improve arterial compliance. This means they relax the walls of arteries and thus help to improve blood flow and prevent high blood pressure. A study of red clover isoflavones (marketed as Promensil) in postmenopausal women demonstrated improved arterial compliance comparable to estrogen use (Nestel 1999). Nestel's study was limited, however, in that it only looked at a few cardiovascular risk end points, so it is premature to recommend isoflavones as a substitute for estrogen replacement (see Chapter 4 for the known cardiovascular benefits of estrogen). Nevertheless it is a good example of the kind of study that needs to be done to evaluate the effects of a huge variety of unregulated isoflavones currently being aggressively promoted to the American public as food supplements.

In a randomized control trial investigating the effect of soy on estrogen deficiency symptoms, it was found that 34 milligrams of soy protein once or twice daily was effective. Hot flashes were significantly reduced, total cholesterol and LDL came down 6 percent and 7.5 percent respectively, and the twice-daily supplement reduced diastolic, but not systolic, blood pressure. Dietary equivalents of 34 milligrams of soy protein include one half-cup of tofu, tempeh, or cooked soybeans, or one cup of soy milk (Washburn 1999).

CAUTION! According to the American Soybean Association, isoflavones levels in soy fluctuate widely. A high soy diet in some women acts like unopposed estrogen, and abnormal uterine bleeding can result. Other plant sources also vary widely in the amount and potency of their estrogenic effects.

Estrogen Skin Creams

European women have been using estradiol cream for estrogen replacement in a gel form they rub into the skin once daily. After drying in a few minutes, the invisible residue is absorbed into the skin and acts as a time-release mechanism for the estrogen. The blood levels achieved are similar to the skin patch, but without the skin irritation problems of the patch. The cream is not yet available in the United States; but some specialty pharmacists can formulate a similar product (see Appendix).

Another skin cream, estriol-progesterone, is made from soybeans and the wild Mexican yam, so it contains estriol, the weakest estrogen, and natural progesterone (which we talk about later in this chapter). Some researchers are investigating the possibility that estriol may have anti–breast cancer properties. The research is based on the observation that Asian women, who have a low incidence of breast cancer, excrete large amounts of estriol in their urine. This suggests that they have more estriol in their blood, and that maybe that is why they have less breast cancer. Asking for a giant leap of faith, promoters of this cream claim it will help prevent breast cancer and, further, that the progesterone will stop osteoporosis from advancing. Neither of these claims has valid scientific backup, although it is known that progesterone, in adequate oral or injected doses, will indeed halt bone loss. There have been no major studies of osteoporosis prevention by progesterone delivery in a cream, so use of the cream is still a shot in the dark.

Estrogen Vaginal Creams, Tablets, Liquids, and Rings

Conjugated estrogens and estradiol are available in a vaginal cream. Their primary use to date has been to prevent or reverse atrophic changes (thinning) in the vulva, vagina, and bladder. If you find sex painful because of estrogen deficiency or you are suddenly plagued with recurrent bladder infections, you may benefit from vaginal estrogen. If you have decided to start hormone replacement with oral tablets, the use of a vaginal estrogen cream can "jump-start" vaginal rehabilitation—it works faster than the oral route. When your vagina is back to normal, you can usually stop the cream, and the oral tablets will keep things balanced. But up to 40 percent of estrogen-deficient women cannot keep their vaginas sufficiently estrogenized with the usual HRT methods, so it might be necessary to use vaginal estrogen long-term.

In more frequent and/or larger doses, estrogen from vaginal cream enters the bloodstream in measurable amounts, usually about one-quarter to one-half of the equivalent dose taken orally. There is interest among some researchers in whether this might be an effective route for estrogen replacement. At the present, no products are available to use this route as a sole source of HRT. It seems that micronized estradiol suspended in saline (salt water) and placed in the vagina by douching results in a blood level four times higher than the cream route. Micronized estradiol vaginal tablets are also well absorbed, and can be a convenient method for those who have side effects, such as nausea, from oral tablets (Reichman 1996).

An estrogen-containing vaginal ring, called Estring, is available. It is inserted much like a diaphragm and constitutes a continuous-release estrogen source that lasts three months. Its primary use is for restoring vaginal and urinary tract thinning (atrophy). A small amount of estrogen gets into the circulation, but not enough to influence the uterine lining, so progesterone is not needed. The vaginal ring is better tolerated than estrogen cream, and the continuation rate of usage is much better since it is convenient to use (Ayton 1996). For women who do not have a cervix, the ring is more difficult to retain.

The creams and the vaginal ring work well for treatment of estrogen deficiency of your vagina or bladder, but they do not deliver adequate dose levels for other estrogen deficient parts of your body. To accomplish that, you need the oral tablet form or the skin patch.

To Pill or to Patch, That Is the Question

The differences between the estrogen pill and the skin patch have to do with how the body handles them. Oral estrogen is absorbed into your bloodstream from the intestine. Then it passes through the liver (called first-pass metabolism) where it is reconfigured largely into estrone for safekeeping, as we described earlier in the chapter. Estrogen's first pass through the liver also has a beneficial effect on your lipoproteins, raising HDL and lowering LDL. Triglycerides, a form of fat derived from food, are an independent risk factor for heart disease in women; they are sometimes elevated by oral estrogens, which is undesirable. Other first-pass metabolic changes are the production of a liver protein called sex hormone binding globulin which binds some of the estrogen and makes it less useable. Oral estrogen increases blood-clotting factors, a risk if you have a prior history of coronary heart disease or a blood clot in your legs or lungs. Oral estrogen can raise blood pressure in about 5 percent of users (Wild 1996).

In contrast, estrogen delivered by patch initially bypasses the liver and immediately starts being used in tissues. There is a delayed beneficial effect on lipoproteins of three to six months, but it eventually kicks in. Because estrogen in this form initially bypasses the liver, triglycerides are not elevated by the patch (Nieto 2000). Estrogen from the patch does eventually pass through the liver, but there are advantages to avoiding first-pass metabolism. There is less negative effect on the liver's functioning, and the liver has less negative effect on the estrogen. (Note: If you are also using progesterone, you must still take it every day in pill form; but, as an alternative, a progesterone patch called CombiPatch has become available, which contains both estrogen and progesterone). Here are some factors to help you decide whether the pill or the patch is the right choice for you.

Consider the pill if:

- The patch fails to deliver acceptable estradiol blood levels. This is especially important if you have risk factors for heart disease or osteoporosis, because you may fail to receive estrogen's beneficial effects under these conditions. Skin thickness, which varies from one woman to the next, influences how well estrogen is delivered into your bloodstream.

- Your lipoprotein profile is unfavorable, and you do not wish to risk the three- to six-month delay in improving your HDL and LDL levels. Knowing your cardiovascular disease risk factors is important to this decision.

- The patch won't stick because you live in a hot climate or sweating is a problem.

- The patch causes intolerable skin irritation.

- You are taking progesterone pills and prefer to take both hormones at the same time, although the CombiPatch can solve that problem.

Consider the patch if:

- You have high triglycerides.

- You took oral estrogen and it raised your blood pressure. The patch does not do this.

- Taking oral estrogen causes nausea.

- You have had abnormal clotting disease in the past such as a blood clot in a leg or in the lung (called a pulmonary embolus).

- Taking the pill aggravates your migraine headaches.

- The pill does not maintain a steady enough estrogen level to relieve your estrogen deficiency symptoms, such as hot flashes, mood swings, and short-term memory loss.

- You are a poor pill-taker and often forget to take them.

Other Options

Two methods of estrogen supplementation that we haven't mentioned yet are estrogen pellets placed under the skin and estrogen shots. Pellets provide steady estrogen levels for three months, when new ones must be added. They have the same advantages as the patch in terms of avoiding the first-pass effect. The disadvantage of pellet use is that they must be placed under the skin with a large-bore tube called a trocar. This requires local anesthesia and stitches afterward. It's easy to see why they are not in widespread use.

Estrogen shots are generally discouraged because they can cause uneven estrogen levels from one shot to the next. Nevertheless, estrogen shots may be the only option for women whose bodies do not absorb oral preparations and who have reasons not to use the patch. And the highs and lows that occur with injectable estrogen can be reduced by more frequent, smaller injections.

Designer Estrogen—Raloxifene

Raloxifene is a form of estrogen that was designed by cellular biologists in such a way that it will attach to bone receptors, but not to estrogen receptors in breast or endometrial (uterine lining) tissue. It therefore helps build bone density while avoiding potentially adverse effects that estrogen can cause in breasts and the uterus. Raloxifene (trade name Evista) is FDA-approved for prevention and treatment of osteoporosis in women who must not use estrogen because of risk factors for breast cancer. Raloxifene is categorized as a selective estrogen receptor modulator (SERM).

In a three-year trial with raloxifene in women with osteoporosis, the drug produced a 2 percent increase in bone density. Researchers found a 30 percent reduction in vertebral fractures, but no effect on hip fractures (Ettinger 1999. Reduction of Vertebral Fracture). That's good, but not as good as estrogen can do. A small study revealed no reduction in CVD risk factors for postmenopausal women taking raloxifene (Walsh 1998). It also appears that this designer estrogen does not attach to brain receptors, since hot flashes occur with its use. The evidence to date indicates that raloxifene should not be regarded or used as an estrogen substitute. Nevertheless it is an option for women who wish to protect their bones and reduce the risk of breast cancer, but are unwilling to or must not use estrogen.

As mentioned in Chapter 6, raloxifene has been shown to reduce the risk of breast cancer by 76 percent in postmenopausal women even if they are not at high risk. Several more SERMs, such as idoxifene and droloxifene, are in the research pipeline and being tested to determine their effects in preventing bone loss, improving blood lipids, and reducing breast cancer risks (Harvard Women's Health Watch 2000). As they are refined and studied, they may provide an astonishing breakthrough that can perhaps lay to rest the concerns you may have about the ill effects of estrogen replacement.

Alternatives to Estrogen Use

Breast cancer survivors, women with a strong contraindication to use of estrogen, and those fearful of taking estrogen are candidates for alternatives to estrogen replacement. The statin (anticholesterol) drugs mentioned in Chapter 4 appear to be as effective as estrogen for prevention of heart disease. It is now recommended that women with coronary heart disease use statins rather than estrogen replacement therapy for lowering abnormal blood lipid levels (Harvard Heart Letter 2000). Useful drugs to prevent osteoporosis include the bisphosphonates, calcitonin, parathyroid hormone, raloxifene, and tamoxifen (Santen 1999). Hot flashes respond, but not dramatically, to vitamin E (Barton 1998), clonidine, megestrol acetate, venlafaxine (Effexor), and some phytoestrogens, but none of them is as effective as estrogen. For thinning of urogenital structures, vaginal moisturizers and lubricants help about 60 percent, but estrogen reliably treats 100 percent. Newer methods of delivering estrogen to the vagina without significant absorption into the system include the vaginal estrogen ring (Estring) and low-dose vaginal creams.

Estrogen with Progesterone

Now let's take a look at another female hormone, progesterone. The main reason for adding progesterone to estrogen in HRT is to protect the uterus from developing endometrial cancer. As we mentioned earlier in this chapter, use of unopposed estrogen increases the risk for that type of cancer between five and eight times. When progesterone is added, however, the cancer risk is reduced to about the same level as in nonusers (Gershenson 1996). If your uterus has been removed, you don't need to take progesterone.

Until recently, progesterone has only been available in a variety of synthetic forms called progestins. Natural progesterone is now available as well. Natural progesterone supplements are inactivated in the intestine and poorly absorbed, so it was not useful in hormone replacement. Recently natural progesterone has been micronized, or broken into very fine particles that are easily absorbed. Both forms of progesterone (progrestin and micronized progesterone) are quite useful in hormone replacement.

What Does Progesterone Do?

You know that progesterone protects the lining of your uterus from overstimulation by estrogen because it is an antiestrogen. But what about estrogen's role in prevention of heart disease and osteoporosis? Does progesterone prevent the prevention? As it turns out, for the most part, it doesn't. Let's see what effects it does have in terms of risk factors.

Cardiovascular Disease

Estrogen lowers cholesterol, raises "good" HDL, and lowers "bad" LDL; that's well known. Does progesterone's antiestrogen effect negate estrogen's good deeds? It does, but not much. The net effect is that the rise in your HDL is slightly less than with unopposed estrogen, and there is no effect on LDL. Even the slightly adverse HDL effect diminishes with time, and makes no clinically significant difference in cardiovascular protection (Speroff 1994. Estrogen and Cardiovascular).

Progestins and natural progesterone have been found to lower triglycerides (Writing Group for the PEPI Trials 1995). That is a welcome benefit because high triglycerides are closely related to heart disease in women.

Osteoporosis

Progesterone is active in bone metabolism. When progesterone is combined with estrogen, new bone formation is enhanced slightly (Cauley 1995). Even used alone, progesterone stops bone loss, but it is not nearly as effective as estrogen.

Depression and Mood

Progesterone lowers serotonin, one of your "feel-good" brain chemicals, and decreases the absorption of its precursor, tryptophan. Both of these changes may cause mild depression when progesterone is in your bloodstream. Progesterone levels are normally highest in the second half of the menstrual cycle, when depression is a common emotion. Between 5 and 10 percent of women have depressive feelings or other adverse side effects (mentioned below) as a result of using any form of progesterone, natural or synthetic. Some women become severely depressed (dysphoric) when exposed to progesterone. These are women who could not take birth control pills when they were younger and find that they cannot use progesterone replacement therapy as they age (Leventhal 1997).

Breast Cancer and Combined HRT—a Controversy

Several studies have been published on combined estrogen-progesterone HRT and breast cancer, but so far the results have not been in agreement. In 1995, an analysis of the Harvard Nurses' Health Study was published in the New England Journal of Medicine and gained national headlines (Colditz 1995). That study showed a 30 to 40 percent increase in breast cancer for women over fifty-five who had been on combined HRT more than five years. The study predicted that in following 200 such women over a period of ten years, instead of the seven breast cancers that would be expected, there would be ten if all 200 had been on HRT more than five years.

A month later, a study from the University of Washington was published in the Journal of the American Medical Association (JAMA) citing more statistically significant (meaning scientifically reliable) figures, and it found no increase in breast cancer for women taking combined HRT (Stanford 1995). As a matter of fact, the women in this study who had used HRT for eight or more years had a decreased risk for breast cancer, but the media ignored this.

Well, here's yet another of those scary stories. In January 2000, the JAMA published a frightening article (Schairer 2000) which suggested that progestin plus estrogen replacement therapy (PERT) raises the risk of breast cancer more than estrogen replacement therapy (ERT) used alone. This observational retrospective study involved 46,355 women, a significant portion of whom were included in the study by telephone interviews. This is a technique for gathering data that is fraught with error. Breast cancer was identified in 2,082 women. Only 10 percent of the 46,355 women had ever taken PERT and among these, they found 77 women with breast cancer, meaning 1 percent of PERT users. From such small numbers, nothing can be concluded that is statistically significant or clinically useful, and that should have ended it. But the authors went on to compare breast cancer in PERT users with body weight and finally found twenty-six cases in thin women who had used PERT more than six years but less than sixteen years. A subanalysis of these meager data finally revealed an increased risk for breast cancer in long-term PERT users who were thin. This number of cases is far too small to make meaningful conclusions. Nevertheless, the article was written and the JAMA published it, resulting in front-page headlines and major news stories in the broadcast media. Millions of women were frightened all over the country. Dr. Sarah Berga (2000) called the Schairer article "simplistic to the point of being both wrong and irresponsible." Berga went on to say that we must demand better reporting from our medical journals. This is yet another example of manipulated data tortured to a conclusion that isn't supported by the data collected.

Two weeks after publication of the above article, a second observational study on PERT was published (Ross 2000) reaching similar conclusions, and also based on "over interpretation of relatively weak epidemiological results" (Speroff 2000).

The point is that the links between combined HRT (using progesterone) and breast cancer have not come even close to being proven. The current consensus among researchers on estrogen and breast cancer after dozens of studies is that if a risk for breast cancer exists, it is in a small segment of the female population that has not yet been identified; the same may be true when estrogen and progesterone are combined in HRT. The Women's Health Initiative is studying this issue. The American College of Obstetricians and Gynecologists does not recommend a change in clinical practice based on these two studies (ACOG 2000). Meanwhile, physicians and patients alike are caught in the crossfire of a hormone information war that isn't proving anything credible or useful.

Types of Progesterone and Progestins

A number of types of progesterone and the progestins are available, and we take a look at them here.

Medroxyprogesterone acetate (MPA)

MPA (Provera, Cycrin) is a progestin, or synthetic progesterone. The Women's Health Initiative is using it in their study. Most other progestins are derivatives of testosterone, but MPA is derived from progesterone. It is available in a variety of doses for flexibility in using it in cyclic or continuous HRT regimens. Side effects such as moodiness and bloating may occur with MPA, so the lowest dose possible should be used. Researchers have found over past years that we can safely lower the dosage of progestins to reduce side effects and still maintain endometrial protection (Woodruff 1994). MPA and other progestins do prevent HDL from rising to as high a level as it would with unopposed estrogen, but there is no effect on LDL. In spite of this, there is no apparent long-term adverse effect on heart disease (Speroff 1994. Estrogen and Cardiovascular).

Norethindrone Acetate

Norethindrone acetate (Aygestin), a progestin, is derived by chemically changing testosterone by changing molecules. It produces no male-like effects. Norethindrone acetate behaves much like MPA in the bloodstream, declining after about twenty-four hours. The tablets are scored so they can be broken in half for lower dosages. Side effects are about the same as for MPA, or perhaps a little less. The effect on lowering HDL is the same as for MPA.

Norethindrone

Norethindrone (Micronor, Brevicon) is the "Mini-Pill." It is similar to norethindrone acetate, but it provides a very low dose compared to norethindrone acetate. The primary use for this hormone has been as a progestin-only (no estrogen) birth control pill. It is currently being used with estrogen in the continuous HRT regimen (taking a pill every day, 365 days a year).

Natural Micronized Progesterone

Natural progesterone, unlike progestin, is derived from wild Mexican yams, soybeans, and peanuts. It is micronized for easy absorption from the intestine. The molecular structure of micronized progesterone (MP) is identical to the progesterone produced by your ovaries. Oral MP has been used in France since 1980, and until recently was only available in the United States from specialty pharmacies and mail-order companies (see Appendix). The problem with the U.S. sources is that potency and consistency can vary from batch to batch. Since 1998, MP has been available in the U.S. from several pharmaceutical companies under trade names Prometrium, Progestan, and

Lugesteron. The FDA has approved a new vaginal progesterone, called Crinone Gel, for prevention of endometrial hyperplasia, the cancer precursor. Use of Crinone does not raise blood levels of progesterone, so no side effects are experienced. At a cost of $50 for a month's supply, Crinone is about four times more expensive than the oral forms.

Megestrol Acetate

Megestrol acetate (Megace) is a progestin that has been used primarily for treatment of recurrent cancer of the breast and endometrium. It is a very potent progestin, supplied in 20 and 40 milligrams tablets. For women who cannot take estrogen or who are having hot flashes from tamoxifen use in breast cancer (see Chapter 6), megestrol acetate can relieve hot flashes with a dose of 20 milligrams twice daily. This progestin has also been shown to increase bone density at these doses, which is a plus (Reichman 1996). A minus is that it may have an adverse effect on lipids if used long-term. Megestrol is a special-use drug, and more research needs to be done on it.

Side Effects?

Taking progesterone can make some women feel awful. Progesterone is the hormone that reaches high levels in the second half of the menstrual cycle, and it can give you sore breasts, lower your energy level, cause water retention, increase your appetite, make you feel bloated, and make you depressed.

Only 30 percent of women experience these side effects. If you do have adverse side effects, you can change the type of progesterone you use, the schedule on which you take it, or the dosage itself.

Synthetic Progestins versus Natural Progesterone

Several studies have shown that the antiestrogen effects of synthetic progestins have adverse metabolic and vascular effects. These include mild inhibition of the estrogen-mediated rise in good HDL (Writing Group for the PEPI Trials 1995), altered insulin sensitivity (Elkind-Hirsch 1993), prevention of blood vessel dilation (Sorensen 1998), and microscopic changes in artery walls that could lead to plaque formation (Adams 1995). As yet, none of these changes has been linked to harmful consequences. On the other hand, in human and animal studies of natural progesterone none of these metabolic or vascular side effects were observed so long as recommended dosages were followed. Therefore, natural progesterone may have a better risk-to-benefit profile than the synthetic progestins (de Lignieres 1999).

Androgens (Male Hormones)

Guess where your estrogen comes from. Give up? Male hormones. Your ovaries, as well as your adrenal glands, start with androgens (male hormones)

Alphabet Soup	
T	Testosterone
ASD	Androstenedione
DHEA	Dehydroepiandrosterone
DHEAS	Dehydroepiandrosterone sulfate

and the follicles in your ovaries convert them to estrogen. The same thing happens in fat cells: Cholesterol is converted first to an androgen and then to estrogen. Both genders make female and male hormones. The fundamental difference is that one of them is very dominant in each gender.

There are five different androgens. Your ovaries make two of these five: testosterone (T), a strong androgen, and androstenedione (ASD), a weak one. Both T and ASD are made in the interior cells of the ovary, called the stroma. They are then converted to estrogens by the follicle cells near the surface of the ovaries as they mature every month and prepare an egg cell. Small amounts of the androgens remain unchanged, however, and enter your circulation. There they perform certain important functions, such as maintaining your energy level, improving your sense of wellness, and activating the sexual circuits in your brain. Your adrenal glands also produce ASD, as well as dehydroepiandrosterone (DHEA), another weak androgen, which enter your bloodstream. Your ovaries can pick them up and convert them to estrogens too (a sort of backup supply source). Some of these androgens remain unchanged by your ovaries, though, and make their rounds in your body, where they may be later converted to estrogens by whatever tissue they visit: fat cells, muscles, skin, brain, kidneys, and others. About 25 percent of your T supply comes from ovarian androgens, another 25 percent comes from your adrenal gland androgens, and the remainder is derived from fat, skin, and muscle cells that convert ovarian and adrenal androgens to testosterone.

Estrogen-Androgen Ratios

The net result of all the reconfiguration and conversion we just described is that a stable ratio between blood levels of estrogen and androgen is maintained in your body from puberty to menopause, but estrogen levels exceed androgen by a huge margin. With time, ovarian follicles diminish in number, so production of estrogen and testosterone (T) both decline. By menopause your follicles are sufficiently diminished in number that estrogen declines sharply, by 80 to 90 percent. T levels only go down by about 50 percent, however, because the cells in the stroma of your ovaries can still make androgen, as can your adrenal glands (Rosenberg 1988). There are just not enough follicles left to convert the testosterone to estrogen, and this distorts the ratio of estrogen to T: There is a net loss of both hormones, but there is relatively more T than before. This relative T increase results in an increased sexual desire for about 50 percent. Unfortunately, it is short-lived because by about the fourth or fifth year after menopause, T production will have declined further (Kaplan 1993).

At menopause, androgen is less suppressed by estrogen, and it may express itself in malelike ways. You may notice more facial hair, a deeper voice, and a changed body fat distribution. Body fat distribution changes from a "pearlike" female concentration about the hips, to the "applelike" male shape around the waist. Weight gain in midlife is not from estrogen use as the popular myth would have you believe. It is from the changed balance of estrogen and androgen, with the additive effect of reduced physical activity and food consumption that is increased to more than an age-related lowered metabolic rate justifies. The androgen imbalance also creates a risk for other, unfavorable malelike changes, such as rising blood pressure, higher cholesterol, lowered HDL, and raised LDL. These changes can start in your forties; as a transitional woman, you should know some things about recognizing the imbalance and correcting it if needed.

Symptoms of Androgen Deficiency

Male hormones have important functions in terms of maintaining muscle tissues, building bone, and keeping an optimal energy level, but they also have a potent influence on how your brain works. Too much testosterone can cause hyperactivity, a shortened attention span, scattered thoughts, aggressive, violent dreams, and abnormally increased sexual desire. When male hormone levels decline, you may experience a deterioration in these areas. Also, loss of muscle mass may be noticeable in the unwelcome appearance of flabby arms and other parts of your body. Your skin may become dry and your hair thinned. You may notice that you just don't have your customary get-up-and-go. Your interest in sex may have slipped several notches on your list of "great things to do at every opportunity." Or you may simply feel that "something is wrong," but you just can't put your finger on it. If symptoms of estrogen decline are also present, such as hot flashes, sleep disruption, disturbed concentration, moodiness, and so on, then think about the possibility that your body is experiencing not only an estrogen decline, but a low testosterone level as well.

Should You Really Take Male Hormones?

Not every woman needs to take male hormones, but a number of situations might justify your considering them, usually in combination with female hormones:

- **Both ovaries surgically removed:** This procedure immediately drops the bottom out of androgen and estrogen production. If symptoms from sudden estrogen loss (hot flashes, moodiness, short-term memory loss) are combined with the symptoms of androgen deficiency (loss of energy, slowed thinking, absent sexual desire, diminished sense of well-being), you may need both hormones to get back on an even keel. Androgens in women are basically psychotropic (affecting the mental state) hormones that influence the way you feel: They act as an antidepressant. This is consistent with the observed effects of androgen deficiency. Estrogen replacement therapy should be the first treatment for estrogen deficiency symptoms. Then, if symptoms of androgen deficiency persist, male hormone replacement should be added.

- **Hysterectomy:** If your uterus is removed, even if the ovaries are not taken out, you have a 30 percent chance of becoming menopausal within four years (Cutler 1990). It has to do with compromised blood supply to the ovaries as a result of the surgery. Estrogen replacement is, of course, important for all the reasons we've discussed. Male hormone replacement is an option if androgen deficiency symptoms are also present.

- **Loss of sexual interest:** Male hormones exert the major influence on female sexual desire. Estrogen is primarily involved with sexual responsiveness, such as lubrication, arousal, and orgasm, but testosterone is the engine of desire, fantasies, and the motivating forces that make you want to have sex. Sexual interest can be blunted by estrogen deficiency symptoms such as hot flashes, moodiness, and vaginal dryness. If your loss of interest in sex does not improve with estrogen replacement, though, and is not related to other problems like hypothyroidism, depression, or relationship problems, adding testosterone can make the difference.

- **Loss of energy:** A general loss of energy may well be due to things like anemia, hypothyroidism, other chronic diseases, or just a frantically busy lifestyle. If these aren't factors, supplements of male hormone may put the zing back into your life.

- **Vertebral osteoporosis with compression fractures:** This is a problem seen in postmenopausal women who have done little to prevent osteoporosis. Adding testosterone to HRT can help prevent more fractures, but a good prevention program starting now is a much better option.

- **Breast tenderness:** Women taking female hormones often complain of breast tenderness. If you have been hormone-deficient for several years, your breasts may be more sensitive when you start HRT. Adding testosterone helps reduce the pain.

There are a lot of negative myths about androgen use in women and the virilizing effects it might cause: "You'll get a mustache and a beard plus acne, you'll look like a muscle-beach volleyball player, your voice will deepen, you'll get liver damage, you'll become a sex-starved maniac." Like most myths, there is a kernel of truth in them, but problems like these are related to the dose and type of male hormone used. With low doses, less than 5 percent of women experience virilizing effects (Sherwin 1996). Androgen sensitivity varies from woman to woman, so its use in therapy must be individualized.

Types, Dosages, and Administration

Several types of preparations of male hormones are available. They come in varying dosages, and they are administered in a number of ways.

Types of Preparations

Synthetic hormones are chemically compounded in a laboratory to resemble what the body naturally produces. Testosterone can be made exactly the way your ovaries make it, but it is not well absorbed from the intestine. To get around this, a methyl group is added to the molecule. This makes it more potent than natural testosterone, so small doses are necessary. Methyltestosterone (Android, Estratest) is being used less and less in recent years. Fluoxymesterone (Halotestin), another synthetic, has largely supplanted it. Fluoxymesterone is better tolerated, lasts longer in the body, and has fewer side effects. Synthetic preparations are commercially available in tablets, pellets, patches, and injectables. Several products (Estratest, Depo-Testadiol) are now available that combine estrogen and methyltestosterone in a single tablet or injectable. With a prescription, a knowledgeable pharmacist can prepare skin creams, skin gels, and vaginal suppositories. Testosterone enthanate (Delatestryl) is often used as a monthly injection.

Natural testosterone from soybeans and wild Mexican yams is poorly absorbed, so it is micronized in the laboratory. It is available in tablets of varying strength from specialty pharmacy companies (see Appendix).

Dosage

Proper dosage is important in the use of androgens. This is another situation where one dose doesn't fit all. Each woman's dose should be individualized and fine-tuned as necessary. Typically, treatment starts with a low daily dose and gradual increases over time until your androgen deficiency symptoms improve. If symptoms (lack of energy, slowed thinking, absent sex drive, depressed mood) are unimproved with a moderate dose, you probably don't need the testosterone you are taking, and another source of your persisting symptoms should be investigated. Indeed, before agreeing to a higher dose, you should insist that your blood level of free testosterone be checked first. An adequate blood level of free testosterone indicates that a higher dose is not the way to proceed.

If laboratory testing of your testosterone (T) is done, it is important to measure both your total T and free T. The reason for this is that circulating T is normally bound to a protein called sex hormone binding globulin (SHBG) and only a fraction of it is free to influence your tissues. With slowing of ovarian function, SHBG is less occupied by estrogen molecules and relatively more of it binds testosterone. This results in less and less free T available. A total T level could well be within the normal range, while free T is abnormally low. Not knowing this can mislead your doctor to advise you that you don't need testosterone.

Testosterone testing is expensive. This is probably a factor in the emerging practice of giving a trial dose of androgens at first, rather than checking blood levels in the laboratory. If the desired benefits are not obtained with a trial of use, tests can then be ordered.

Routes of Administration

Androgens are usually taken orally. Tablets were originally designed for men, in doses generally too high for women, but lower-dose tablets are now available. A good way to get androgens into your system is by letting the tablet dissolve under your tongue. Lozenges are available; but the smallest one contains way too much testosterone for a woman. Skin gels are being tried, but not much is known about them as yet. Many women find a combination estrogen-testosterone tablet the most convenient way to take both hormones.

CAUTION! If you are taking estrogen and testosterone in combination, you still need progesterone; androgen does not protect your endometrium from the unopposed effects of estrogen.

Injectable preparations cause wider fluctuation in blood levels than tablets, which makes it more difficult to keep your symptoms controlled. Unwanted side effects are more common because it is more difficult to find the right dose. Too much male hormone can result in the development of coarse facial hair. Once a hair follicle is stimulated by male hormone, it continues to be dark and coarse, even after the hormone is stopped. Electrolysis or laser therapy is then required to remove the unwanted hairs. (No amount of plucking or waxing will get rid of them.) Injectables sometimes wear off without notice, causing significant fluctuations between there being too little and too much male hormone in your system. On the other hand, injectables have the advantage of bypassing the liver and intestinal tract, which avoids the potential for partial hormone inactivation by SHBG. Long-acting injectables (Depo-Testadiol) may be useful once an appropriate dose has been established through the use of tablets.

Androgen pellets are also available. Placed under your skin, pellets provide a constant male hormone level, without the ups and downs of oral or injectable testosterone (Notelovitz 1993). The dosage is always within the normal testosterone range, so excessive hair growth and acne are rarely a problem. The disadvantage of this method of male hormone administration, however, is a big one: Placement of new pellets to keep the hormone level constant requires a small incision and stitches every three months. Biodegradable pellets are being developed for other hormone supplementation and may be a future source for androgens. A recent study of pellets used to increase sexual desire showed that desire returned to normal within three months, compared to no improvement in women who used placebo pellets (Leventhal 1997).

The testosterone skin patch is available for men, but it delivers far too much testosterone for use in women.

If you decide to take androgens, keep in mind that your body is different from that of every other woman. Your symptoms and needs are yours alone. You are the only one who knows how you feel and the only one who knows when you feel better. Androgen use requires a close working relationship with your doctor, and individualization of your dosage. Don't settle for less.

Other Androgens: DHEA and DHEAS

Some links have been drawn between DHEA (dehydroepiandrosterone) and the aging process. This hormone is produced by the adrenal gland, as we mentioned earlier in the chapter. Humans and other primates are the only species capable of making large quantities of DHEA and DHEAS. At birth, we all have high levels of these hormones. Then they decline until puberty, when they begin to rise again, reaching a peak in the late twenties. From that time on, a slow steady decline ensues, and about 80 percent of DHEA and DHEAS is gone by the seventies.

DHEA is one-hundredth as potent as T. Some of it circulates in the bloodstream in its free form, but most of it is bonded to a sulfate, becoming DHEAS, which is one-thousandth as potent as T (Luthold 1993). This weak androgen can be converted to testosterone if needed. Some studies have suggested that DHEA has an antiaging role, in addition to acting as a reservoir for conversion to testosterone. The question arose as to whether the human aging process is influenced by the steady drop that occurs in these hormones. Low levels of DHEA and DHEAS in men have correlated with an increased risk for heart disease, but an apparent gender difference exists, because in women, the highest risk for CVD was in those who had the highest levels of DHEA and DHEAS. People with Alzheimer's disease were observed to have a 50 percent decrease in their expected levels of both forms of the hormone (Nestler 1995).

Researchers next turned to the question of whether supplements of these hormones would act as an antiaging drug. Men and women were given a high dose on a daily basis. The men did fine, with improvement in their lipoproteins, but women did poorly: They had worsened lipid profiles with lower HDL; they became insulin-resistant, which caused weight gain; and they developed the "apple body" male pattern of obesity.

Then, a small group of women and men were given a significantly smaller amount daily, just enough hormone to restore the DHEA and DHEAS to the levels of their youth in about two weeks. There were initial benefits in raised testosterone and lessened insulin resistance, but these were lost within six months of continued use. Even DHEA blood levels went back to the pre-treatment range within six months of continued use. In addition, good HDL levels remained adversely affected in spite of the return of DHEA blood levels to normal (Casson 1998).

Other small studies have noted positive benefits in both women and men:

- No decrease in insulin sensitivity, a common trait of aging (Bates 1995)

- Increased activity of natural killer cells, suggesting that immune competence was improved (Araneo 1995)

- Improvement in major depression (Wolkowitz 1995)

- Better sleep, memory, and mood (Baulieu 1995)

- Increased energy

- Improved ability to handle stress

- Improved sense of well-being and improved sexual desire (Arlt 1999)

These were all small studies, but the prospect of slowing the adverse effects of the aging process is exciting. If DHEA and DHEAS supplements can be shown to prevent the usual age-related loss of immune competence, a reduction in the cancer rates associated with aging can be expected. More studies will, of course, be needed. Since there have been no large, long-term clinical trials to back up these claims, there is no FDA approval for using DHEA in humans for any reason. Even though there is no scientific evidence indicating that it should be a part of the human diet, this hormone is currently being sold without prescription as a food supplement (Skolnick 1996). It will be interesting to see what further research reveals.

Hormone Replacement Regimens

We've taken a pretty detailed look at the effects of taking estrogen, progesterone, and androgen. Now you are ready to understand how they are put together in a treatment plan. There are several approaches, and none of them works for everyone; the one that works for you may be quite different from that of other women you know. Your decision on whether to take HRT and, if so, in what form, should be based on your understanding of why it is recommended and the form in which you are comfortable using it.

A national study of women who received prescriptions for HRT revealed that 20 to 30 percent never even got their prescriptions filled (Ettinger 1996). Another study found that 38 percent discontinued HRT in less than a year. Within six months of starting HRT, 63 percent were using the hormones "from time to time," and this spotty use was up to 90 percent after two years. After seven years, only 10 percent were still taking hormones (Berman 1996).

There are many reasons for such low numbers:

- On the part of women, fear of cancer and irregular bleeding were the most frequently cited reasons for declining HRT (Speroff 1994. Managing Bleeding).

- Side effects (bleeding, bloating, fluid retention, sore breasts) are intolerable for some.

- Physicians and health-care providers of all stripes have failed to educate American women about hormonal decline in general and on the value of HRT. Part of this is because perimenopausal and menopausal understanding is not widespread enough in the medical community. Part is because we haven't made a strong enough effort to educate you.

- Preventive health care is a hard sell. Until confronted with an adverse health problem (obesity, heart disease, osteoporosis, high blood pressure, cancer), many people are not motivated to do much of anything about averting the problem.

- Fear of aggravating prior health problems (breast cancer, uterine cancer, blood clots in legs or lungs)

- Some women decide that HRT is unnatural and regard it as experimenting with their bodies.

The regimens we describe in the following sections are those currently in use. It cannot be said that one is superior to the others; there are reasons for using each. One of them will likely meet your hormonal needs, your life schedule, and your comfort zone.

Unopposed Estrogen

We discussed the risks of unopposed estrogen use earlier in this chapter. It has practically disappeared as a way of treating women, except for those who do not have a uterus. Today, a common source of unopposed estrogen is herbs, such as ginseng, dong quai, and black cohosh, which contain phytoestrogens. It is not yet known whether consuming these herbs increases cancer risk.

There has been a rising interest in and use of estrogen only, but with the addition of progesterone for two weeks every three months (Ettinger 1994). This method is actually called quarterly cycling, rather than truly unopposed estrogen. There is now evidence that the endometrium may not be protected after the first year on quarterly cycling. An unreported study is underway to investigate using progestin every six months in women using low-dose estrogen (Ettinger 1999. Personal Perspective).

CAUTION! Chances of developing an endometrial cancer are quadrupled with as little as six months of unopposed estrogen use (Grady 1995).

Cyclic HRT

There are two methods for accomplishing cyclic HRT. The classic regimen uses both estrogen and progesterone in a cyclic fashion, with five days off each month. The other is to use estrogen continuously but progesterone cyclically. The cyclic methods may be the best to use for women who are estrogen-deficient but still having menstrual periods, or for women who have just recently become menopausal.

Cyclic Estrogen and Progesterone

In a course of treatment involving cyclic estrogen and progesterone, you typically take estrogen each month from day one through day twenty-five. Progesterone is added for the final twelve to fourteen days of estrogen use. Then both are stopped until day one of the next month. During the five or six off days (depending on what month it is), you have a menstrual period.

With this method, menstrual periods continue as always, which can be either reassuring or a nuisance, depending on your point of view. A further disadvantage for some women is that during the five or six days off, estrogen deficiency symptoms may return, such as hot flashes, mood fluctuations, and fragmented sleep.

Cyclic HRT may be the best method in late perimenopause or early menopause because less breakthrough bleeding occurs than with continuous methods (see the next sections). Nevertheless, it can take three to four months for your body to fall into the rhythm you are imposing on it. During this time you may have episodes of light breakthrough bleeding. For the large majority of women, this situation resolves itself. If the bleeding is heavy or continuous, though, be sure to contact your doctor. You could have an endometrial problem.

Continuous Estrogen and Cyclic Progesterone

In the second cyclical treatment plan, estrogen is taken continuously, 365 days per year. Progesterone is added for twelve to fourteen days of each month. It is a popular method for HRT because it eliminates the "off" days experienced with the first method. With this method, it also takes three to four months for your body to become accustomed to the cycle. Once that has happened, bleeding should occur only when you are off progesterone. Any other type of bleeding should be reported to your doctor.

Continuous Combined HRT

With continuous HRT, both estrogen and progesterone are taken daily, 365 days per year. The progesterone dose is half that used for the cyclic methods. The rationale for continuous progesterone is that it provides continuous protection of the endometrium. With this method, the uterine lining eventually becomes thin, and the glands inactive. With nothing to shed, there is no more uterine bleeding. That sounds like good news, but 30 to 40 percent of women will have breakthrough bleeding at unannounced intervals for about the first four months. After a year, 80 to 90 percent of women using this method will have stopped all uterine bleeding (Reichman 1996). This pattern (or more accurately, nonpattern) of bleeding is most likely to occur in women who are fewer than three years past their menopause. The cyclic regimens tend to work best during these years. Nevertheless, if you are unwilling to put up with monthly bleeding, the continuous method may be for you.

CAUTION! If bleeding is heavy or continuous, or if you have no bleeding for several months and it resumes, call your doctor.

Some doctors have started using the continuous regimen on a Monday-through-Friday schedule. This seems to lessen the problem of initial breakthrough bleeding. The total estrogen dose is reduced by about 30 percent with this weekend-off method, so CVD and osteoporosis protection may be compromised. Your blood lipoprotein levels should be monitored, and you should have a yearly bone density scan if you use this method long-term.

Low-dose Estrogen

Studies on this issue suggest physicians have been wrong to regard the minimum effective estrogen dosage of conjugated estrogen as 0.625 milligrams or its equivalent (Ettinger 1999. Personal Perspective). Evidence is accumulating that shows estrogen's effect is linear, as opposed to all-or-nothing at a presumed threshold level of 0.625 milligrams. This means some of the benefits are diminished with lower doses, but so are the risks. Nevertheless, if conjugated estrogen is used in a 0.3 milligrams dose, the protective benefit on the cardiovascular system is undiminished. For women on half-dose estrogen, 1,500 milligrams of supplemental calcium daily is recommended to improve its effect on bone. There are no data regarding low-dose estrogen and breast cancer other than to suggest that lower doses pose lower risk.

Estrogen deficiency symptom control is less effective on low-dose regimens, so it is recommended to use "standard" doses during the early years of estrogen depletion. The dose can then be reduced in three to five years after menopause with no recurrence of symptoms.

Since many women decline to use current standard estrogen dosages because of cancer fear or side effects, low-dose estrogen may be more acceptable. Ettinger's position is that a low dose is better than no dose.

Summary

Two decades ago, this would have been a very short chapter, but the past twenty years have brought many changes to hormone replacement therapy. Scientific advance is often fraught with controversy, and HRT has certainly been no exception. If your aim is to decide on whether or not to use HRT, numerous studies suggest that the first five years can be a free trial. You can see how you like it without incurring an increased risk for breast cancer. You can also see if it makes enough difference in bone density to protect you from osteoporosis, and whether it reduces your risk factors for heart disease. Meanwhile, newer and safer options will likely emerge from the community of researchers who are contributing to making hormone decline a safer passage for women.

Your primary responsibility to yourself regarding HRT it to become as fully informed as you can before you make a decision about using this therapy. You have a choice to use it or not to use it, but your choice is one of the most important health-care decisions you will make in your lifetime. If you are in the early stages of perimenopause, the information in this chapter may not apply to your immediate needs, but it should help make your future choices easier. The decision you make about using HRT should be the result of considering the benefits of symptom relief, CVD protection, osteoporosis prevention, reduced risk of colon cancer, and protection of age-related brain deterioration; and weighing them against the risks of uterine or breast cancer and potential side effects. Your final decision should then be based on a composite of your knowledge, your trust in your health adviser, your intellectual perceptions, and your own body wisdom.

O O O O

8

Integrative (Alternative) Medical Disciplines: Are They a Good Choice for You?

Women who are experiencing the symptoms of diminishing hormone production that can accompany perimenopause tend to seek out a health-care provider who can provide relief. The choices sort themselves out to traditional and integrative (a.k.a. alternative) medical care. The term "alternative medical care" is now out of favor, so we will go with the flow and call it "integrative." We've already looked at the benefits and the risks of HRT. If you choose not to take hormones, there are alternatives for managing the symptoms of estrogen decline. A problem you may run into is that practitioners of both traditional and integrative medicine tend to disparage each other's disciplines. The loser in this case is you. Both traditional and integrative medical practices have benefits. If you make a choice to exclude one at the expense of the other, you may be throwing the baby out with the bathwater.

Acute-care Western medicine is unequaled in saving lives and in relieving immeasurable pain and suffering. It is in the treatment of chronic diseases and persistent adverse symptoms, however, that integrative therapies can claim their niche. Our culture perceives a growing need for healing that supports people's efforts to reconnect mind, body, and spirit in the pursuit of wellness. Nearly one of every two adults aged thirty to forty-nine used at least one integrative therapy in 1997, and spent $21 billion out of pocket for this care (Eisenberg 1998). This chapter looks at a variety of integrative medical disciplines that are legitimate approaches to alternative forms of healing. The remedies offered vary from medicine prescribed by licensed physicians to a huge number of naturally occurring plant and animal derivatives available without prescription, as well as nonmedicinal therapies. There are far too many options to include in the confines of this book, so we've chosen the ones we think are representative—the ones hormone-deficient women tend to seek most frequently. They include traditional Chinese medicine, herbal therapies, homeopathy, acupuncture, naturopathy, holistic medicine, and mind/body techniques. (Other alternatives we haven't included in our discussion include ayurveda and yoga, massage and bodywork, chiropractic, relaxation and meditation, hypnotherapy, spiritual healing, and energy work.)

Traditional Chinese Medicine (TCM)

Traditional Chinese medicine (TCM) has been practiced for five thousand years. When Western medicine was having its beginnings, TCM was already ancient, and Chinese medicine has been successful in treating many areas of illness over the centuries. However, Western medicine has surpassed it in some well-known areas, such as control of infection, vaccine prevention of disease, treatment of acute illnesses such as heart attacks, and surgical emergencies.

A basic tenet of Chinese medicine is that good health requires that you remain in harmony with the world around you at all stages of life. The further belief is that your body is divided into five energy centers, controlled by five organs: kidneys, lungs, liver, heart, and spleen. In classical theory, a life force, called qi (pronounced "chee"), flows from one control center to the next, in twelve channels. The channels are like meridians that intersect to form a grid or meshlike pattern all over your body. More recent theory is that fifty-nine energy channels exist (Fugh-Berman 1997). Each channel has its own distinct pulse, which can be monitored to assess health status. If the flow of qi is too much or too little in any channel, an imbalance is created in the network, which in turn increases your risk of disease. A finite amount of qi exists in your body. It can be depleted by various problems in life, but qi can also be restored by the use of herbs, diet, acupuncture, and relaxation techniques. In addition to qi, there are two other major components of living organisms: blood and moisture. In order to determine the cause of illness, a TCM practitioner looks for imbalances in moisture/dryness, cold/heat, and excess/deficiency of the three main components (qi, blood, and moisture) in each of the five organ networks (kidneys, lungs, liver, heart, and spleen). Treatment utilizes herbs, acupuncture, acupressure, and physical exercises such as t'ai chi and qidong to promote health.

The yin and yang relationship is another Chinese concept fundamental to understanding energy balance. Yin and yang are opposite but balancing energies that are present in your body and, for that matter, throughout the universe. If one is at a low level, the other fills in the void and reestablishes the balance by becoming high. Yin is feminine, considered as representing things that are cold, dark, still, and heavy. Yang is masculine, and it is associated with things that are hot, bright, mobile, and lightweight. A fever is yang, and a chill is yin. Low energy is yin, and hyperactivity is yang.

Your uterus and ovaries are in the energy sphere of your kidneys. Hormone deficiency problems are considered a kidney deficiency in yin energy. Since qi flows from your kidneys to your liver, you also get a liver-yin deficiency. Now you have a yang excess in both energy centers as opposing balance is restored. A yang excess makes hot things—like hot flashes—happen. Yin deficiency causes insomnia and poor sleep. The liver qi is associated with anger, so a yang excess here causes rising emotions and irritability. Anger and irritability in turn cause stagnation of liver qi, which results in distention and bloating (Bienfield 1991). Are any of these symptoms starting to sound familiar?

Chinese Herbal Medicines

Once your energy imbalance has been diagnosed, treatment may take a variety of forms. Chinese herbal treatments are usually a mixture of plant, mineral, and animal extracts, even though they are all called herbs. A tea is brewed or a liquid extract is prepared as an oral tonic. The preparations are directed at a specific deficiency that is producing specific symptoms. The herb *Rehmannia glutinosa* is the main yin tonic. Other herbs are added to it to increase its potency or decrease side effects (Bienfield 1991). With a variety of formulations, hot flashes with night sweats, irritability, and headaches may all be treated. If a yang deficiency is perceived to be the problem, dodder is added to Rehmannia to treat a diminished libido. Insomnia, heart palpitations, and nervousness are thought to be from altered flow of qi between the heart and kidneys, so a Rehmannia preparation called Emperor Tea is used to treat it. As you can imagine, with hundreds of herbs available there are many, many more combinations of herbs for other specific situations. If you decide to use herbs, do it on the advice and under the supervision of an experienced herbalist. There are no data available as to whether you will have less cardiovascular disease or osteoporosis as a result of using herbal treatment for perimenopausal symptoms.

A license is not required to practice Chinese herbal medicine. Therefore it is appropriate to ask practitioners about their training, and where they went to school, and to request references from prior patients. Practitioners should also be members of local and national Chinese acupuncture professional associations. See the Appendix for information resources on Chinese medicine.

Acupuncture and Acupressure

Intersections of the energy channels near your skin surface form the basis for acupuncture treatment. Originally, about 365 acupuncture points were recognized, but now there are over 2,000 (Fugh-Berman 1997). Acupuncture involves the insertion of tiny needles into specific exterior body locations for therapeutic purposes. Selection of the appropriate point is important, of course; but so is the angle and depth of insertion. Differences in angle and depth at the same acupoint can cause opposite effects. The needle is sometimes twirled to maximize the effect being sought.

At the sites where these meridians cross one another, the flow of qi can be enhanced, diminished, or redirected by the insertion of acupuncture needles. Acupuncture points have been shown to have differing electrical resistance. The needles stimulate electrical impulses, causing release of neurotransmitters, which in turn raise the endorphin levels in your brain as well as peripherally in your tissues. Endorphins are your own internal pain relievers. They are opiumlike chemicals that can produce sedation and a sense of well-being. (The "high" you feel after vigorous exercise results from endorphins.) Changing the flow of qi can aid a faltering organ system. Acupressure techniques, also known as shiatsu, tsubo, and jin shin jyutsu, are a means of using massage at known locations to accomplish the same results as acupuncture. Some practitioners also use electrical stimulation at acupuncture points.

Acupuncture and acupressure are primarily directed at symptoms. Relief from symptoms is widely reported by both patients and practitioners. Hundreds of studies of acupoint stimulation have been done, but generally they suffer from inadequate description of study design, or poor controls, are too small, or are scientifically inadequate in other ways. Nevertheless, acupuncture and acupressure have been variably successful in treating a variety of symptoms such as hot flashes (Wynon 1995), low back pain (Coan 1980), migraines but not tension headaches (Vincent 1989; Vincent 1990), nausea and vomiting due to morning sickness (De Aloysio 1992), postsurgical nausea (Barsoum 1990), chemotherapy nausea (Yang 1993), and motion sickness (Warwick-Evans 1991). It has also been helpful in substance abuse detoxification (Brewington 1994), stroke rehabilitation (Hu 1993), and enhancement of athletic performance (Ehrlich 1992). Acupuncture at specific points on the ear contributes to appetite suppression and weight loss (Integrative Medicine 2000).

When properly performed, acupuncture is quite safe, but it is capable of inflicting serious trauma (such as collapsed lung, damaged blood vessels, or cardiac compression) if performed by inexperienced or poorly trained practitioners. If acupuncture is licensed in your state, you can locate a practitioner in the yellow pages. In states where licensing is not required, be sure to look for acupuncturists who are certified by a national board and have "Dipl Ac" (Diplomate of Acupuncture) after their names. See the Appendix for more information resources.

Homeopathy

Samuel Hahnemann, a German physician and chemist, founded the medical discipline called homeopathy in the late 1700s. Its premise is that the mind and body are inseparable and mutually dependent. Homeopathy involves administration of minute doses of substances that in a healthy person are capable of producing symptoms like those of the condition to be treated. Symptoms are regarded as a signal that something has changed and that the mind/body is trying to heal itself. For example, hot flashes are a symptom of hormone depletion, fever is a symptom of infection, and a mood change is a response to an external or internal stress. In homeopathy, symptoms are regarded as more important than the disease process that may be producing them. For this reason, homeopathy is not used for disease prevention.

The goal of traditional Western medicine is to identify and eliminate the cause of illness. Chinese medicine seeks to strengthen the body's ability to deal with disease by harmonizing its energy forces. Homeopathy tries to provoke the body to strengthen its vital forces and heal itself.

"Like is cured by like" is the basic tenet of homeopathic treatment. If you are having adverse symptoms produced by a toxic substance, the cure results from using an extreme dilution of that same offending substance. Homeopaths call this potentization by dilution or succussion. The theory is that these minuscule doses will stimulate your body to marshal its defense mechanisms and attack the source of your symptoms. Some of the remedies are so diluted that not even a single molecule of the original substance remains. Homeopaths believe that even if no molecules remain from the original substance, a message or "ghost" is imprinted on the diluting liquid. Even when laboratory analysis cannot detect the "ghost," it is claimed that its presence is proven by the response of the person who takes the remedy (Fugh-Berman 1997). Homeopaths remind critics that just because you don't know how something works doesn't mean it doesn't work.

Homeopathic remedies typically cause an initial exaggeration of symptoms. With continued use in progressively increasing doses, however, your body eventually overcomes the toxic effect, and health is restored. Allergists use a similar principle in desensitizing you to things like pollens and bee stings. Because of the extremely small amounts used, the substance prescribed is not regarded as having cured you. Rather, your improvement is believed to have come from your mind/body being stimulated to heal itself.

Homeopathic practitioners are interested in all aspects of your life: age, occupation, general health, diet, moods, lifestyle habits, relationships, and other external and internal factors. The homeopath integrates this information with your original complaint and selects a remedy. All the substances used occur naturally in plants or animals. Sometimes, two or three attempts are needed before the right remedy is found. Homeopaths emphasize that you must be committed to this mode of treatment to achieve success; homeopathic healing is a process, not just an office visit and a prescription. Typical homeopathic thinking is that nothing is incurable; it is simply a matter of selecting the right remedy. No specific training is required to prescribe homeopathic remedies, but most practitioners are licensed health-care providers such as nurses, physicians, and acupuncturists.

Homeopathic remedies are sold over the counter at health stores and supermarkets, but since selection of a remedy is so highly individualized, these preparations are likely a waste of your money. As with traditional Chinese medicine, your hormone deficiency symptoms may be relieved with homeopathy, but there is as yet no body of scientific evidence that homeopathic remedies will protect you against cardiovascular disease or osteoporosis.

Naturopathy

The philosophy of naturopathy is taken from Hippocrates: "The body heals itself, and the task of the physician is to support this inherent healing potential." There are six basic principles:

- Respect the healing power of nature: the practitioner's responsibility is to remove the impediments to healing and bolster the body's inherent capability to heal itself.

- Treat the whole person: wellness is a result of interactions of physical, mental, emotional, spiritual, genetic, environmental, social, lifestyle, and other factors.

- Do no harm.

- Use the least invasive treatment that will help.

- Identify and treat the cause of illness, meaning not simply causative agents such as bacteria but also factors such as lifestyle, dietary habits, and emotional states.

- Prevention is the best cure.

Naturopaths see their role as educating their patients and encouraging them to take responsibility for themselves. These practitioners use any number of modalities, including clinical nutrition, therapeutic manipulation, massage, herbal medicine, homeopathy, and psychological counseling. In Germany, naturopathic services have been found to be so cost-effective that traditional physicians and pharmacists are required to receive education in naturopathy and botanical medicine (Collinge 1996).

So naturopaths take the best of many disciplines and treat the whole person. They feel there are several important transitions or "gateways" in a woman's life where they can be helpful: puberty, establishing a stable personal relationship, pregnancy and childbirth, and perimenopause/menopause. Any of these transitions can result in great change to a woman's health and personality. If you maintain wellness during these transitions, you will more fully enjoy the next phase.

There are two accredited naturopathic medical schools in the U.S., (Bastyr University in Washington and the National College of Naturopathic Medicine in Oregon) and their graduates are licensed in about a dozen states (Jacobs 1994).

Holistic (Integrative Medicine)

Holism refers to a system of preventive medicine that takes into account the whole individual, the individual's responsibility for personal well-being, and all influences (social, psychological, environmental) that affect health, including nutrition, exercise, and mental relaxation. The basic premise is that all medical disciplines can be integrated and used to complement each other. These include homeopathy, herbal therapy, acupuncture, nutritional therapy, stress management techniques, and conventional medical practices such as X-ray, surgery, laboratory testing, and prescription medicines. Integrative medicine is practiced by licensed medical doctors whose orientation is patient-centered as opposed to disease-centered. Conventional medical practices and techniques are regarded as secondary alternatives and are used only if necessary.

Herbal (Botanical) Treatments

The ads sound great: "Herbal Remedies Can Boost Your Energy, Improve Your Memory, Reduce Stress, and Strengthen Your Immune System." The Dietary Supplement Health and Education Act of 1994 stipulates that herbal preparations may not be marketed by a supplier for the diagnosis, treatment, cure, or prevention of any disease. Since the Federal Drug Administration (FDA) does not have regulatory jurisdiction over botanicals as drugs, herbal remedies have become a major factor in American health care almost overnight. Spared the stringent FDA rules for proving effectiveness and safety, suppliers are free to make controversial claims based on minimal evidence. Sales are doubling every four years (Physicians' Desk Reference for Herbal Medicines 1998). Herbs are moving out of the health food stores into supermarkets and drugstores, accelerating the trend toward self-medication with "natural" supplements. The fact is that many people are using them as drugs, not as dietary supplements. As the use of unfamiliar botanicals spreads, it is increasingly important for health-care professionals and the general public to become familiar with the truly useful preparations as well as the ineffective and dangerous ones.

A common public perception is that herbs cannot cause harm because they are "natural"; but so are many poisons. It is true that herbal preparations are less concentrated than pharmaceutical prescription medications, because most prescription drugs contain but a single active ingredient. The argument is that herbal preparations are buffered by the many other compounds contained in them and are therefore safe. Indeed, a staggering variety of active ingredients may be present in an herb and these can have profound effects, both good and bad. Some herbs produced in areas other than Europe or the United States may contain dangerous levels of lead or other heavy metals, making them toxic and extremely dangerous. Interaction of herbs with other prescription drugs being taken can seriously increase a drug's effect, resulting in overmedication, or block its effect.

A major problem with botanicals is standardization. Many labels say "standardized" and suggested doses are usually specified. The problem is there may be many active ingredients in a single herb, and with no existing legal definition of standardization for botanicals, many dosage suggestions represent guesswork. The techniques for standardizing a botanical active ingredient are new and expensive and if multiple active ingredients exist, standardization is a daunting task. This is further complicated by the fact that not all of the active ingredients may be known; for some herbs no active ingredient has been shown to exist. Since manufacturers are not required to prove either the safety or the effectiveness of botanicals, there is little incentive to adopt the rules governing standardization of drugs. Nevertheless, you are better off if the label bears the words "standardized" or "German standards." (German experience with botanicals is quite extensive.)

If herbs are recommended by your health adviser, be certain to disclose any drugs you are taking. The reverse is also true: Tell any prescribing physician of herbs you are using. You and your health adviser need to know what you are doing if herbs are to make a valuable contribution in preventive health care. Herbs need to be properly identified (mistakes are common), capable of maintaining their potency (many do not), clearly labeled for proper indications and contraindications, and prescribed as well as used in proper doses. Contact this Web site for a government compendium about food supplements: www.nal.usda.gov/fine/IBIDS.

A number of herbs with phytoestrogens are available to treat the symptoms of hormone deficiency. There are two main families: the isoflavone family includes biochanin A, genistein, formononetin, daidzin, daidzein, equol, coumestrol, and prunetin; the lignan family includes matairesinol, secoisolaricresinol, enterolactone, and enterodiol. We realize these names may be unfamiliar to you, but they appear on the package labels, so you should look for them. The estrogenic action of these compounds ranges from one-hundredth to one-thousandth that of native human estradiol. Phytoestrogens are not found just in soy. Indeed, they are found in more than 300 plants, including apples, plums, carrots, oats, potatoes, sunflower seeds, olive oil, and coffee. Herbs of current interest to perimenopausal women include:

- **Ginseng:** Ginseng is a widely advertised herb with estrogenic properties (which are not so widely advertised). Some herbalists combine it with dong quai (see the next item) and use the combination for menstrual disorders, depressed sexual desire, depression, insomnia, nervousness, hot flashes, chronic fatigue, and general old age. One Web site advertises ginseng to treat a dozen different ailments, including the common cold, HIV infection, and Alzheimer's disease. Reliable science about the medicinal benefits of ginseng is lacking, although the chemical properties have been identified. The principle active ingredients are called ginsenosides, and thirteen different types are known. Many other compounds are also present, including sugar, fats, B vitamins, minerals, phytohormones (plant hormones), and volatile oils. A major problem for ginseng is lack of quality control. Of several dozen commercial products tested, 60 percent had very little ginseng and 25 percent had none at all (Wellness Letter 2000. Herb with a thousand faces). At present, there is no consistent scientific evidence to support the use of this herb.

CAUTION! Used in large amounts, ginseng can cause abnormal uterine bleeding, breast soreness, high blood pressure, and ovarian cysts (Scheidermayer 1998; Reichman 1996). Use ginseng with great caution if you have had breast cancer or have high risk factors for endometrial cancer. Large doses over a prolonged period of time provide a significant amount of unopposed estrogen, which carries risks for endometrial cancer (see Chapter 7). Ginseng should not be used with estrogen or corticosteroids (cortisone derivatives) because of the potential additive effects.

- **Dong quai:** The estrogenic potency of dong quai is far less than that used in hormone replacement therapy or birth control pills; if an estrogenic effect is desired, large doses are used. It is used to treat menstrual cramps, menstrual irregularities, and hot flashes. You should avoid it if you have heavy menstrual periods, fibroids, or diarrhea, since it can enhance these problems. The precautions regarding the use of unopposed estrogen apply to treatment with dong quai (see Chapter 6).

- **Ginkgo biloba:** This herb is thought to have antioxidant properties, which protects brain cells from damage by oxygen free radicals. In addition, it improves blood circulation in the brain. Many people take this herb to improve their vigilance, thinking, and memory (Hornig 1998). It isn't widely known, however, that ginkgo has anticlotting effects. It can cause bleeding gums or uterine bleeding, particularly if you are taking aspirin or other anticoagulant medicines, such as warfarin (Coumadin), or other herbs with anticlotting properties, such as ginger, garlic, ginseng, or feverfew (Wellness Letter 2000. Wellness made easy). It may increase migraine headaches. Buy only ginkgo that includes a standardized extract known as EGb761.

• **Black cohosh:** Black cohosh, also known as squaw root, is an herb Native Americans have used traditionally for menstrual cramps. It is thought to have substances that relieve pain and act as sedatives. There is sufficient estrogenic activity to improve hot flashes and diminish vaginal atrophy. The estrogenic activity is even strong enough to lower FSH (follicle stimulating hormone) levels, just as birth control pills do. Black cohosh is also a vasoconstrictor, which accounts in part for the relief it provides from hot flashes. In a double-blind study of hot flash control at Purdue University School of Pharmacy, black cohosh was compared with conjugated estrogen (Premarin) and with a placebo. Black cohosh was found to be superior to both Premarin and the placebo for control of hot flashes and other estrogen deficiency symptoms. Nevertheless, other studies contend that this herb is as yet unproven for general treatment of estrogen deficiency (Baker 1999). Because no studies exist on the risk for endometrial cancer with this herb, it is recommended that it be used not longer than three to six months (Tyler 1997). Remember from Chapter 6 that as little as six months of treatment with unopposed estrogen increases the risk of endometrial cancer fourfold, and the increased risk lingers for several years.

• **St. Johns wort:** This very popular herb is being used for mild depression and depressive moods. Studies show it is equally effective as standard antidepressants, with fewer side effects (Ernst 1995; Philipp 1999). It has at least ten compounds that can have druglike actions. Some of them affect the way the liver metabolizes drugs, resulting in blood levels that are too high or too low. In the elderly, if combined with the antidepressants called MOA inhibitors, or with SSRIs (Prozac, Zoloft, Paxil), St. Johns wort can cause dizziness, confusion, and very high blood pressure. It reduces the effect of blood thinners such as aspirin and warfarin (Coumadin). Interaction with oral contraceptives may cause breakthrough bleeding or reduce their effectiveness in preventing pregnancy (Wellness Letter 2000. Worry wort). In addition, St. Johns wort has an adverse effect on the tumor suppressor gene BRCA1, this effect can increase the risk of breast and ovarian cancer in women who inherit a mutated form of this gene. This herb can cause photosensitivity, meaning bright light may be irritating and that you can get sunburned easily.

• **Red clover:** Although red clover, marketed as Promensil, contains phytoestrogens, when compared to a placebo for control of hot flashes and lowering of cholesterol, there were no significant differences (Baber 1999; Knight 1999). This is because it binds to estrogen and progesterone, reducing their availability to tissues (Zava 1998). Red clover has been shown to be comparable to estrogen in improving arterial compliance, which lowers blood pressure (Nisly 1999). A caution with red clover is that warfarin, a blood thinner, was originally derived from this plant, so there may be a potential for abnormal bleeding problems or stroke.

- **Chasteberry:** Chasteberry gets its name from the belief that the plant would inspire chastity. Monks in ancient Mediterranean cultures would eat it to suppress their sexual desire. It has been used in Europe for many years to treat female reproductive tract disorders such as menstrual abnormalities, premenstrual syndrome, estrogen deficiency complaints (hot flashes), and infertility (Robbers 1999). This implies that it has a strong estrogenic component, which may be why it helps hot flashes. Unopposed estrogen precautions apply.

- **Garlic:** This botanical is promoted for lowering blood pressure and cholesterol. One of its phytonutrient sulfur ingredients, ajoene, acts like a blood thinner to decrease platelet agglutination and therefore the tendency for clot formation. Garlic should be used cautiously by people taking blood-thinning medicines like warfarin or other anticlotting herbs such as ginger, ginkgo, or feverfew. Garlic is being studied for its potential to enhance the immune system and possibly aid in cancer prevention. Odorless garlic and aged garlic have little of the sulfur compounds allin, allicin, scordinin, or ajoene, the most active ingredients.

- **Echinacea:** This herb is taken to boost the body's immune system and its resistance to common winter infections. It can aggravate autoimmune disorders such as rheumatoid arthritis, lupus, AIDS, or multiple sclerosis. People subject to hayfever and allergic skin reactions may have severe allergic reactions. If taken for more than eight weeks, echinacea can be toxic to the liver (Harvard Women's Health Watch 2000). Echinacea in the whole or tincture form may be more effective than in tablets or capsules.

- **Valerian root:** Surveys place valerian root as the tenth most popular herb in the United States (Brevcort 1998). It is a mild and effective sedative and sleep aid that is generally recognized as safe. Different valerian species are not equivalent, so the European variant, *Valeriana officinalis L*, is the type most often used (Hardy 1999). Valerian root should not be used with barbiturates or other sedatives since it can cause excessive sedation.

- **Cooling Herbs:** Some herbs are used alone or in combination to cool the body if you are having hot flashes. These include chickweed, elder flower, and violet. They are said to change the body's thermostat, although very little in the way of scientific study exists.

CAUTION! If you are considering a future pregnancy, it may be important to avoid echinacea, St. Johns wort, saw palmetto, and gingko biloba. Under laboratory conditions, all have been shown to adversely affect sperm and egg cells in hamsters, preventing penetration of the egg by sperm (Ondrizek 1999).

Herbs and surgery don't mix. Gingko biloba, ginseng, garlic, feverfew, and ginger have anticlotting properties that can lead to excessive bleeding. St. Johns wort (an antidepressant) and kava kava (a relaxant) may prolong the sedating effects of anesthesia. The American Society of Anesthesiologists recommends you stop taking all herbs at least two weeks before elective surgery (Women's HealthSource 2000).

For information about dietary supplements and herbal interactions with other drugs, go to http://vm.cfsan.fda.gov/~dms/supplmnt.html.

Homeopathic Remedies for Perimenopausal Symptoms

Earlier in this chapter we described the principles of homeopathy. Let's take a look at what's available for treating the undesirable symptoms of perimenopause.

- **Sepia:** Sepia is derived from the inky secretions of the cuttlefish. It is one of the most commonly used homeopathic remedies for fatigue, irritability, low sex drive, and vaginal dryness (Ullman 1991).

- **Evening primrose oil:** Evening primrose is a roadside weed that particularly favors railroad tracks. The fatty acids of this oil develop a more effective cell membrane for diffusing metabolic products, and this is said to improve function of the brain, adrenal glands, eyes, and reproductive organs (Ullman 1991). This active ingredient is also found in seed oils of corn, wheat germ, sesame, sunflower, and safflower plants. Evening primrose oil is also used to treat menstrual cramps and PMS symptoms. However, several placebo-controlled studies have shown that it has no beneficial effect on PMS (Khoo 1990; Kleijmen 1994). It does not help hot flashes, but because of its weak estrogenic qualities, it may delay the age at which they first appear. Unopposed estrogen precautions are advisable.

- **Lachesis:** This substance is derived, believe it or not, from the poisonous venom of the American bushmaster snake. The venom is highly diluted and has no toxic effects. It is used for hot flashes, palpitations, and headaches. Candidates for treatment with lachesis are characterized as women who are overbearing and demanding and who have fits of rage and strong libidos (Ullman 1991).

- **Pulsatilla:** Pulsatilla comes from the windflower. To homeopaths, the "pulsatilla type" is said to be women who are shy and nonassertive, weep easily, have low energy and low sexual desire, and have hot flashes around the face (Ullman 1991).

- **Nux vomica:** Made from the poison nut, nux vomica helps nausea, backache, disrupted sleep, perfectionistic tendencies, and chronic anger (Ullman 1991).

- **Bioflavonoids:** There are over 400 types of bioflavonoids. They are derived from soybeans, oriental spices, green tea, citrus fruits, and citrus rinds. They are mildly estrogenic, with a chemical structure that resembles estradiol. Women who have a high bioflavonoid intake in their diet have few symptoms of estrogen decline. Japanese women, for example, average about 5,000 milligrams of bioflavonoids daily, compared to the American diet of 800 to 1,000 milligrams (Ojeda 1995).

If you are being treated for estrogen deficiency symptoms with any botanical product, ask the prescribing practitioner if the remedy has estrogenic qualities. You and your health adviser must both have a clear understanding of the adverse effects of treatment with unopposed estrogen if unintended results, such as abnormal bleeding or endometrial cancer are to be avoided.

Areas Where Botanical (Plant) Therapies Must Improve

With the increasing use of botanicals, the general public's interests would be better served if the following could be implemented:

- More good science is needed, meaning randomized, controlled trials. One difficulty in designing trials for botanicals is that study results are hampered by the inability to conduct trials of "single" therapies. By their nature, herbs are complex, containing many nutritional and pharmacological compounds, which are often unpredictable.

- Standardization of product preparation by industry suppliers must improve. It is inadequate because the botanical product industry is unregulated. In a $30 billion-per-year market, shortcuts are inevitable. At present, it is probably best to buy standardized botanicals from German companies; they are more closely regulated and therefore more reliable.

- Special problems with herbs are related to the soil type and other conditions in which they grow, which plant parts are used, and processing methods. Reliable data on related dangers must be gathered and analyzed.

- The public belief that "If it is natural, it is safe" is often untrue and therefore unsafe, so responsible public education by the industry and health practitioners is essential.

- Traditional and integrative health practitioners must acknowledge each other. Mutual mistrust results in patients' becoming reluctant to inform their health adviser of ongoing therapy by another practitioner of a different discipline. This leads to unintended interactions between therapies.

Dietary Alternatives for Diminishing Hot Flashes

Some foods aggravate hot flashes and others diminish them. Consumption of hot foods and drinks, alcohol, and spicy foods should all be minimized to avoid food-related hot flashes. To lessen hot flashes, you can add more phytoestrogens to your diet. Japanese women have few complaints of hot flashes (only 1 percent), so their diet was studied by Finnish researchers in 1988. The typical Japanese diet is high in soybean products, which contain phytoestrogens. Because of their dietary habits, the women studied had 1000 times more phytoestrogens in their urine than women on a Western diet (Aldercreutz 1991).

The primary phytoestrogens in soybeans are proteins called genistein, daidzein, matairesinol, and secoisolaricresinol. The Finnish study of soy protein showed that taking 25 to 50 grams daily (instead of animal protein) lowers cholesterol, raises HDL, and lowers LDL in both women and men. There is speculation that genistein may also have a positive influence on a woman's risk for breast cancer (Shao 1998). The Japanese diet includes about 20 grams of soy foods per day (Aldercreutz 1991). One study showed that half a cup of tofu, tempeh, or cooked soybeans or one cup of soy milk daily will supply 34 milligrams of soy protein (Washburn 1999). More than 300 other food plants also contain phytoestrogens, although few have quite the estrogen benefit you can get from soybeans.

Mind/Body Medicine

The thread running through most of the integrative treatment disciplines we've discussed is what is often called mind/body medicine. Dr. Deepak Chopra, in his book *Quantum Healing: Exploring the Frontiers of Mind/Body Medicine*, describes a nonorthodox and non-Western mind/body approach to healing. The premise of quantum healing is that in each of us is a package of intelligence, which happens to be contained in a body. All cells of the body use neurotransmitters to stay in constant communication with each other. (Hormones are a good example of this.) Everything is under the control of the intelligence pool, the mind. In this sense, mind means more than just the brain and the nervous system. It includes the intelligence that resides in each of the trillions of cells of the entire body. If something goes wrong, such as a certain cell turning into a rogue cancer cell, the intelligence network is immediately aware of it, and healing is set in motion. According to Chopra, we may cure ourselves of cancer hundreds of times during a lifetime this way. Sometimes, though, the internal healing commands become overwhelmed by certain illnesses, such as cancer or infection, and the battle is lost. The challenge is to learn how to tap into this intelligence deliberately and consciously, rather than leaving it to work at the subconscious level, where it normally operates. The mind could turn out to be a very efficient healer, given its huge database of information and its capacity to fashion defenses to disease. This approach to medicine may, in time, make traditional and current integrative medical strategies seem crude.

Mind/body medicine is being seriously explored by many talented people who have achieved remarkable success in improving a broad variety of ailments. Examples of currently used mind/body techniques are transcendental meditation, biofeedback, visualization/guided imagery, hypnotherapy, massage therapy and bodywork, spiritual healing, yoga, and behavior modification. (We take a look at some of these in Chapter 11.) As with most medical regimens, universal success is difficult to achieve. Nevertheless, mind/body medicine is now a field of endeavor rather than a concept. As application of these techniques improves, future successes may be astonishing.

Summary

Traditional versus integrative, orthodox versus nonorthodox, mainstream versus fringe, Western versus Eastern. These are all terms tossed about by the proponents of each of these schools of thought. Whether or not you believe in the integrative therapies discussed in this chapter, and others we didn't discuss, their safety and effectiveness need to be studied as an issue of public health—because they are being used by an increasingly large segment of the population. Consumers deserve this information. Meanwhile, rather than choosing one of these categories of care over the others, it makes sense to seek a middle ground. All of these approaches to treatment have much to offer toward the goal of wellness, and to each other. It also makes sense to seek a total approach to your health care, integrating techniques of traditional Western medicine with those of integrative medicine and other ancient healing approaches.

Your body is an exquisitely sensitive machine that demands balance to function properly and maintain wellness. The balance can be achieved in different ways and with different tools that traditional and integrative medicine can each supply.

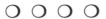

9

Wellness for a Change: Good Nutrition and Exercise

Wellness is much more than the absence of disease. Wellness also means feeling vigorous, alert, robust, fresh as a daisy, and having the sense that you are in control of your body and your life. If you want to achieve and maintain wellness, you must assume the helm, guiding your lifestyle in ways that will ensure your goal. Wellness is also more than being conscientious about seeking care when you get sick. Contemporary health care is generally thought of as a problem-solving system: You go along day to day until you get sick, and then you rely upon your doctor to make it all better. You may get well from your disease this way, but your lifestyle may have been the cause of your illness. Antibiotics and a cough medicine will clear up your bronchitis, for example, but smoking may be the underlying reason you are susceptible to it. Physical therapy and an anti-inflammatory agent may help your backache, but a sedentary lifestyle and being overweight may be causing it.

Maintaining wellness involves becoming focused not just on the symptom that distresses you, but also on the larger issues that influence your overall health. These issues include adequate nutrition, a balanced diet, and exercise. These are the topics of this chapter. Weight control, limitation of destructive lifestyle habits, and management of stress are also involved in wellness. They arc the topics of Chapters 10 and 11. Our goal is to show you how you can utilize these elements, how they are interrelated, and why they are necessary to your achieving wellness. If you have been thinking about losing weight, getting in shape, quitting smoking, and eliminating some other destructive lifestyle habits, your perimenopausal years represent an excellent time to start making these changes. This chapter and the next two are not just about making you live longer, but about your living well while you do it.

Nutrition

Protein, carbohydrate, and fat are the three principal categories of food. Water can be considered a fourth category. Each of these types of food, called macronutrients, contains varying amounts of vitamins and minerals, and each serves an important role in a balanced diet. Over the years, nutritionists and other food scientists have studied these ingredients and their various effects on our bodies. As a result, they have been able to make recommendations for the most healthful combination of protein, carbohydrate, and fat in the diet. First, let's consider the individual nutritional value of proteins, carbohydrates, fats, minerals, and vitamins. Then we'll put them together in a nutritional plan.

Protein

Your body makes protein by assembling amino acids into chains. There are twenty-two known amino acids, and your body can make all but nine of them. These nine are known as essential amino acids, and they must be supplied by your food intake. A complete protein is one that supplies all nine essential amino acids. Meat and dairy products are complete proteins, but fruits and vegetables are not.

Protein is second only to water as the most abundant substance in your body. It forms the basic structure of all parts of your body, including your bones. Muscle is mostly protein. Hormones, enzymes, and antibodies are all made from protein. When you are growing tissue or repairing it, protein is the essential ingredient. Protein in your body is also an energy source; but your body doesn't use it for this purpose as much as it uses carbohydrate and fat, unless your body is deficient in them. (This is what happens during starvation.)

While most nutritionists agree that only 30 percent of your diet should be protein, most Americans consume much more than that. If your protein intake is more than 50 percent above daily needs, you lose calcium in your urine (Notelovitz 1993). And guess where the calcium comes from: your bones. This loss is not good for prevention of osteoporosis. Another risk is that the typical American diet derives most of its protein from meat and dairy products, which are high in fat. High fat intake increases your risk for cardiovascular disease, obesity, and certain cancers. So not enough protein is bad, too much is bad, and just right is just right. To see where you stand in protein consumption, calculate how much protein you need each day, at 0.42 grams per pound of your body weight. Then look over Table 9.1 for a list of commonly consumed protein foods to get a rough estimate of whether you meet the recommended intake. If you are a vigorously active woman (daily aerobics, proficient athlete), a calculation using 0.5 to 1.0 grams per pound would be more appropriate.

Table 9.1. Daily Protein Needs for Women		
Formula using weight in pounds: _____lbs x 0.42 = _____grams per day		
Food Source	**Serving**	**Protein in Grams**
Chicken	4 oz	36
Beef	4 oz	32
Fish	4 oz	28
Wheat cereal with milk	1 cup	28
Beans with rice	1 cup	17
Eggs	2	14
Cottage cheese	½ cup	14
Milk	1 cup	9
Cheddar cheese	1 oz	7
Beans	½ cup	7
Pasta	1 cup	5
Potato	1 medium	5
Whole wheat bread	1 slice	3

Adapted from: Ojeda 1995.

Carbohydrates—Pure-Burning Fuel

Carbohydrates consist of sugars, starches, and fiber. They are your primary energy source, with assists as needed from fat and protein. From your brain cells to your muscle cells, carbohydrates are the first thing your cells go for when they want to get something done that requires energy. Carbohydrates circulate in your blood as glucose, and this is your body's first choice when it comes to energy needs. Blood glucose can get used up quickly, though, so your liver converts some of it into a substance called glycogen and stores it for stoking the fire when necessary. If you have been really "carbing out," however, carbohydrates are converted to fat by insulin and tucked away in places that are not always inconspicuous.

Your body can make carbohydrate from components of protein and fat, so there aren't any essential carbohydrates (that is, carbohydrates you can only obtain through diet). The three types of carbohydrates are worth discussing, though, because they have differing effects on your body and your health: simple sugars and refined carbohydrates; complex carbohydrates; and fiber.

Simple Sugars and Refined Carbohydrates

Simple sugars appear naturally in honey, fruits, and unrefined sugar (sweets). They are absorbed directly into your bloodstream without any significant digestive alteration, which is why you get such a quick energy surge from them. Refined carbohydrate foods are those made from white flour, refined sugar, and white rice. They are low in vitamins and minerals, and they don't contain fiber. (We'll talk more about fiber in a moment.) Sugar is a great source of instant energy, but it is also a source of quick fatigue. When you load up on sugar, your blood glucose rises rapidly. This causes your pancreas to pour out insulin to get your blood glucose under control. Insulin production often overshoots the mark in reducing your blood sugar, and you end up with too little glucose. Now you feel tired and weak again, so another shot of the sugar source seems irresistible.

Over time high blood glucose levels may require higher than usual insulin levels to control them. This is called insulin resistance. With larger amounts of insulin circulating to stanch the glucose tide, more glucose is converted to fat and stored. Obesity results, which in itself increases the risk of diabetes. But too much insulin in your bloodstream over the years is also closely related to hardening of the arteries, high blood pressure, heart attacks, strokes, and accelerated aging of all your body's cells. Insulin resistance increases with aging, so moderation in your use of sweets during perimenopause is prudent.

Complex Carbohydrates and Their Fabulous Fiber

Carbohydrates that need to be digested to be absorbed are called complex (rather than simple) carbohydrates. Complex carbohydrates are chiefly starches found in potatoes, rice, pasta, corn, grains, and beans (such as lima, navy, and kidney beans), but also in fruits and vegetables. When you eat them in an unrefined or unprocessed state, they provide abundant vitamins, minerals, and especially fiber. Complex carbohydrates should constitute 40 to 55 percent of your daily caloric intake (Bland 1999; Daoust 1996), but in the typical American diet, this is far from the case.

Dietary fiber is the indigestible part of these foods. It is found in the plant cell walls, and it does not become absorbed into the bloodstream. There are two types:

- **Water soluble fiber:** This type of fiber is found in whole grains, oat-bran cereals, beans, and barley, as well as in many fruits and vegetables. Soluble fiber aids in lowering cholesterol, triglycerides, and low-density lipoproteins (LDL).

- **Insoluble fiber:** Insoluble fiber is predominantly found in whole-wheat products, wheat bran, corn and rice bran, and the skins of fruits and vegetables. This is the fiber that softens stools and prevents constipation. Consumption of insoluble fiber bulk also results in a form of intestinal calisthenics, keeping the muscles of your gastroin-testinal tract toned.

Nutritionists recommend 25 to 30 grams of fiber each day, which is in stark contrast to the average fiber-depleted American diet of 10 to 15 grams. There are numerous benefits to an adequate fiber intake:

- **Decreasing the risk of coronary heart disease:** An analysis of the Harvard Nurses' Health Study found that higher intake of dietary fiber significantly reduces the risk of heart disease. Women who consumed an average of 22.9 grams of fiber each day had a 27 percent lower risk of developing heart disease than those who ate an average of 11.5 grams. Only whole-grain cereal fiber, but not fiber from fruits or vegetables, was protective. It takes five or more cereal breakfasts per week to attain this level of consumption. Although cereal fiber was not shown to have a substantial beneficial effect on cholesterol, it does decrease insulin resistance and reduces triglycerides. Good sources of cereal fiber are oat bran, oatmeal, and cold breakfast cereals (Wolk 1999). Fiber is only one beneficial component of whole grains. A 1999 report from the Nurses' Health Study found that whole grains in breakfast cereal, brown rice, oatmeal, and bran reduce heart disease risk to an extent that can't be explained by fiber content alone. Women who ate an average of 2.5 servings of whole grains per day had 30 percent lower risk than those who had only 0.13 servings. A serving is one slice of bread, one ounce of ready-to-eat cereal, or a quarter-cup of cooked cereal, rice, or pasta (Harvard Heart Letter 2000).

- **Controlling moods:** Complex carbohydrates may reduce some of the negative moods associated with PMS. Carbohydrates raise the brain level of the amino acid called tryptophan, which is converted to the neurotransmitter called serotonin. Serotonin influences sleep patterns, pain perception, and hormone secretion and has an overall calming effect. Inadequate serotonin levels are associated with depression. So start your PMS day with a large bowl of a high-carbohydrate cereal, even if you hate the cereal, hate the bowl, hate the spoon, and hate the skim milk you pour over it. Chances are good you'll feel better within an hour or so.

- **Decreasing the risk of diabetes:** Fiber takes longer to be broken down than other food components, so it slows the absorption of glucose into your bloodstream. This aids in blood sugar control, and decreases the likelihood of glucose being stored as fat. It also decreases your risk of developing diabetes and helps blood sugar regulation in those who are already diabetic.

- **Decreasing cancer risks:** As we pointed out in Chapter 6, a high-fiber diet has been associated with decreased incidence of colon cancer, although a recent study has cast doubt on this benefit. It may lower the incidence of other cancers as well.

- **Controlling weight:** High-fiber foods are lower in calories and fat than low-fiber foods. In addition, digestion of fiber is slow, which contributes to your feeling fuller longer.

- **Controlling intestinal problems:** Fiber prevents constipation because it absorbs water, creating a softer stool. (Stool softeners like Metamucil are powdered fiber.) Soft stools from an adequate fiber diet prevent the formation of diverticuli, which are little outpouchings from the wall of the colon. These can become inflamed and painful, causing a condition called diverticulitis.

When you increase your fiber intake, do it gradually. A big jump can result in gas and bloating. Be sure to drink plenty of water (six to eight cups a day) with your increased fiber diet. (There will be more bulk in your intestine; without water accompanying it, you can become constipated.) Also be aware that fiber can prevent or decrease the absorption of calcium and iron. If you are using these supplements, do not take them at the same time as a high-fiber meal. Table 9.2 lists the fiber content of common foods. When you select breads and cereals, stick to whole-grain products. Refining of these grains removes 60 to 90 percent of the vitamins, minerals, and fiber (Willett 1994).

Table 9.2. Fiber Content of Various Foods		
Type of Food	**Serving**	**Fiber in Grams**
Cereals		
All Bran with extra fiber	½ cup	14.0
All Bran	½ cup	12.9
100% Bran	½ cup	10.0
Raisin Bran	¾ cup	5.3
40% Bran Flakes	½ cup	4.3
Oat bran, cooked	¾ cup	4.0
Oat bran cereal, cold	¾ cup	2.9
Corn flakes	¾ cup	2.1
Special K	¾ cup	1.2
Cream of Wheat	¾ cup	0.5
Rice Krispies	¾ cup	0
Breads		
Pita bread, whole wheat	1.5" pocket	4.4
Pumpernickel	1 slice	2.7

Whole wheat	1 slice	1.5
Bagel, plain	1	1.4
White bread, French, Italian	1 slice	0.6
Croissant	1	0

Legumes (Beans & Peas)

Black-eyed peas, cooked	¾ cup	12.3
Kidney or pinto beans, cooked	¾ cup	14.0
Kidney beans, canned	¾ cup	4.7
Lima beans, cooked	½ cup	3.5
Lentils, cooked	½ cup	5.2
Split peas, cooked	½ cup	3.1
Peas, canned	½ cup	2.8

Fruits

Apple, large, with skin	1	4.7
Apricots, dried	10	3.6
Orange	1 medium	3.0
Pear, with skin	1 small	2.9
Peach, with skin	1 medium	2.0
Prune, dried	3 medium	1.7
Rasberries, fresh	½ cup	1.7
Grapefruit, medium	½	1.4
Pineapple, canned	½ cup	1.2
Banana, medium	1	0.7
Raisins	2 tbsp	0.4
Grapes, green, fresh	½ cup	0.4

Vegetables

Peas, green, cooked	½ cup	4.3
Potato, baked + skin	1 medium	4.2
Brussels sprouts, cooked	½ cup	3.8
Corn, whole, cooked	½ cup	3.0
Carrots, raw	1 medium	2.3
Broccoli, cooked	½ cup	1.5
Spinach, raw	1 cup	1.4
Tomato, cooked	½ cup	1.0
Lettuce, iceberg	1 cup	0.6

Adapted from: Ojeda 1995; Cutler 1992

Glycemic Index for Foods

Carbohydrates differ in how fast they get into your bloodstream as glucose. Simple carbohydrates leap into your blood because they do not require significant digestive action by your intestine. On the other hand, complex carbohydrates, especially if laden with fiber, take longer. But that's not the end of the story. Some complex carbs are quicker than others to enter your blood. Those that enter the blood quickly can create a high blood glucose level, called hyperglycemia. The glycemic index is a method of rating the speed of this transition from consumption to blood entry (Wolever 1997). Glucose and white bread are the benchmarks, and are rated at 100. All other foods are compared to them. The higher the glycemic index number for a food, the faster it raises your blood sugar. And conversely, the lower the glycemic index, the slower your blood sugar will rise.

The obvious importance of rating foods with a glycemic index is to give you an idea of how severely your insulin levels will respond to handle the glucose load created. The more insulin you have circulating in your blood, the greater its adverse influence on your long-term health. Rating a food for its glycemic index is a rather complex process. It depends on the type of sugar in the food, the amount of fiber (the most important glycemic influence), amount of protein and fat, and the method of cooking or processing the food. Not all foods have been rated, but you can get a handle on unrated foods: The more fiber, protein, or fat, the lower its glycemic index. High glycemic foods are typically high in refined sugars or flours and/or are highly processed. Look over Table 9.3 for the glycemic index of some common foods. Notice especially how processing and cooking influence glycemic index ratings.

The glycemic index is a good research tool, but it is difficult to put into practice in planning a diet, because a food's score changes according to what foods are eaten with it, and other characteristics such as ripeness and food preparation. Nevertheless, an awareness of a given food's glycemic rating can be a general guideline in selection.

Table 9.3.   Glycemic Index (GI) of Common Foods

Food	GI		
Fruits		Grapes	45
Apple	49	Orange	59
Apple juice (unfiltered)	55	Orange juice	71
Apricot	73	Peach	25
Banana	82	Pear	34
Cherries	23	Plum	25
Dates	95	Prunes	52
Grapefruit	26	Raisins	93

Cereals

All-Bran	74
Cornflakes	121
Oat bran	85
Oatmeal (instant)	89
Oatmeal (slow-cooked)	49
Puffed rice	132
Puffed wheat	110
Shredded wheat	97

Dairy Products

Custard	59
Ice Cream (full-fat)	59
Ice Cream (fat-free)	90+
Milk (whole)	44
Milk (skim)	46
Yogurt (plain, full-fat)	52
Yogurt (fruit & sugar)	90+
Yogurt (fruit & artificial sugar)	63
Yogurt (frozen, fat-free)	90+

Sugars

Glucose	100
Fructose	26
Honey	126
Lactose	57
Maltose	150

Snack Foods

Corn Chips	99
Potato Chips	77
Rice Cakes	132

Grains

Bread (white)	100
Bread (wheat)	100
Bread (rye, pumpernickel)	68
Baguette (French bread)	131
Buckwheat	78
Macaroni (boiled 5 min)	66
Rice (brown or white)	81
Rice (instant, boiled 1 min)	65
Rice (instant, boiled 6 min)	121
Rice (polished, boiled 5 min)	58
Rice (polished, boiled 10-25 min)	83
Rye crisp crackers	45
Spaghetti (white, boiled 15 min)	67
Spaghetti (white, boiled 5 min)	45
Spaghetti (brown, boiled 15 min)	61
Pasta (protein-enriched)	38
White flour	100
Whole meal	100

Vegetables and Legumes*

Artichoke (cooked)	25
Asparagus	22
Baked Beans	70
Beets	68
Broccoli (raw)	23
Brussels sprouts (raw)	23
Carrots	92
Cauliflower (raw)	21
Corn (sweet)	76
Chick peas	64
Kidney beans (canned)	71
Kidney beans (dried)	43
Lentils (green, dried)	36
Lentils (green, canned)	74
Lima beans	46
Peas (green, dried)	50
Peas (frozen)	65
Potato (mashed)	117
Potato (new, white, boiled)	80
Potato (new, red, boiled)	70
Potato (russet, baked)	116
Soy beans (canned)	22
Soy beans (dried)	20
Yam	74

Nuts**

Almonds	15
Peanuts	15
Walnuts	15

---

*   Generally low GI because of fiber   **   Low GI from high fat and protein

The Skinny on Fat

Your body needs fat, but there's a limit. Fat is a very concentrated source of energy; it contains nine calories per gram, as compared to four calories per gram in both proteins and carbohydrates. Fat stores represent a valuable portable warehouse for energy and water to which your body can turn when your metabolic machine is running a little short. Fat insulates your body from cold and cushions vital organs from injury. Dietary fat aids in the absorption of the fat soluble vitamins A, D, E, and K. Fat makes your food taste good. Because it digests more slowly than other foods, fat also gives you that pleasant feeling of fullness after a meal. That was the good news. And now, the rest of the story.

Americans consume about 34 percent of their daily calories from dietary fat (McDowell 1994). Some have estimated the level to be as high as 40 percent. The number should actually be about 25 to 30 percent to meet your body's needs and maintain health. The American fat epidemic makes the news often enough, and maybe you have already cut back on your use of butter, and started to trim the fat off your meat and drink low-fat milk. If so, you are heading in the right direction; but remember that there are fats in many everyday foods. You probably already know that items like cheesecake, potato chips, and nuts are high in both calories and fat. Also watch out for fast foods and TV dinners, cream soups, lunch meats, avocado, cheese, and desserts like donuts and chocolate. These foods are high in calories, too, which end up as reserve stores of fat if they exceed your body's needs.

Dietary fat is more readily converted to body fat than either carbohydrates or proteins, so it gets distributed to places you don't want it, like your hips and thighs and around your middle. As we described in Chapter 7, perimenopausal women tend to have pear-shaped bodies. Postmenopausal women accumulate fat about the abdomen, as men do (the apple shape). Not only does a high-fat diet contribute to obesity, it raises your risk of cardiovascular disease, high blood pressure, diabetes, and certain cancers.

What about Cholesterol?

Cholesterol isn't really a fat. It is a waxy substance, called a lipid, found in animal foods and dairy products. We talked about cholesterol in Chapter 4, and about the role it plays in cardiovascular disease. Cholesterol itself, however, is not harmful; indeed it is vital to your existence. Cholesterol helps build cell membranes (all three trillion of them). It is also the basic building block for hormones. Your body uses it to make vitamin D. Cholesterol also forms a protective sheath around nerves, which facilitates transmission of impulses, and it serves many, many other important biologic functions. Your body can manufacture all the cholesterol it needs, but you add to the supply from the foods you eat, and there's the rub: If your cholesterol intake is too high, your blood level of cholesterol rises. Then you start parking the excess

Table 9.4. Calories, Fat, and Cholesterol in Foods

Food	Serving	Calories	Fat (grams)	Cholesterol (mgs)
Candy				
Milk chocolate bar	1 oz	150	9.2	5
Cheese				
Cheddar	1 oz	112	9.1	30
Cottage, 2% fat	½ cup	100	2.2	9
Monterey jack	1 oz	105	8.5	30
Swiss, pasteurized	1 oz	95	7.1	26
Cheese Whiz spread	1 oz	80	6.0	15
Condiments				
Mayonnaise	1 tbsp	100	11.0	5
Diet mayonnaise	1 tbsp	45	5.0	5
Miracle Whip	1 tbsp	70	7.0	5
Dairy Products				
Whole milk	1 cup	150	8.1	34
Low-fat milk	1 cup	122	4.7	20
Skim milk	1 cup	89	0.4	5
Yogurt, nonfat	1 cup	127	0.4	4
Yogurt, whole milk	1 cup	141	7.7	30
Egg, whole	1 med	78	5.5	250
Egg yolk	1 med	59	5.2	250
Egg Beaters	¼ cup	25	0	0
Fats & Oils				
Butter	1 tbsp	108	12.2	36
Margarine	1 tbsp	108	12.0	0
Vegetable oil	1 tbsp	120	13.5	0
Butter Buds	1 oz	12	0	0
Molly McButter	1 tsp	5	0	0
Seafood				
Crab, king	3½ oz	93	1.9	60
Fish sticks, frozen	3½ oz	176	8.9	70
Lobster	3½ oz	91	1.9	100
Mackerel	3½ oz	191	12.2	95
Oysters	3½ oz	66	1.8	50
Salmon	3½ oz	182	7.4	47

Continued on the following page

				Table 9.4. cont.
Food	Serving	Calories	Fat (grams)	Cholesterol (mgs)
Seafood (cont.)				
Sardines, canned in oil	3½ oz	311	24.4	120
Shrimp	3½ oz	91	0.8	100
Tuna, canned in oil	3½ oz	197	8.2	63
Tuna, canned in water	3½ oz	127	0.8	63
Breads				
English muffin	1	133	1.0	0
Pita, pocket	1	145	1.0	0
White	1 slice	68	0.8	0
Whole wheat	1 slice	61	0.8	0
Meats				
Beef, trimmed, cooked	3 oz	192	9.4	73
Ground beef, 27% fat	3 oz	251	16.9	86
Ground beef, 10% fat	3 oz	213	11.9	86
Lamb chop	3 oz	188	8.9	82
Pork chop	3 oz	219	12.7	80
Spareribs	3 oz	338	25.8	103
Bacon	1 slice	40	3.0	5
Ham, 3% fat	3 oz	120	6.0	45
Chicken, light, no skin	3 oz	153	4.2	66
Chicken, with skin	3 oz	210	12.6	75
Turkey, light, no skin	3 oz	153	4.2	66
Turkey, with skin	3 oz	210	12.6	75
Veal, lean only	3 oz	120	2.7	84
Beef liver	3½ oz	140	4.7	300
Beef brain	3½ oz	106	7.3	2100
Bologna	1 oz	88	8.1	15+
Canadian bacon	1 oz	45	2.0	13
Liverwurst	1 oz	139	9.1	35
Salami	1 oz	112	9.8	22
Hot dog	1.6 oz	142	13.5	23
Salad Dressing				
Blue Cheese	1 tbsp	71	7.3	4–10
Russian	1 tbsp	74	7.6	7–10
French	1 tbsp	66	6.2	0
Italian	1 tbsp	83	9.0	0

Adapted from: R. E. Kowalski. 1990. *The 8-Week Cholesterol Cure.* New York: Harper & Row; W. Cutler 1992. *Menopause: A Guide for Women and the Men Who Love Them.* New York: Norton.

amounts of this waxy substance along the walls of arteries, which leads to hardening of your arteries, high blood pressure, and coronary heart disease. In other words, cholesterol is a "good guy" who can do bad things. You probably know people like that.

Cholesterol performs its marvels in your body's cells by being carried to them in your bloodstream. The carrier substances, called lipoproteins, are manufactured in your liver by combining fat and protein, to which cholesterol is attached for a free ride. Well, not always free—you may pay a price in the form of cardiovascular disease if your lipoproteins get out of whack. Don't get discouraged, though; you can control your lipoproteins. Table 9.4 lists the amount of cholesterol in many common foods.

Which Fat Is Which?

There are several types of dietary fat. Too much of any of them is not good for you, but some are worse than others. All fats are composed of fatty acids, which are chemicals that are put together in a variety of ways to make each type of fat. Saturated fats and hydrogenated fats are the main troublemakers. Monounsaturated and polyunsaturated fats are less harmful. Triglycerides are another form of fat that your liver makes from the food you eat. We discuss each of them below.

Saturated Fat

Saturated fat is dietary enemy number one. You get it from animal foods and dairy products. Cholesterol has gotten a bad name because of saturated fat. A diet high in cholesterol does not necessarily raise the blood cholesterol if saturated fat intake is low. It's okay to eat one or two eggs per day as long as your consumption of saturated fat and trans fatty acids is low (Hu 1999. A prospective study). (We discuss trans fatty acids in a minute.) On the other hand, a high saturated fat diet raises bad LDL cholesterol and significantly increases the risk of CVD.

Saturated fats are usually solid at room temperature. Examples include butter, cheese, lard, meat fat, and chocolate. Some are liquid, like coconut oil, palm oil, and cream. Less than one-third of your daily fat intake should be saturated fat (Dreon 1990; Daoust 1996). Your body does not have a biologic need for saturated fat; it can derive all the essential fatty acids it needs from unsaturated fat, which we talk about shortly.

Hydrogenated Fat (Trans Fatty Acids)

Hydrogenation is a chemical process that converts naturally occurring oils like coconut and peanut oil to saturated fat. These are the oils used in many processed products, such as corn chips, baked goods, potato chips, and french fries. Margarine and shortenings use hydrogenated fat. A tablespoon of margarine has 2 grams of saturated fat plus about 2 grams of hydrogenated fat, for a grand total of 4 grams of "bad" fat. Trans fatty acids are just as bad as saturated fat in raising your bad LDL, but they also lower your "good" HDL, which saturated fat does not do. There is a 66 percent higher risk of heart disease in women who used margarine four or more times daily compared to women who used it almost not at all (Willett 1993).

TIP! Manufacturers were not required to list the amounts of hydrogenated fat in their products until about mid-2000. The label will usually identify it as "partially hydrogenated vegetable oils."

Polyunsaturated Fats

Polyunsaturated fats are generally liquid at room temperature. They include vegetable derivatives of cottonseeds, corn, safflower, sunflower, soybeans, and wheat germ. Polyunsaturated fats lower blood levels of cholesterol, but they also lower HDL as well as LDL, so it's a mixed blessing. Monounsaturated oils are considered safer.

Monounsaturated Fats

Monounsaturated fats have no undesirable effects on cholesterol. As a matter of fact, they make LDL cholesterol more resistant to oxidation, which reduces the tendency of cholesterol to be deposited as plaque on artery walls. This is a definite plus. Monounsaturated fats are vegetable products contained in olive oil, peanut oil, and canola oil. Mediterranean cultures consistently follow a diet that derives 30 to 40 percent of calories from fat, yet the heart attack rate is half that of the United States (Bland 1999). It is believed that this is due, in part at least, to their fondness for olive oil. Other genetic and cultural factors may also be involved, of course. If you are choosing between olive oil and butter, go for the olive oil; but don't make olive oil a net addition to your fat intake. If you are going to emphasize olive oil in your diet, cut back on something else, like meats and poultry. Too much fat is too much fat, no matter what form it takes.

Triglycerides

Triglycerides are another form of fatty acid that your body gets primarily from food. You store it in fat cells for energy use as needed. Most foods that contain fat have triglycerides. High levels pose much more of a risk for coronary heart disease for women than the same levels in men (Lapidus 1986).

Fish Oils

There's been a lot of hoopla in recent years about omega-3 fatty acids, a polyunsaturated fat found in a large variety of fish. Studies of the Inuit people showed their traditionally high-fish diets resulted in less than half the heart attack rate of that experienced in the continental forty-eight states (Kromhaut 1985). Eskimos have about the same cholesterol levels in their blood as we do in the continental U.S., but they have lower triglycerides than we do. This benefit was traced to the omega-3 fatty acids in fish oil. These fatty acids lower triglyceride levels quite effectively. They also have a beneficial influence on clotting factors, which is thought to be part of the reason for the lowered heart attack rate in the study. In addition, dietary fish has been associated with a reduced risk of sudden cardiac death, thought to be due to prevention of abnormal heart rhythms which lead to cardiac arrest (Albert 1998).

Does this mean you should eat a lot of fish? Sort of. A Harvard study of middle-aged male professionals (women were not studied, unfortunately) demonstrated that eating as little as one or two servings of fish a week conferred as much protection as a high-fish diet (Albert 1998). Fish oil is available in capsules, several of which must be taken each day. The experts who have studied fish oil capsules have sounded a different note on this issue. They found that concentrated fish oil use will lower your triglycerides, but it may actually raise your undesirable LDL. The recommendation is to avoid fish oil capsules, and to rely on fish consumption for the known benefits (Notelovitz 1993). Sardines are very high in omega-3 fatty acids; other excellent sources with lesser amounts are sockeye salmon, Atlantic mackerel, albacore tuna, herring, and halibut (Bellerson 1993).

In terms of heart health, the type of fat women eat is more important than the amount of fat. Nurses' Health Study researchers found that the saturated fats in meat and dairy products and the trans fats in margarine as well as many baked goods were more harmful than monounsaturated and polyunsaturated fats. Replacing a mere 5 percent of saturated fats with calories from unsaturated fats such as canola oil, olive oil, and nuts was estimated to reduce the risk for coronary heart disease by 42 percent. Even better, replacing only 2 percent of trans fat with calories from unhydrogenated, unsaturated fats was estimated to cut the risk by an amazing 53 percent (Hu 1999. Dietary fat intake).

Isoflavones in Beans for Lowering Cholesterol

The principle isoflavones in beans are genistein and daidzein. Studies show that one or two servings per day of soy protein (not the whole bean) containing these isoflavones reduce total cholesterol, LDL cholesterol, and diastolic blood pressure. The benefit can come from processed soy protein ingredients including isolated soy protein, soy protein concentrate, soy flour, and texturized soy protein. You may be surprised to know that in these processed forms, soy products have ten to fifteen times more fat than most other beans, but soybeans also have more protein. Beans with lower fat content include lima, kidney, and fava beans and lentils. In spite of the higher fat content, the FDA has approved products containing 6.25 grams per serving of soy protein as eligible for a label claim that it may reduce the risk of coronary heart disease if combined with a diet low in saturated fat and cholesterol (Duke 2000).

Plant Phytosterols for Lowering Cholesterol

In addition to replacing saturated fats with unsaturated fats to improve your health, total cholesterol and LDL can be lowered 10 to 15 percent by two new margarines derived from plant phytosterols (Hallikainen 1999). These are naturally occurring plant substances known as stanol and sterol esters. Stanol esters are derived from wood and marketed as Benecol, while sterol esters come from soybeans and are marketed as Take Control. Each of these products is available as a spread and a salad dressing. When used two to three times daily, they are equally effective. Neither can be used in cooking. They are high in calories, so if you use them they should be substituted for currently used fatty foods rather than as a net addition to your fat intake. Because stanols are not absorbed, they might provide an advantage over the sterols, whose systemic hormonal effects are not yet known. It also appears that stanols are safe and effective in combination with the prescription statin drugs in lowering serum cholesterol levels (Szapary 2000).

Vitamins and Minerals

Vitamins are essential in small amounts for regulation of your metabolism and for normal tissue growth and function. There are thirteen known vitamins, and they sort themselves into two categories: fat soluble and water soluble. The fat soluble vitamins—A, D, E, and K—are dissolved by fat in the intestine and stored in your body, sometimes for surprising lengths of time. Vitamin A, for example, can remain in your liver for up to two years. Because these vitamins are stored, it is possible through the use of supplements to accumulate much more than you need and suffer serious toxic side effects. Water-soluble vitamins, such as the B vitamins and C, do not pose this risk because they are not stored, and any excess is passed in the urine.

With aging, your metabolic rate slowly falls. Caloric needs decline while vitamin needs increase. Adjusting your daily diet to make up for the shortfall of vitamins can become a complex operation, so it makes sense to take a daily multiple vitamin supplement that provides a balanced regimen without providing megadoses. As you will see in a moment, however, the recommended dietary allowance (RDA) for several of the vitamins and minerals in a standard multivitamin preparation may be inadequate for you.

Antioxidant Vitamins and Minerals

Nutritional research has shown that oxygen, although it is necessary for survival, can actually cause you harm. At the cellular level, oxygen is used in the chemical reactions that produce energy and a host of useful metabolic products. A by-product of this molecular activity with oxygen is the release of particles called oxygen free radicals. The problem with free radicals is that they have either one electron too many or too few to remain stable. They go whizzing around in their molecular soup looking for that missing electron. In the process, they smash into the cell wall and other molecules, leaving a trail of damaged, largely misshapen proteins and damaged genes. This damage at the cellular level speeds up the aging process in all cells of your body. Free radical attacks on LDL change it into plaque, which attaches to artery walls and clogs them. They may even damage the cellular genes, causing a mutation and setting up the cell for future cancerous activity.

Don't think you have to cut back on your oxygen consumption, though. Antioxidants can help solve the problem. The antioxidant vitamins are A, C, and E. Selenium, zinc, magnesium, and copper are antioxidant minerals. Their beneficial function is to gather up the cavorting free radicals and bind them into harmless, stable molecules that cause no cellular damage. The question, though, is whether your diet can supply you with enough antioxidant vitamins, or whether you need to take supplements. Let's look at each of these vitamins.

Vitamin E

Vitamin E occurs naturally in foods such as bran, wheat, nuts, seeds, sweet potatoes, fish, crab, and cold-pressed vegetable oils. It has been shown in a variety of studies (Stampfer 1993; Jandak 1989; Kardinaal 1994; Diaz 1997) to have benefits in the following areas:

- **LDL cholesterol:** Prevents oxidation of LDL and subsequent plaque deposits on artery walls. This reduces hardening of the arteries, high blood pressure, heart attacks, and strokes.

- **Platelets:** Decreases the stickiness of platelets and thus reduces the risk of blood clots forming in plaque-damaged vessels. This also means fewer heart attacks and strokes.

- **Cell membranes:** Neutralizes free radicals inside the cell so they cannot attack the fatty acid components of the cell wall. This reduces cellular aging and, among other things, the brown marks on the skin known as "liver spots."

- **Cognitive function:** Improves memory and delays age-related memory impairment (Schmidt 1998).

- **Vitamins A, C, and B complex:** Protects them from oxidation and inactivation.

- **Immune system:** Enhances this system's ability to resist genetic mutations and cancer formation.

- **Chromosome damage:** Together with vitamin C, reduces damage to chromosomes from carcinogens and radiation.

- **Muscles:** Improves muscular efficiency in using oxygen.

- **Cancer prevention:** An Iowa study showed a 70 percent reduction in colon cancer for women on high-dose vitamin E supplements (Reichman 1996).

Part of the Nurses' Health Study at Harvard was an eight-year follow-up of 87,000 women, ages thirty-four through fifty-nine, who took 100 to 250 IU (international units) of vitamin E daily. This level is six to fifteen times the RDA for Vitamin E (Bland 1999). Those who used it for two years or more had a 40 percent reduction in risk factors for coronary heart disease. Those who took 30 IU or less also benefitted, but with slightly less than a 25 percent reduction in risk factors (Willett 1994; Diaz 1997). The Heart Outcomes Prevention Evaluation (HOPE) study looked at more than a mere reduction in risk factors for heart disease. HOPE was a randomized, five-year trial using vitamin E and a placebo to evaluate whether the death rate from CVD was decreased (Yosuf 2000). Alas, it found no difference in vitamin E users and the placebo group.

So should you take a vitamin E supplement? The answer is: maybe. More research needs to be done for a solid recommendation, but there are no data suggesting that it's bad for you. Toxic levels are reached at about 3,000 IU a day, but the beneficial dose is only 200 to 800 IU a day. Reaching that level requires a supplement, because you just can't get that much from eating foods rich in vitamin E, such as sunflower seeds, filberts, and cucumbers, for example.

Vitamin A and Beta-Carotene

Vitamin A is a fat soluble antioxidant derived from carotenoids in plant and animal sources. Carotenoids are contained in vegetable pigments, particularly in carrots, and their most noteworthy member is beta-carotene, from which vitamin A is made. About one-quarter of dietary beta-carotenes are converted to vitamin A, and the rest are stored in fat tissues in your liver for later use, or passed out of your body through the intestine. Animal vitamin A sources are fish, beef liver, and fish liver oil.

Vitamin A is essential in bone and tooth formation, growth and repair of tissues, maintenance of healthy skin, and normal night vision. When researchers found that vitamin A could halt the growth of breast cancer cells in laboratory cell cultures, studies got under way to see if this was true in real life. The Nurses' Health Study data showed a 25 percent higher risk for breast cancer in diets low in vitamin A or beta-carotene. Supplements of vitamin A did not affect the breast cancer risk in women whose diets were adequate in beta-carotene, suggesting that dietary beta-carotene sources are all that is needed for this benefit (Hunter 1993). In lung cancer and heart disease studies, a different story unfolded. The Beta-Carotene and Retinol Efficacy Trial (CARET) studied people at high risk who were smokers, former smokers, and asbestos-industry workers. CARET found an increase in both lung cancer and coronary heart disease with vitamin A supplements or beta-carotene pills (Wellness Letter 2000. Beta-Carotene Pills). Some studies have shown a reduction in heart disease with vitamin A use, but not in megadoses (Reichman 1996). Another study (Krasinski 1989) reported that vitamin A supplements in megadoses caused liver damage, and the higher the dose, the worse the damage. Even high dietary intake of vitamin A is associated with decreased bone mineral density and a doubled risk for hip fracture (Melbus 1998). Bottom line: It's better to get vitamin A and beta carotene from food than from pills. You can get what you need from dietary fruits and vegetables, and your body can store vitamin A for as long as two years. Good sources of vitamin A include beef liver, carrots, sweet potatoes, spinach, and cantaloupe.

CAUTION! If you are planning to become pregnant, note this: A large study of 22,000 pregnant women found that supplemental vitamin A (not beta-carotene) in doses over 10,000 IU daily was associated with fetal malformations (Reichman 1996).

Vitamin C (Ascorbic Acid)

Vitamin C is an antioxidant found in most fruits and vegetables. It is far and away the most widely researched of the vitamins. The RDA for vitamin C is 60 mg, but doses up to 10,000 milligram have been recommended in conditions of stress (Levine 1987). The FDA is increasing the RDA to 120 milligram. Since it is water soluble, vitamin C is not stored in your body. Indeed, most of it is excreted in urine within three to four hours after you take it. Foods rich in vitamin C include orange juice, kiwi fruit, broccoli, and raw tomatoes. They must be consumed soon after they are cooked or otherwise prepared (sliced, pureed, juiced) because the vitamin quickly evaporates. Cooked foods that are stored quickly lose their vitamin C.

Vitamin C's health credentials are impressive:

- **Cardiovascular disease:** As an antioxidant, vitamin C prevents oxidation of LDL cholesterol and reduces the risk of plaque formation on artery walls. RDA levels are not sufficient for this protection (Hallfrisch 1994).

- **Bones:** Vitamin C facilitates absorption of calcium from the intestine and therefore assists in bone formation.

- **Toxic effects of alcohol:** If you have red wine with a red meat dish, the tannin in the wine will prevent the iron in the meat from being absorbed. As little as 250 milligrams of vitamin C during such a meal appears to prevent this. A tomato salad does nicely. Vitamin C also seems to help prevent hangovers (Zannoni 1987).

- **Nitrosamines:** Vitamin C inhibits formation of nitrosamines, cancer-promoting free radicals that result from the oxidation of nitrites in cooked meats, especially hot dogs, bacon, and other processed meat products (Ojeda 1995).

- **Cancer:** According to Lohman (1987), vitamin C reduces the risk of death from all cancers by 14 percent. It has been shown to favorably influence the immune system in responding to several cancers, such as leukemia, advanced breast cancer, and colon cancer, as well as precancers, such as high-grade abnormalities in cervical cells.

Studies have also shown that vitamin C helps prevent cataracts, promotes wound healing and iron absorption from the intestine, and plays a role in the formation of adrenaline, your stress-reaction hormone.

Vitamin C is depleted in your body if you have a wound, a fever, are under high stress, or are taking aspirin, antibiotics, or steroids. Smoking also depletes vitamin C. In these situations, you need more vitamin C than the RDA of one hundred-twenty milligrams. A daily supplement of 250 to 500 milligrams is recommended (Wellness Letter 2000. Vitamin C). Up to 10,000 milligrams a day in divided doses may be taken, usually without ill effect. This varies from person to person, as well as with the severity of the situation producing the vitamin C depletion. If your body needs vitamin C, it will absorb it; but if not, the excess is eliminated through bowel movements. The signal that you are taking more than you need is loose stools (Pauling 1986). So if diet alone doesn't supply the amount of vitamin C you need in a specific situation, take a supplement.

Although smoking depletes vitamin C, a recent study found that smokers taking vitamin C increase their risk for heart disease rather than diminish it. Smokers were observed to have a two-and-one-half times increased thickness of artery walls on 500 milligrams per day (Wellness Letter 2000. Does this Mineral)

Antioxidant Vitamin Summary

Numerous observational studies have shown that high dietary intakes of vitamin E, beta-carotene, and vitamin C are associated with lower heart disease risk but randomized trials have not. The American Heart Association reviewed the existing literature on antioxidants and heart disease and recommends, pending more research, that you get these nutrients by consuming antioxidant-rich produce and whole grains instead of supplements (Tribble 1999).

Deeply colored fruits and vegetables have the best antioxidant ingredients. Look over Table 9.5 for a list of highly pigmented foods rated for their antioxidant potential. The foods are listed in descending order for their ORAC (oxygen-radical absorbance capacity). Fresh, frozen, or dried foods are better than processed forms.

B Vitamins

The B vitamins are water soluble like vitamin C, but they are not antioxidants. The seven B vitamins are B_1 (thiamin), B_2 (riboflavin), B_3 (niacin), B_5

Table 9.5.   Best Antioxidant Foods
(ORAC Scores for 3.5-ounce servings

Fruits		Vegetables	
Prunes	5770	Kale	1770
Raisins	2830	Spinach	1260
Blueberries	2400	Brussels sprouts	980
Strawberries	1540	Broccoli florets	890
Raspberries	1220	Beets	840
Plums	949	Red bell peppers	710
Oranges	750	Yellow corn	400
Red grapes	739	Eggplant	390
Cherries	670	Carrots	210

(pantothenic acid), B_6 (pyridoxine), B_9 (folic acid), and B_{12} (cobalamin). Food sources include green vegetables, whole grain cereals, liver, and brewer's yeast. Your body also makes its own B vitamins, in your intestines. You can't store B vitamins, so your body needs a daily supply. They play a different role than the antioxidants, but they are no less important:

- **Energy:** B vitamins convert carbohydrates from food you eat into glucose for direct and immediate energy. They also provide your backup energy source by converting glycogen stores in your liver and muscles into glucose.

- **Fat and protein:** B vitamins are essential for metabolizing both fat and protein.

- **Vascular disease:** B_6, B_{12}, and folic acid are necessary to prevent the conversion of one amino acid, called methionine, to another amino acid, called homocysteine. Evidence exists that elevated homocysteine levels are an independent risk factor for cardiovascular disease. As estrogen levels fall in women, homocysteine levels rise, so transitional women must maintain an adequate daily intake of these vitamins (Stampfer and Willett 1993; Selhub 1999; Eikelboom 1999). Multivitamin supplements are an adequate source of these vitamins, but many cold breakfast cereals are also fortified with them.

- **PMS symptoms:** Vitamin B_6 is instrumental in the formation of serotonin. Taking 100 to 150 milligrams of B_6 a day helps many PMS sufferers. Permanent neurological damage has occurred with doses over 200 milligrams. (Reichman 1996; Ojeda 1995).

- **Central nervous system:** Folic acid is concentrated in your spinal fluid and is necessary for proper brain functioning. It is also necessary for proper brain development and to prevent neural tube defects in a growing fetus. If you are planning to become pregnant, your baby's best protection comes from your being on 0.4 milligrams of folic acid at the time of conception (Medical Research Council 1991 ACOG 1992).

- **Red blood cells:** Folic acid is needed to form the protein that, combined with iron, is used in your red blood cells as hemoglobin.

Vitamin D

Vitamin D is the last of the fat soluble vitamins. In the strictest scientific sense, vitamin D is neither a vitamin nor a nutrient; it is instead a hormone (Harvard Women's Health Watch 1999). Manufacture begins in the skin from the influence of sunlight, continues in the liver, and is completed in the kidneys. Dietary sources are fatty animal products, such as fish liver oils, beef liver, tuna, salmon, butter, milk, and eggs. Milk, the most common dietary source, is now artificially fortified with vitamin D in the U.S. Sunlight exposure of about fifteen minutes per day allows ultraviolet rays to convert cholesterol molecules in your skin to vitamin D. It is also made synthetically and included in multiple vitamins or as a separate product. For ingested vitamin D to be absorbed from your intestine, fat, bile, and vitamin A are necessary. Once aboard, vitamin D can be stored in your liver and other organs.

As discussed in the osteoporosis section of Chapter 4, vitamin D is needed to absorb calcium from the intestines for incorporation into your bones. If your diet has sufficient vitamin D (400 IU) from foods and you get daily sun exposure, you, like most people in our culture, are probably not deficient in this vitamin. In older women, it may take 800 IU daily to protect against hip fracture. The safe upper limit for vitamin D is 2,000 IU per day.

Vitamin D is also associated with reduced risk for colon cancer. Additional evidence suggests that vitamin D may be involved in breast cancer prevention. Researchers have found the frequency of breast cancer is less in women who live in sunnier areas like the American Southwest.

Calcium

Chapter 4 took a thorough look at the various roles calcium plays in your body's functioning. The bottom line is that you need about 1,000 milligrams of this mineral daily during your perimenopausal years and 1,200 milligrams after menopause.

Several foods and drugs can reduce your calcium absorption and utilization:

- Excessive protein intake (50 percent above daily needs) increases calcium excretion. This is not an unusual amount of protein consumption in the U.S., so be alert to your dietary intake.

- Caffeine, nicotine, and alcohol all increase calcium loss in your urine.

- Phosphorus found in processed foods (especially soft drinks) causes the parathyroid gland to remove calcium from your bones and excrete it in your urine.

- High fiber intake binds calcium in your intestine and diminishes absorption. Stool softeners such as Metamucil cause this problem, so don't take them with your calcium supplement.

- Tetracycline antibiotics, cortisone derivatives, anticonvulsants, and cholesterol-lowering drugs (lovastatin, niacin, colestipol) interfere with calcium absorption and should be taken separately from your calcium supplement.

- Foods high in oxalates (spinach, chard, collards, turnip greens, parsley, rhubarb, peanuts, tea, cocoa, legumes) contain substantial calcium, but it is bound by the oxalates and therefore unavailable for absorption. The oxalates can also bind other calcium sources you consume at the same time. It's okay to eat these foods for other nutrient value, but it is best to avoid taking a calcium supplement for several hours afterward.

Iron

It turns out the conventional wisdom that perimenopausal women should supplement iron was wrong. Ionized iron is actually an oxidant, and oxidants, as we've been discussing, do bad things to you. A Finnish study in 1992 correlated high iron levels with an increased rate of heart attacks in the 1931 men they studied (Notelovitz 1993). They postulated that part of the reason for women having few heart attacks before menopause is their relatively low iron stores during the menstrual years. When menstrual periods stop, iron levels rise in postmenopausal women, and so does the risk for heart attacks. You are probably getting all the iron you need in your diet, so don't supplement (aside from a multivitamin) unless you are proven to be iron-deficient.

Magnesium

Magnesium is a trace mineral, about 70 percent of which is located in your bones. It has functions similar to those of calcium in your body, with involvement in muscle contraction, nerve-impulse transmission, and heart muscle contraction. Magnesium is necessary for activation of enzymes that metabolize carbohydrates and amino acids. It is also part of tooth enamel.

You need magnesium to absorb calcium. These two minerals work together in a reciprocal fashion. Too much magnesium inhibits calcium absorption, and too much calcium does the same to magnesium. The current nutritional recommendation is that they stay in a constant ratio of two to one, calcium to magnesium (Ojeda 1995). For you as a transitional woman, your daily calcium intake of 1,000 milligrams should be balanced with 500 milligrams of magnesium. After menopause, if your calcium needs increase to 1,200 to 1,500 milligrams, your magnesium should go up accordingly.

Like calcium, magnesium absorption is decreased by an excess of protein, oxalic acid foods (dark green leafy veggies), and alcohol. Use of diuretics also depletes magnesium. The FDA has set the RDA for magnesium at 280 milligrams, but this fails to take into account the increased calcium needs of midlife women and the two to one ratio needed between the two minerals. If your diet is low in fish, milk, grains, and green vegetables, it makes sense to use a magnesium supplement at half the level of your calcium intake.

Selenium

This antioxidant is a trace mineral found in many foods. You don't need much; a mere 200 micrograms (a microgram is one millionth of a gram) daily is regarded as adequate, but that tiny amount is essential. A lack of selenium impairs the immune system's ability to protect you from cancer, but high doses don't seem to improve immunity in healthy people. A daily supplement of 200 micrograms reduces the risk for colon, lung, breast, liver, and prostate cancer. More than 400 micrograms daily can cause nausea, vomiting, hair loss, and tooth loss. Dietary sources include grains, Brazil nuts, seafood, chicken, and meats. A small serving (three ounces) of red snapper contains 150 micrograms; a similar serving of beef contains 33 micrograms. Fruits and vegetables contain very little selenium. Supplements are not recommended, but if you do take them don't go over 200 micrograms (Wellness Letter 2000. Does this mineral prevent cancer).

Let's Plan a Diet

This section is about using nutritionally healthful principles to fashion a diet that you can stay with for the rest of your life. It is not a plan of deprivation and denial that will leave you hungry all the time; we know that won't work.

In 1995, the U.S. Departments of Agriculture and Health and Human Services published the Dietary Guidelines for Americans, which made these recommendations.

- Eat a variety of foods. More than fifty nutrients are required, which means a variety of foods is necessary.

- Balance the food you eat with physical activity to maintain or reduce your weight.

- Include plenty of grain products, vegetables, and fruits in your diet.

- Choose foods low in saturated fat and cholesterol.

- Choose foods moderate in sugar content.

- Choose foods moderate in salt and sodium content.

- If you drink alcoholic beverages, do so in moderation.

Since you want the second half of your life to be vibrant and enjoyable, following these recommendations is important.

Eating in America is a risk factor in itself for promotion of disease. Our diet has now been linked to high blood pressure, heart attacks, obesity, diabetes, cancer, gastrointestinal diseases, skin problems, and accelerated aging. These are some of the so-called "diseases of civilization."

According to a U.S. Department of Agriculture (USDA) food consumption survey, only 3 percent of the population eats a balanced diet. Seventy-five percent of women over thirty-five fail to consume the RDA of calcium (Block 1991). The dietary lifestyle you establish is as important as anything you can do in determining your future health. Not only that, eating for wellness influences how you feel and appear right now. Physical fitness is an equal partner in this effort, and we'll get to that in the next section.

Before you plan your new diet, it makes sense to take a look at your current diet to see where you may need to change. According to Dr. Linda Ojeda (1995), you should avoid consuming any of the following more than four times each week. Some say you should eliminate them altogether (Schwartzbein 1999):

- Fried or deep-fried foods

- Canned foods

- Frozen, prepackaged, or instant foods

- White bread and white rice

- Processed meats

- Fast foods

- Chips and dips

- Desserts, candy, and ice cream

- Mayonnaise, sour cream, and syrup

As for beverages, avoid more than two cups of coffee a day, more than four alcoholic drinks a week, and soft drinks, tea, or diet drinks more than five times weekly. You should also examine your general eating and exercise habits. Do you often skip one or more meals? Are you on a diet of fewer than 1,000 calories per day? Are you sedentary (no regular exercise program)? Is there continuous stress in your life? Do you smoke? If you tend to go overboard in any of these areas, you owe yourself a major reevaluation of your habits, an overhaul of your diet, and probably some nutritional supplementation.

As the years pass, your metabolic rate slows, which means that if you continue to eat the same way as you did in your younger years, you will probably gain weight—the infamous "middle-age spread." You need fewer calories to maintain your weight now. You still require the same amount of nutrients, but to avoid weight gain, they need to be contained in foods that add up to fewer calories.

Proportions of Food Types

In 1956, the USDA issued its "basic four" food groups, with which you probably grew up. The recommendation was for more or less equally balanced portions of meat, dairy products, grains, and fruits and vegetables. Nutritional scientists began having another look at the basic four when it became apparent that as a nation, we were becoming too fat. In 1992, the USDA came out with the Food Guide Pyramid (Figure 9.1), which represented current scientific thought about the proportions of the basic foods we should eat. The focus of the Dietary Guidelines for Americans is on foods rather than nutrients, and the food pyramid reflects this. It defines six food groups instead of four, with emphasis on complex carbohydrates, fruits, and vegetables as the staples. Meat and dairy products have been relegated to a far smaller role. A "balanced diet" meant a balance that reflected the proportions in the food pyramid. The pyramid was to be regarded as a guideline for deciding what proportions of each type of food you should incorporate in your diet. It turned out to be 55 percent of daily calories from fruits, vegetables, and complex carbohydrates, 30 percent of calories from fat, and 15 percent from protein.

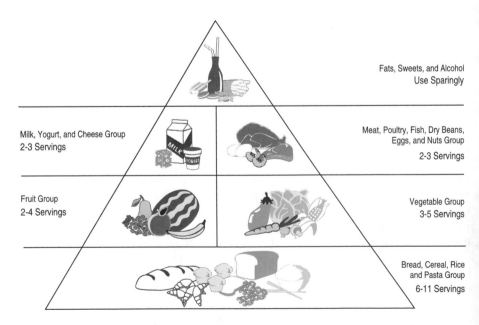

Figure 9.1.   The Food Guide Pyramid

In spite of this USDA advice, and a general population trend to follow it, we have continued to become fatter as a nation. Nutritionists began to have another look at these recommendations to determine what was wrong. It turned out that we are eating more fat than ever, but it is a smaller percentage of the total diet because of the huge recommended increase in carbohydrate intake. This strongly suggested that the proportions recommended by the government's food pyramid needed to be revised. Food scientists launched more studies and a flurry of new diets began appearing. We discuss these new concepts in Chapter 10 where weight control is covered.

Amount of Calories You Need

How many calories should you consume each day? A formula for determining your caloric needs is summarized in Table 9.6. The calculation is based on your knowing your ideal weight. You can determine this by calculating your body mass index discussed in Chapter 10.

Table 9.6. Daily Caloric Needs for Women	
General Activity Level	**Daily Calorie Intake**
Sedentary	Ideal weight x 11
Moderately active	Ideal weight x 14
Active	Ideal weight x 18
Adapted from: Ojeda 1995	

Basic Rules for a Healthy Diet

It's important to educate yourself about food. Read all you can about healthful foods—including both how to select them and how to prepare them. The bookshelves and magazine racks are awash in excellent literature. Also, read food labels. The front of the package may shout "No cholesterol," but the nutritional facts label may reveal that it is loaded with fat, or that the recommended serving size may only fill a thimble.

Here are four principles for creating a healthy diet, along with some specific suggestions:

- **Select foods of high nutritional value that are not highly processed:** These include fresh fruits and vegetables that are harvested when they are ripe. Processing of foods, such as milling of grains, removes up to 90 percent of fiber. Try to consume five servings of fruits or vegetables daily.

- **Reduce fat in your diet:** Red meat is a great source for protein, but it's laden with fat. Try skinless chicken breast instead. Think of meat as an additive rather than a main course—for example, use it in soups, stews, casseroles, and salads. Use low-fat or nonfat dairy products. (Try mixing whole milk and skim milk products until you get used to the new tastes.) Try low- or nonfat substitutes, such as evaporated skim milk instead of cream where possible, and eat low-fat snacks (fresh veggies in ice water, fresh fruit, low-fat baked crackers, whole grain crackers). To be labeled "low-fat," a food must have 3 grams of fat or less per serving; "nonfat" or "fat-free" must be less than 0.5 grams (Wellness Letter 2000. Low-Fat Foods).

- **Increase your fiber intake:** To increase your fiber intake, start with raw or lightly cooked fruits and vegetables. When your digestive system is able to tolerate them (when there's not much gas), add more high-fiber cereals and breads to the mix. Then add beans, most of which are both high in fiber and a good protein source. Beans are a good foundation for a meatless dinner, but be sure to drink about eight cups of water each day when you are eating a higher-fiber diet to avoid constipation.

- **Increase antioxidants by eating more fruits and vegetables:** This includes green and yellow vegetables, citrus fruits, and wheat. As already discussed, vitamin C supplements may be needed from time to time. Regarding the need for vitamin E supplements, studies reviewed by Harvard researchers show that dietary intake of vitamin E provides good cardiovascular disease protection without supplements (Rexrode and Manson 1996). In spite of this, and because vitamin E is so well tolerated, it is widely recommended as a supplement (Bland 1999).

So have at it. Give some honest thought to whether or not your diet measures up to healthful standards. If it doesn't, take steps now to change it, and you will be protecting your future health.

Exercise

Exercise should share equal billing with nutrition in your program for achieving wellness. In the twenty-first century, it's no longer necessary to carry water from the well or hunt for or grow your own food. Simple, ordinary walking has been replaced with automobiles, elevators, escalators, and "people movers" like those in airports. We can access the whole world with our fingers on telephones, computers, and television. Even our TVs have remote control. Strong muscles are no longer necessary for much of what you encounter in the average day.

The price of these work savers is what have been called "diseases of civilization." It is estimated that 25 percent of all deaths from chronic disease can be laid at the feet of physical inactivity (Reichman 1996). An osteoporotic hip fracture sentences a woman to a sedentary existence, and three to six months later she may be dead from pneumonia because of inactivity. Chronic heart disease may be so disabling that exercise is difficult or impossible, and that can bring on an earlier death from the disease. In other words, don't wait until exercise must be an element of your rehabilitation from a health problem. Work at avoiding the development of such problems by including regular exercise in your plan for wellness.

Among many other benefits, exercise helps hot flashes by increasing the endorphins in your brain. A decrease of this brain opioid is associated with inactivity and more hot flashes, so the more you exercise and raise your endorphins, the fewer hot flashes you will have. Women who exercise aerobically three hours each week have far fewer hot flashes than women who are sedentary.

Do You Really Need to Exercise?

Let's look at the benefits of exercise so you can make an informed decision. It is common knowledge that exercise plays a major role in weight control. You probably know that it also contributes to strong muscles and sturdy bones. There's more to this story, though. Exercise benefits every part of your body—every organ, tissue, and cell. Further, your mind and your spirit become more agile and energized by the upbeat feeling that exercise brings with it. Exercise can help save your life; without it, your body deteriorates.

Weight Control

The short answer to the question of how exercise fits into weight control is that exercise burns calories. It builds muscle, which is the most biologically active tissue in your body. The more muscle tissue you have, the more calories you burn; but you don't need to become a muscle-bound behemoth to benefit. You just need more muscle than you probably have at the moment and exercise will accomplish this for you. Exercise speeds up your metabolic rate, which is why it burns calories. Exercise also decreases your appetite and therefore the number of calories you take aboard to be burned in the first place.

With adequate muscles, which, with your bones and organs, are part of your lean body mass, you burn more calories even at rest. The term for this is resting metabolic expenditure (RME). The larger your lean body mass, the greater your RME. Indeed, 60 to 75 percent of the calories you burn every day result from your resting metabolic expenditure (Leibel 1995). This is true whether you are sleeping or just hanging out.

You can lose weight with a diet-only program, but if exercise is combined with it, you do not need to limit yourself to constant dieting. As a matter of fact, if you are exercising, it is not a good idea to severely restrict your diet; you need adequate calories for the energy your exercise consumes. Include nutritious foods; just avoid eating them with both hands.

Stress Control

Vigorous exercise brings oxygen to every cell in your body by stepping up circulation. This creates energy and improves your capacity for handling stress. Beta endorphins, your body's "feel-good" drugs, are released during vigorous exercise, leaving you feeling relaxed and at ease afterward. Also, exercise helps you to sleep soundly, because your body is more tired. Researchers at Harvard have found that regular exercise reduces depression and is a practical means of handling the emotional stress of everyday living (Benson 1993).

CAUTION! Avoid exercising just before bedtime. The stimulation may actually prevent your getting to sleep.

Longevity

Regular exercise can prolong life. A large study at the Institute for Aerobics Research found that the death rates from all causes were reduced by 44 percent in women (and men) who exercise regularly (Blair 1989). This list includes heart disease, cancer, and even accidents. The reduction in heart attack deaths was 50 percent.

Cardiovascular Disease

The dramatic reduction in heart attack deaths with exercise results from improving several cardiovascular disease (CVD) risk factors:

- It lowers your total cholesterol level, lowers bad LDL, lowers triglycerides (an independent risk factor for women), and raises good HDL. All winners.

- It lowers blood pressure.

- Exercise reduces the risk of blood clots by decreasing the stickiness of platelets and by increasing components of your blood that dissolve small but dangerous blood clots.

- It lowers the insulin level in your bloodstream by burning glucose, which diminishes the necessity for insulin. Too much insulin in your blood for too long a time promotes the formation of plaque on artery walls. This leads to hardening of the arteries and high blood pressure.

- It improves the strength of your heart muscle and its pumping efficiency; your heart pumps more blood per heartbeat. When your exercise plan results in cardiac fitness, your heart can have up to 36,000 beats a day fewer than an unfit heart (Reichman 1996). That works out to nearly 200 million saved heartbeats during your transition years alone!

Bone Strength

We made the case for preventing osteoporosis in Chapter 4. Weight-bearing exercise not only prevents bone loss, it has been shown to stimulate the formation of new bone in women who have low bone density. If you have risk factors for osteoporosis, get your bone density checked. Exercise is crucial for you if your bone density is below normal. If it turns out to be normal, however, just thank your lucky stars, and get (or keep) going with an exercise program to keep it that way. Exercise has a more beneficial effect for you as a perimenopausal woman in building bone than it will after you reach menopause. After menopause, exercise works mainly to keep the bone you already have. The point is this: Don't wait until menopause to start exercising. You want to arrive at menopause with a sturdy skeleton.

Estrogen Deficiency Symptoms

Exercise has been shown to be one of the best methods of relieving hot flashes. An old study (Wallace 1982) showed that a moderate-intensity exercise program actually increased estrogen levels. Some researchers feel that low levels of endorphins in sedentary women are in part responsible for hot flashes. As you now know, exercise increases your level of this brain chemical.

Intestinal Function

Less constipation results from regular exercise because your intestinal tract is stimulated, along with the rest of your body. Physical activity stimulates digestion and a more complete absorption of nutrients.

Cancer Risks

Former women athletes who continue to exercise have a 50 percent decreased incidence of breast cancer and a 60 percent decrease in cancers of the cervix, ovaries, uterus, and vagina (Frisch 1989). That's impressive.

Brain Changes

Physically fit people are protected from several central nervous system changes that have traditionally been thought to be due to aging. Exercise increases blood flow to your brain and increases the release of brain chemicals called neurotrophins. These chemicals act like a fertilizer in your brain; they increase the number of connections between brain cells. This improves your ability to process and retain new information. In addition, your physical reaction time is improved (Brink 1995). These abilities are best protected with complex physical activities such as aerobic dancing, racquet sports, and swimming. Aerobic walking works also, but not quite as well. The ideal aerobic activity for brain improvement is one that also involves some decision making during the exercise, such as tennis and dancing. "Brain fade" and slowed physical reaction time may not be an inevitable consequence of time; fitness has a role in preventing these changes.

A vibrant life can be yours if you exercise because you can look better, feel better, think better, and have a biological age that can be significantly less than your chronological age. From all of the above, any fair-minded person would have to conclude that exercise is crucial to achieving wellness.

Coming Up with a Fitness Plan

Now that we've listed all the reasons exercise is good for you, it's time to make some decisions. There are many forms of exercise, so you have choices. Keep in mind that the type of exercise you choose is not as important as the fitness level you achieve, so your selection should be an exercise plan that will realistically fit into your life—one that's based on the goals you set, and your age and current level of fitness. Goal-setting is probably one of the most important preliminaries to starting an exercise program. If you decide what you want out of it first, there is a greater likelihood that you will achieve it. These are the goals you might consider.

- Cardiovascular fitness
- Weight control
- Muscular strength
- Improved flexibility
- Coordination and balance
- Osteoporosis prevention
- Better brain functioning
- All of the above

Please don't regard these goals as just another wish list. Give sober and serious thought to them. What you decide for yourself should be something you really want to pursue. Cardiovascular fitness and weight control tend to be the most common choices. Don't regard your exercise plan as a temporary inconvenience, like a fad diet. This is going to become a new part of the rest of your life, so make it something you can realistically incorporate into your life and enjoy.

The Formula

Since the 1980s, the recommendation of most fitness experts has been to exercise three to four times weekly at a level that keeps your heart rate within a specified target zone (explained below) continuously for 30 to 60 minutes at a time. The formula calls for aerobic conditioning, muscle strengthening, and flexibility exercises (Pollack 1990). This works quite well, but it takes a lot of planning to incorporate it into a busy life. In spite of the proliferation of health clubs, new athletic shoe and clothing designs, and exercise gadgetry, not enough Americans do anything about putting regular exercise into their lives.

A slightly different approach from the traditional one has been recommended by the Centers for Disease Control and Prevention, and the American College of Sports Medicine. They found that acceptable physical fitness could be accomplished by moderate-intensity physical activity if it was carried out for half an hour a day. In addition, they found that the activity does not need to be continuous. If you accumulate thirty minutes of exercise in eight- to ten-minute minute segments every day (or most days), you can become moderately fit. You just need to incorporate activities that burn 200 calories per hour for a total of thirty minutes.

How can you figure out how many calories you're burning? Some examples may help. Brisk walking on level ground, cycling under ten miles an hour, using a power lawn mower, general housecleaning, and playing golf all burn four to seven calories each minute. More strenuous activities, such as walking uphill, moving furniture, cycling over ten miles an hour, and using a hand mower burn over seven calories a minute. With the above choices, you may not need to bear the expense of a health club or buy a lot of special equipment to arrive at moderate physical fitness. Try cycling to work, walking briskly to lunch, and using the stairs instead of the elevator. Three ten-minute events performed at about the same pace as brisk walking can get it done for you.

It's clear then that you can achieve fitness by many means, great and small. Without too much disruption of your average daily schedule, you can easily weave these things into your life. Just remember that moderate physical fitness will significantly decrease your chances of future illness and premature death. If you want to be more than moderately fit, then go for it. More effort is required, of course, but the payoff in better health and wellness is worth it.

Exercises for Perimenopausal Women

The three basic forms of exercise are aerobic conditioning, muscle strengthening, and stretching exercises. Each category includes a wide variety of activities from which to choose, so you can avoid becoming locked into a set routine.

Aerobic Conditioning

Aerobic exercise means systematic physical activity designed to increase oxygen consumption. The main objective is to increase the amount of oxygen your body can process in a given amount of time. This is called aerobic capacity. By improving your ability to utilize oxygen in aerobic exercise, you improve the functioning of your respiratory and cardiovascular systems, as well as increase muscle tone. This type of activity involves your body's large muscles, which speeds up your metabolic rate, increases your heart rate, and delivers more blood and oxygen to every cell in your body. Calories are burned in the process, too. Aerobic capacity reflects not only the condition of your muscles, but also the condition of your vital organs, so in that regard it is the best measure of your body's physical fitness.

Aerobic activity can be anything from running to dancing to climbing stairs to raking leaves. Your choice of activity should be based on your current level of fitness, how it will fit into your lifestyle, and the fitness goals you have set for yourself.

CAUTION! High-impact aerobic exercise is widely known to result in damage to tendons, muscles, and joint surfaces. This means any activity in which you are off both feet at the same time (jogging, jumping, aerobic dancing). Low-impact exercise does not provide as much cardiovascular conditioning, but it is still sufficient in this regard and is less likely to result in injury.

Your built-in speedometer for aerobic conditioning is your heart rate. The recommended training rate for any aerobic exercise is 60 to 80 percent of the maximum recommended heart rate for your age. The simple formula for determining your personal training rate is to subtract your age from 220 and multiply by 0.6 to 0.8. For instance, for age 40 it's 220 – 40 = 180 x 0.6 to 0.8 = 108 to 144. Do whatever level of exercise it takes to keep your heart rate in this range while you are exercising. As your fitness improves, you will find that you can tolerate more exercise. As a matter of fact, once your physical reserves have increased, you will notice that it takes more aerobic activity to keep your heart rate in the 60 to 80 percent target range. This is a convenient way to track your progress, and it provides a potent motivation to keep you interested and involved.

To check your heart rate during aerobic exercise, slow down enough to feel your carotid artery pulse. (You can feel your carotid pulse by pressing your fingertips into the soft neck tissue just below the angle of your jawbone.) Count this pulse for six seconds, and add a zero to whatever number you get to determine your beats per minute.

If you are a beginner, start in the lower part of your target heart range and work up gradually to the 80 percent level, but do not exceed the upper limit. Excessive exercise levels that put you beyond your target training heart rate only subject you to needless injuries, and result in sore muscles. For your exercise to be aerobic, it must be continuous for the duration of your specific program. This can be a mere ten minutes if you are making three short aerobic efforts each day, or a continuous thirty to sixty minutes three to five times weekly.

Muscle Strengthening

The value of stronger muscles to you as a perimenopausal woman is that they will protect you from joint and tendon injuries, which become increasingly common with disuse of your muscles. Strengthening your muscles and increasing their size dramatically increases your ability to burn calories and control your weight. A by-product of the effort this takes is the improvement in bone density that results from weight-bearing exercise. Stronger muscles translate to more competence in the way you use your body. You will be more agile and more graceful, and have better posture and a confident gait. This leads to fewer of the clumsy accidents we all hate.

For a muscle to be strengthened, it must be contracted against resistance. Most aerobic exercise involves some form of weight-bearing muscular activity. The majority of aerobic exercises (walking, jogging, dancing, step climbing, and so on) stress using lower body muscles; it might be a good idea to use hand-held weights during these activities to acquire upper-body muscle strengthening. You can target more specific muscle groups with free-weight training and weight training machines like Nautilus. Isometric exercise (active contraction of muscles against steady resistance), elastic resistance, and body-weight resistance (push-ups, pull-ups) are also effective for muscle strengthening. Swimming is great for upper body training, and it is fantastic aerobic work.

TIP! Don't worry that muscle-strengthening exercises will turn you into a middle linebacker. You don't have enough testosterone to get that kind of muscle bulk.

Stretching Exercises

Stretching exercises promote flexibility. As the years pass, inactivity results in loss of elasticity in muscles, tendons and joints. We stiffen up. A program of stretching exercises, though, can keep you flexible. Stretching also will improve your posture and help relieve back pain.

There is risk of injury in stretching exercises, so be sure to get expert advice before venturing into a program on your own. Learn how to stretch properly—not herky-jerky and bouncy, but slow and sustained. A stretch should be sustained for about 20 seconds to be effective. Your muscles must also be "warmed up" before you stretch them if you are to avoid injury. This means that you must not start a workout with stretching. If you are an exercise walker, for example, do some slow walking first to warm up your muscles, and then stretch them before you set out on the vigorous part of your exercise program. Stretching your muscles again at the conclusion of your routine, while they are still warm, will contribute to your being supple and prevent post-exercise soreness.

Yoga is an excellent method for improving and maintaining flexibility. Hatha (pronounced ha-ta) yoga, which is a catch-all term meaning physical yoga, has enjoyed a recent reincarnation in our country as more people interested in fitness recognize that it is not merely a cultural fad. From glitzy gyms and spas to local YWCAs, yoga is shaping new trends in exercise and diet (Davis 1996).

Components of an Ideal Workout

There are four components to the ideal workout:

- **Warm up and stretching:** This is an important part of the exercise routine for every age, but it is especially important for you at midlife. If you have been sedentary, your chances of injury are much increased if you don't spend a few minutes on mild activity to increase the blood flow to your muscles. This can be as simple as a few minutes on the rowing machine or some moderate walking. Once your heart rate has increased somewhat or you have broken into a slight sweat, do your stretching exercises to get your muscles ready for increased range of motion and stepped-up activity.

- **Aerobic workout:** As we said, your choice of aerobic exercise can be any type of activity that gets your heart rate into the desirable target range for your age and level of physical fitness. You can vary it depending on your personal schedule of work and family obligations. Working out with a friend or your partner or in a class can add variety and interest.

- **Muscle strengthening:** These are good exercises to add after your aerobic workout, when your muscles are warm and supple. Ideally, they should include all major muscle groups. An alternative is to do these exercises on one or two days when you are not doing aerobic work. This can add some variety to your program and prevent the boredom of doing the same thing every time you exercise.

- **Cool-down and stretching:** This is the opposite number of the warm-up; but it is of equal importance. A gradual slowdown of your heart rate allows the increased blood flow to your muscles and skin to subside. The cool-down can be as simple as slowly walking around until your heart rate is back to normal. This is an ideal time to do some more stretching exercises to prevent muscle stiffness.

CAUTION! After exercising, avoid a cold shower until your heart rate has slowed. Cold water on blood-engorged skin can force massive amounts of blood back into your central circulation by constricting the blood vessels in your skin. This puts a huge strain on your heart. Also, wait to cool down before using a sauna or hot tub; additional heat on blood-engorged skin can draw even more blood out of your central circulation into your skin, which may result in fainting.

Summary

Wellness involves conducting your life in a fashion that decreases your chances of disease and enhances your verve for living. This chapter has shown you the principles of good nutrition, how to plan a healthful diet, and the value of exercise. The next chapter puts all these elements together in considering another aspect of wellness that has a profound influence on the second half of your life: weight control.

O O O O

10

Wellness from Lifestyle Changes: Weight Control, Plus Detoxifying Your Body and Mind

"If I had known I was going to live this long, I would have taken better care of myself." This famous lament of the elderly does not need to be yours. What you do to your body now, while you are young, will have a major impact on your future health. We know that destructive behaviors are responsible for many illnesses—and we're talking major diseases like high blood pressure, heart disease, diabetes, stroke, emphysema, osteoporosis, and cancer. Habits that seem innocent and apparently harmless in the beginning can cause monstrous problems a few years down the road. It's better to have never started overeating, smoking, or using alcohol or recreational drugs, but what if you did? You still have time to protect your health. Changing a long-ingrained behavior is not easy, but the physical and psychological benefits are powerful. This chapter will give you the reasons to try, and some of the ways to get it done.

Weight Control

Americans spend over $33 billion annually on weight-loss services and products, but it is not helping. The percentage of overweight adults, both women and men, is increasing by nearly 1 percent per year. Sixty-one percent of American adults and 25 percent of American children are now overweight

(Women's HealthSource 1999; Centers for Disease Control and Prevention 2000).

Are you sure you have a weight problem? If you think so, it is probably based on what your bathroom scale tells you, or on a standard weight chart that uses your height and frame size to determine your "ideal" weight. The problem with this method is that it only tells you your weight. It fails to distinguish between overweight and overfat. There's a difference. Too much body fat is the real culprit when it comes to obesity-related health risks for high blood pressure, heart disease, diabetes, and certain cancers, such as colorectal cancer. It is possible to weigh more than the standards prescribe, yet not be overfat. For example, a trim-looking aerobics class instructor may appear to weigh twenty pounds less than her actual weight simply because she has good musculature and less body fat than usual. On the other hand, a woman of "normal" weight may be considerably overfat if she has a small muscle mass; of the two, she actually has the less healthy body composition.

Determining your percentage of body fat is the most accurate way to assess your body composition of fat versus lean body weight (meaning your total weight minus body fat). This can be done in a variety of ways. One way is to use skin calipers on your upper arm. Another is to take girth measurements of waist and hips, and another is to have your body weighed underwater. Conversion tables are then used to interpret the measurements. Ultrasound, dual energy X-ray absorptiometry (DEXA), CT scans, infrared interactance, and bioelectric impedance scanning are also being used to make these determinations (Roubenoff 1995; Women's HealthSource 1999). These are all rather complicated methods that require third-party help.

Table 10.1. Female Body Composition (Percent Body Fat) By Age				
			Age	
	26–35	36–45	46–55	56–65	Over 65
Good	18–20	20–23	23–25	24–26	22–26
Average	21–23	24–26	26–28	27–29	27–29
Poor	31–33	33–36	35–38	36–38	35–37
Adapted from: Goldring et al. 1989				

Body Mass Index (BMI)

Body mass index is a simpler way to do an estimate of your proportion of body fat. You calculate your BMI using the following formula: (weight in pounds x 700) ÷ (height in inches squared). So if you weigh 130 pounds and are 5 feet 5 inches tall (65 inches), your calculation would be (130 x 700) ÷ (65 x 65) = 21.5.

Table 10.2. Percentage of Overweight Women by Age	
Age	**Percent of Women Overweight**
30–39	34.3
40–49	37.6
50–59	52.0
60–69	42.5
70–79	37.2
80 +	26.2

Source: National Health and Nutrition Examination Surveys 1992

A BMI of less than 18.5 is underweight, 18.5 to 24.9 is normal weight, 25 to 29.9 is overweight, 30 to 34.9 is mildly obese, 35 to 39.9 is moderately obese and over 40 is extremely obese. BMI is now being used as the standard for reference levels of body weight for women and men. The drawback is that it is based on averages and fails to take into account differing frame sizes. Still, it is a reasonable guide to determining whether you may be carrying too much fat.

Fat Distribution

The way your body fat is distributed is another consideration that influences your health. Total weight is important, but the distribution of fat is an added factor. The greatest distribution risk is if your fat is concentrated around your waist as opposed to around your hips (the apple shape versus the pear shape). Such a body fat distribution is an independent predictor for coronary heart disease in women (Rexrode 1998). A simple method of determining this is to measure your waist and hips with a nonstretch tape. Here's how to do it:

1. Measure your waist at the narrowest point (usually at the navel, but this can vary). For women, over thirty-five inches is associated with higher health risks.

2. Measure your hips at the widest point (over your buttocks).

3. Divide your waist measurement by your hip measurement. A normal value for women is 0.8. If the value is 1 or more, your fat is distributed too much in your abdomen.

If a determination of your body-fat composition is available to you through your doctor or your health club, compare it to the norms for your age in Table 10.1. Your percentage of body fat slowly rises as you grow older.

This is important. If you are now forty-five, you don't need to return your body composition to what it was twenty years ago!

Most women gain weight during the transition years, and weight gain is greater after menopause; this is normal. We are concerned here with overgaining; not with the gradual increase reflected in Table 10.1. A study using body mass index standards showed that 38 percent of women between the ages of forty and forty-nine are overweight, and the numbers rose to 52 percent between ages fifty and fifty-nine (Kuczmarski 1994). Although men tend to reach their peak weight gains between thirty-five and sixty-four, women continue their gain even beyond their middle years. See Table 10.2 for the data collected by the National Health and Nutrition Examinations Survey in 1992. This table shows that during the five decades between ages thirty and eighty, an average of 40 percent of American women are overweight. Current figures place those rates higher still. Are you thinking that you are doomed to this weight gain? That it is inevitable? Maybe not, if you know what causes it.

What Causes Overweight?

Fat storage is the fundamental cause of becoming overweight, but things are more complex than that. Several factors are involved in fat accumulation:

- **Aging:** Aging results in a gradual slowing of your metabolism. It seems related to the fact that after age thirty, women start losing about 1 percent of their muscle mass each year as a result of lessened physical activity. By age thirty-five, this amounts to about one pound a year. With each lost pound of muscle, you burn fifty fewer calories per day. If your caloric intake remains unchanged as time passes, you end up taking aboard more calories than you burn, and the excess becomes stored as fat. By the time you have lost as much as five pounds of muscle mass, your body is storing 250 calories a day. If your daily dietary intake remains the same, you can gain up to twenty pounds in a year.

- **Appetite:** The neurotransmitter norepinephrine stimulates hunger; serotonin suppresses it. Overweight results when these regulators of appetite become short-circuited and the wrong signals are sent. This is not specifically a perimenopausal event; it can happen at any age. The only evidence that it has happened in you is a large appetite that you can't attribute to other causes, such as hyperthyroidism. Why does it happen? See the next bullet item.

- **Genetics:** Genes play a role. We have a genetic mechanism that controls how much body fat we accumulate. It operates much like a thermostat, in that there is a "fat setting" in the brain that programs and regulates the amount of body fat you maintain. An "obesity" gene has been located in humans (Baron 1997). Not surprisingly, it has been named "the OB gene." The gene controls production of a protein called leptin, which sends messages to your brain on the status of your overall body fat content. Leptin controls another brain hormone called neuropeptide Y (NPY), a potent appetite stimulator. If the gene is defective or missing, leptin is not produced in adequate amounts, and NPY is free to make you inappropriately hungry. If your brain is insensitive to leptin, the fat setting may be too high, and obesity results. Research is underway to develop products that will increase the brain's sensitivity to leptin.

- **Gender:** The fact that you're a woman is a factor. Women of normal weight have an average of 22 percent body fat, as compared to 16 percent in men. This stems, in part, from the fact that men have a larger muscle mass than women, so men burn 10 to 20 percent more calories than women, even at rest. Because your body burns fewer calories than a man's, it accepts fat more readily, meaning you can gain weight more easily, and it may be more difficult to lose it. Not fair perhaps, but that's a fact of gender.

- **Metabolism:** Your metabolism plays a definite role. One factor is the muscle tissue story we discussed above. The more muscle you have, the greater your resting metabolic expenditure and the more calories you burn. Another metabolic factor is an enzyme in fat cells called lipoprotein lipase (LPL). This enzyme is active in removing triglycerides from your bloodstream and tucking them into fat cells for energy storage. LPL increases during dieting—your body is trying to get the weight back. This supports the genetic theory that we are all preprogrammed to have a certain amount of body fat.

- **Medical problems:** Less than 2 percent of obesity can be attributed to metabolic disorders or hormone imbalances (Women's HealthSource 1999). Hormones can influence your weight, but contrary to popular thought, glandular obesity hormonal problems are rare.

The Part Hormones Play in Weight Changes

Let's take a closer look at the role of some hormones that influence weight.

Thyroid Hormone

Thyroid hormone levels are influenced by what you eat. Levels of T4, the metabolically active thyroid hormone, are lower during fasting. This is one reason your metabolic rate is lower during a weight loss diet. Your body is trying to conserve its energy resources and resist losing tissue, whether it be fat or muscle. Some diet programs use thyroid supplements to counteract this normal effect, but this is at the risk of increasing calcium excretion, which increases the risk of developing osteoporosis. Overeating increases T4, which raises your metabolic rate in an effort to burn some of the excess calories. However, this weak regulatory effort by your thyroid gland does not work well enough to be a major player in weight control.

Insulin

Insulin plays a major role in causing obesity. It has been called the supervillain of overweight (Daoust 1996). Insulin, produced in the pancreas, is necessary to unlock cells for storage of glucose from your bloodstream. Blood glucose is stored as a substance called glycogen in your liver and muscles, from which it can be readily accessed and reconverted to glucose for energy needs. The problem with insulin arises when there is a glucose overload from dietary intake of high glycemic carbohydrates (explained in Chapter 9). An insulin surge occurs in one to two minutes. Since insulin is thirty times more effective in moving glucose into fat than into muscle, carbohydrate excess results in fat storage and weight gain. Over time, cells exposed to high insulin levels become insensitive to it, a condition known as insulin resistance (or, by some writers, "Syndrome X"). The result of insulin resistance is that insulin has nowhere to go and high levels occur in the bloodstream, a condition called hyperinsulinemia. Chronic high insulin levels cause obesity, clogged arteries, high blood pressure, heart attacks, strokes, increased cancer risks, diabetes, and accelerated aging in all cells. So this hormone is the kingpin of the fattening of America, simply because of our high dietary carbohydrate intake.

Glucagon

Glucagon is also a pancreatic hormone that is released in response to dietary protein intake. Its primary function is to regulate the release of glycogen in a steady fashion so blood glucose levels remains stable. But the big story is that it also releases fat for use as energy, so it can be regarded as your friendly fat-burning hormone. Glucagon has an inverse relationship with insulin, meaning a high insulin level results in low glucagon (Schwartzbein 1999). Can you see where this is leading? Too much carbohydrate and not enough protein result in high insulin levels with accompanying fat storage, as well as too little glucagon and less fat-burning capability. Bingo—weight gain. Dietary fat does not influence the insulin to glucagon ratio.

Human Growth Hormone (hGH)

This is a pituitary hormone that is released in response to exercise. It is your body's most powerful fat-burning hormone. Unfortunately none of us exercise for most of our waking hours, so hGH doesn't exert as great an effect on weight control as we might hope. Guess what, though? High insulin levels suppress hGH. Are you becoming convinced that insulin is indeed the supervillain of overweight?

Hormone Balance

With the understanding that insulin minimizes fat burning and glucagon maximizes it, it is easy to see how your dietary balance, or imbalance, of foods can result in an ideal body composition or compromise your health. A high carbohydrate intake turns on insulin, which stores fat and forces glucose to be used for energy. But a moderate carbohydrate diet combined with more protein allows glucagon to release fat for energy and protects your body from the depredations of too much insulin. Hormones regulate virtually everything your body does. All of your body's hormones are interconnected and interdependent upon each other to regulate your functioning in a fashion that maintains optimum health. This includes your sex hormones, estrogen and progesterone, and many others.

You Can Influence Your Genes

Some of the above discussion, especially about gender and genetics, may make it sound as though what you weigh is beyond your control, so why worry? It's a bit late, of course, to choose your gender or your parents, who gave you their genes, but there is still plenty you can do. Obesity is hereditary 50 percent of the time (Baron 1997); the other 50 percent is accounted for by environmental factors such as your diet and how much you exercise. These things, along with psychological and sociological factors, are the ultimate determiners of your weight.

Until recent years, it was thought that the genes you inherit, and their influence on your body, were immutable: You inherited your eye color, the shape of your nose, and perhaps a predisposition to certain diseases and that's your fate. Scientists began to question the permanence of the messages your genes send to your body's cells, with the observation that genetically brain-damaged children, who were initially unable to speak or walk, could be taught new skills. Through environmental influences utilizing physical training and conditioning as well as nutrition, these children were observed to improve their intelligence and physical skills. Their genes remained the same, but the manner in which the genes operated in their bodies—the occurrence known as genetic expression—could be changed. This observation and many other examples of environmentally mediated changes in genetic expression, led to research into whether or not the environmental influence of nutrition can alter the control genes have over our accumulating body fat.

It turns out nutrition does have this ability. It is eloquently expressed by Dr. Jeffrey S. Bland in his book, *Genetic Nutritioneering* (1999). Bland's term, "genetic nutritioneering," means arranging a lifestyle, diet, and environment that enables you to alter the messages your genes send to your cells. You *can* improve the way your genes control your health and vitality. Since we all have different genetic makeups, our bodies differ to varying degrees in the manner in which we respond to dietary influences. The 55 percent carbohydrate, 30 percent fat, 15 percent protein prescription of the Food Pyramid or the 40-30-30 proportions of the Zone concept (Sears 1995) are not appropriate for everyone. Instead, there is a *range* of proportions that work for the large majority. The correct percentages for you vary depending upon how well your body responds, but somewhere between 55-30-15 and 40-30-30 is a diet for you that will result in an ideal body composition and optimum health.

Weight Loss Diets

We've already talked about your "fat thermostat," or internal fat-setting mechanism. The question is, can your thermostat be reset if it is currently too high and you are overweight? It isn't easy, but it's doable. It involves fundamental changes in how you eat, exercise, and think. Let's take them one at a time, starting with diet.

At any one time, approximately 40 percent of American women are on a diet, even if their weight is normal (Horm 1993). The problem is, diets don't work in the long run. The implication of the word "diet" is that it has a beginning and an end. You set out to lose some predetermined amount of weight, lose it on a specific diet plan, and then you're done with the diet. A high percentage will regain most of the lost weight within a year, and all of it within three to five years (Institute of Medicine 1995). Women often end up weighing more than they originally did. Thus, a temporary diet won't succeed in resetting your fat regulator. When you resume normal eating habits, your lipoprotein lipase enzyme, discussed earlier in this chapter, is still programmed to take as many of the triglycerides as possible from the food you eat, refilling those fat cells you so recently emptied. This often leads to another go at dieting, and another cycle of loss and regain—the infamous yo-yo pattern of weight fluctuation.

Part of the reason for this pattern of weight gain is that losing weight does not eliminate fat cells. Your body contains about 30 billion permanent fat cells, which hold about 135,000 calories, and serve a vital energy storage function (Notelovitz 1993). Your fat cells can sustain your body's energy needs for about six to seven weeks, even without any food. When a fat cell is full, it can store up to 95 percent of its volume in pure triglyceride. When all 30 billion of them are full, your body makes more fat cells to accommodate whatever additional storage requirements your diet imposes, and those cells are permanent as well; they're there for life.

The take-home message for you as a transitional woman is to avoid excess weight to begin with. Your children will benefit from your guidance in this regard; you can help them by carefully managing their food intake and training them in habits of healthful nutrition. In this respect, you may be more helpful to them in their future life and wellness than all your other efforts to get them properly educated and prepared to become adults.

Another reason for regaining weight after a weight loss diet is that calorie deprivation reduces your muscle mass. Weight loss from a diet is 75 percent fat (which is good), but 25 percent lean muscle mass (which is bad)

Table 10.3. Serving Size Equivalents	
Food Serving	**Equivalent**
3 ounces meat or fish	Deck of cards
Cup of vegetables	Size of your fist
Medium apple	Size of a baseball
½ cup cooked pasta	Ice cream scoop
1½ ounces cheese	Pair of dice
1 teaspoon butter, jelly	End of your thumb
1 cup dry cereal	Large handful

(Kayman 1990). Since muscle mass helps burn calories, losing some of it lowers your metabolic rate, and your post-diet return to normal eating habits makes it less likely that you will burn the increased calories and much more likely that you will store them as fat.

For all these reasons, chronic or repeated dieting cannot be relied upon to control your weight. This does not mean you should not reduce your caloric intake to lose excess pounds. Calorie cutting is a powerful tool in weight loss. The point, though, is that success hinges on your adopting a weight control program that incorporates foods you will keep in your diet for the rest of your life. This is not a "diet" in the popular sense of the word, because it is not temporary. It is a new way of life. Such an eating program will not shed weight as quickly as crash dieting, but it is a reliable method to lose weight permanently—especially if it is combined with exercise. A continuing and consistent change in your eating habits is your best shot at resetting your body's internal fat-regulating mechanism.

Weight Loss Principles

The key to a weight loss plan is to reduce the total amount of calories you consume; but the proportions of foods in your diet must remain within range of the percentages we discussed above. Calorie counting is a discouraging pain in the neck, so don't bother with it other than to make an initial determination of how many calories your body needs to maintain ideal weight. For example Table 9.6 in Chapter 9 shows that a 130-pound, moderately active woman needs about 1,800 calories per day to maintain stable weight. Next rely on smaller serving sizes for a daily reduction of 500 to 1,000 calories to reduce your weight. Look over Table 10.3 for meaningful serving sizes. None of the macronutrient (carbohydrate, fat, protein) proportions should be radically reduced or increased out of the recommended range discussed earlier. Just eat smaller portions. Your dietary composition must be such that maximum fat burning takes place. To do this, remember that insulin control is the key to avoid fat storage and allow glucagon to release fat for energy use. This means that high carbohydrate intakes must be avoided. It also means you need adequate protein. The Atkins Diet, the Eades Protein Diet, and others that are based on metabolic imbalance may work initially, but they are not safe or effective for long-term use.

As for fat consumption, most American women consume 80 to 100 grams of fat daily (Ojeda 1995). Since fat contains 9 calories per gram, this amounts to 720 to 900 calories. If our 130-pound woman is trying to maintain her weight, she needs only 600 calories from fat (about 67 grams) to do this if 30 percent of her calories are derived from fat. So a 16 to 33 percent reduction in fat is necessary if she is to maintain her weight, but an even greater reduction is needed if weight loss is her goal.

To accomplish weight control or weight reduction, you not only need to eat the right proportions of each food category, but also the right type of each. Refer to the last chapter for discussions of lean protein, low glycemic-index complex carbohydrate, and "good" fats. But remember this: To lose weight, you must eat fewer calories. Rearranging your food proportions so you can maintain a favorable insulin-to-glucagon ratio helps burn fat, but it doesn't fool your body into shedding pounds if your total calories are not reduced.

CAUTION! Do not attempt a diet with fewer than 1,000 calories on your own; it can be very dangerous. Deaths have been reported as a result of severe caloric restriction (Baron 1997). Such diets have been used for extreme obesity, but they must be pursued under the strict supervision of a physician who understands the potential hazards and can recognize serious problems if they arise.

Stick with the following general principles for reliable and safe dietary weight control:

- **Go slow:** Don't cut calories severely. Losing one or two pounds a week is about the right pace.

- **Emphasize foods high in nutrients and low in fat and calories:** The best choices are raw vegetables and fruits, plus complex carbohydrates, such as whole-grain breads and cereals, pasta, legumes, and rice. (Refer to Chapter 9 for more information on nutrition.)

- **Avoid quick-fix diet programs:** If they promise weight losses of more than the recommended one to two pounds a week, they are usually counting on your losing water, not fat. It won't last.

- **Eat most of your calories early in the day:** This increases the likelihood that they will be used for energy during the day. Meals just before bedtime result in more fat storage.

- **Take a multivitamin supplement:** It is unlikely you can get enough nutrients in a weight-loss diet to supply the vitamins you need.

- **Regard your new diet and the accompanying exercise program as a permanent part of your life.** We can't emphasize this enough.

There are many books on the market to help you make up your individual diet. Sonja and William Connor's *The New American Diet System* details their cholesterol-saturated fat index (CSI) to selecting healthful foods. Dr. Jeffrey Bland's *Genetic Nutritioneering* provides good information on rearranging your food proportions to your advantage. Jane Brody's *Good Food Gourmet* supplies a wide array of recipes, and *Cooking Light* magazine is a good source for low-fat menus.

What about Diet Pills?

A number of diet pills on the market successfully suppress appetite, but none of them keep the weight off. They do not change your internal fat-regulating mechanism, even with long-term use. What they can do is give you a reasonable jump-start on losing weight. If you are significantly overweight (more than 30 percent over your desirable weight), appetite suppressant drugs can produce a weight loss in a few weeks that may motivate you to continue on a long-term plan of dietary control. And if you combine such a regimen with exercise, your chances of permanent change are enhanced even more.

Appetite suppressant drugs (ASDs) enhance serotonin, which dampens appetite, or suppress norepinephrine, which stimulates appetite. Two serotonin enhancing drugs, fenfluramine (the "fen" of "Phen-Fen"), and dexfenfluramine (Redux), were withdrawn from the market in 1997 after it was revealed they were associated with leaky heart valves (Langreth 1997; Abenheim 1996). Since then, interest in using ASDs has waned considerably. None of them have proven to be the magic bullet for treatment of obesity.

The post–Phen-Fen era has seen the introduction of additional attempts at weight control with ASDs. Sibutrimine, marketed as Meridia, is a drug that targets both serotonin and norepinephrine. It has been approved for short-term use in people more than 30 percent above their desirable weight. Concerns have been raised about lack of blood pressure reduction in people losing weight on this drug. Orlistat, marketed as Xenical, causes a one-third reduction in fat absorption from the intestine by inhibiting the action of lipase, an enzyme necessary for fat absorption (Davidson 1999). Side effects include gas, cramping, and a bothersome fatty diarrhea. A randomized control trial found those taking Xenical lost an average of nine pounds more weight in a year and kept it off longer than a placebo group (Sjostrom 1998). Xenical reduces the absorption of fat soluble vitamins (A, D, E, and K), so a daily multivitamin is recommended.

The food supplement industry is promoting what it calls "herbal Phen-Fen." This is a mixture of St. Johns wort, a plant derivative, and ephedra, an ancient Chinese herb also known as ma huang. St. Johns wort elevates serotonin levels resembling the effect of fenfluramine and ephedra is a stimulant that mimics the effects of phentermine (the "phen" in "Phen-Fen"). As yet there are no studies supporting the safety or effectiveness of these plant derivatives. Ephedra has been reported to cause states of severe agitation, seizures, heart rhythm irregularities, heart attacks, strokes, and even deaths (Langreth 1997). The FDA is considering regulation of ephedra as a drug. Metabolife 356 is another herbal product that has garnered extensive publicity on prime-time TV. It has eighteen ingredients, with ephedra and caffeine as the main components. Based on its modest benefit, known risks, and lac.k of long-term safety data, Metabolife 356 is not recommended (Barrette 2000).

Pyruvate, a metabolic breakdown product of glucose, is a very highly touted "fat burner" food supplement that appears on many Internet sites. It is said to boost overall weight loss by 37 percent and enhance fat loss by 48 percent. A close look at the early 1990s literature supporting those claims reveals that pyruvate provides, at most, a very small benefit to obese women in a highly controlled bed-rest environment. The small benefits were exaggerated by statistical manipulation (O'Mathuna 1999).

The obesity gene produces a hormone called leptin that attaches to specific brain receptor sites and regulates how much fat your body stores. Obesity results if the receptor sites are insensitive to leptin or if not enough leptin is produced. Leptin (by injection only, unfortunately) is being used in research projects, and several pharmaceutical companies are working (feverishly, we suspect) on drugs to increase the brain's sensitivity to leptin.

Another approach to obesity control involves neuropeptide Y (NPY), a brain chemical that has been shown in laboratory animals to be a potent stimulus to feed. NPY is suppressed by leptin. Researchers are trying to develop a drug that will prevent NPY from attaching to brain receptor sites and thus dampen the desire to eat.

The bottom line for using currently available drugs to combat obesity is that they are unlikely to result in more than a 5 to 10 percent reduction in body weight. Starting a weight reduction program with such drugs may be initially helpful, but long-term success still depends on permanent changes in your dietary lifestyle.

Exercise—a Must for Weight Control

If you cut back on the amount of food you eat, you will reliably lose weight. Eventually, however, your body will start resisting this self-imposed tissue destruction and start slowing your resting metabolic expenditure. You burn fewer calories, and weight loss slows. A major cause of this metabolic change is the loss of muscle that results from food deprivation. If you lose twenty pounds from dieting alone, a quarter of it will have been muscle mass. You already know that a pound of muscle will burn about fifty calories each day, so losing five pounds of muscle cuts your calorie furnace by 250 calories every day. This looks good on the bathroom scale, but your body composition will have been compromised. The answer to this problem is to combine exercise with your new dietary lifestyle. No weight loss program is complete without it.

There are several reasons why exercise plays such a vital role in weight control:

- Exercise burns calories and stimulates production of human growth hormone, a potent fat burner.

- It keeps your muscles from deteriorating by preserving your lean body mass. This is particularly important since your body's resting metabolic expenditure of calories (60 to 75 percent of the total daily energy expenditure) is correlated with lean body mass.

- Exercise suppresses appetite. Total food consumption is less in people who exercise regularly. If exercise is combined with your new way of eating, you can make fewer cuts in your food intake. As a matter of fact, it is important to allow yourself a few more calories to compensate for the energy expended by exercise. Not a bunch more—just more than you would allow yourself on a weight loss program. This, in turn, may make it easier to stick with your new dietary program.

- Exercise helps to diminish the health risks of being overweight, including high blood pressure, abnormal lipid profile (high cholesterol, high triglycerides), diabetes, heart disease, and certain cancers.

- When exercise is combined with a weight loss diet, it becomes the most efficient way to lose weight. It has long been known that neither exercise nor diet alone is as effective as they are in combination (Johannessen 1986).

- Strenuous exercise releases endorphins in your brain, which generates a feeling of well-being and relieves depression. This helps create a feeling of equanimity that can help you accept your new weight control program and stay enthusiastic about sticking with it. When you have reached your target weight, continuing exercise has been shown to increase the likelihood that you will maintain it. Nonexercisers more consistently regain weight. The Harvard studies (mentioned in Chapter 9) of athletes showed that once you have become physically fit, you continue to benefit: You have a higher level of fat-burning enzymes, so keeping your weight under control becomes easier.

What Kind of Exercise?

The decision as to which type of exercise you choose is an important one. Muscle-strengthening exercise will keep you from losing vital muscle mass, so it is an important part of the mix (Butts 1994). On the other hand, while the use of free weights and the machines at the health club make for better muscles, they do little to burn fat. You need aerobic activity to accomplish that. (We described some aerobic activities in Chapter 9.)

With weight control as the goal, you need a type of aerobic exercise that differs from that needed for achieving cardiovascular fitness. It revolves around your need to burn fat. In the first twenty minutes of aerobic exercise, the energy you expend is provided by glycogen, which is stored sugar in muscle tissue and the liver. It isn't until your glycogen stores are exhausted that your body turns to fat for energy. This means that a longer workout, of about forty-five minutes, is necessary. For this reason, select a form of exercise that you can sustain for that length of time, such as cycling or walking. As discussed in Chapter 9, you will need to gradually build up to that level if you are unfit or a beginning exerciser.

Ideal exercises might be brisk walking, whether around the neighborhood or on a treadmill, and cycling around town or on a stationary unit. Platform step-aerobics and aerobic dance are also excellent as long as they remain low-impact. Swimming is good aerobic exercise and great for muscle strengthening, but it is hard to sustain it long enough to get to the fat-burning stage. Watch out for jogging, running, and some forms of aerobic dance; they are high impact and therefore risk injury to your knees, hips, and ankles, especially if you are overweight.

Be sure to alternate aerobic exercise with weight training to maintain your muscle mass. Exercising three to four days a week may be sufficient for cardiovascular fitness, but weight loss needs an everyday, or nearly everyday, commitment (Kayman 1990). Never go to bed without a plan for exercise the next day. If you planned to walk three miles but you wake up at seven instead of six and it's raining cats and dogs, have a backup plan. Never go to bed without planning what you will eat the next day. By having your diet and exercise plan firmly in mind, you are more likely to succeed with both endeavors.

A suitable exercise program can be designed for almost anyone. If you are a beginner, get some advice from your physician. You need to be as sure as possible that the exercise program you are undertaking will not be harmful to you. If you are over fifty, many experts suggest a treadmill electrocardiogram (ECG) to determine whether your heart can sustain the increased workload. A treadmill ECG hooks you up to a machine that monitors your heart while you undergo an increasing workload of walking. It may also be helpful to have your exercise program set up by a professional fitness expert who can steer you around situations that may injure you. This is especially true for stretching exercises. (Many health clubs employ certified training experts.)

The guidelines for weight control exercise are essentially the same as for anybody else (see Chapter 9), with these added precautions if you are overweight:

- **The warm-up phase:** This phase of exercise is especially important, because being overweight tends to make you less flexible. Your muscles and tendons are more easily injured. For these reasons, do some slow walking, cycling, or rowing until your heart rate has increased or you have begun to sweat. Then do your stretching exercises. Don't do any exercise that hurts; wait until you have lost some weight and try again.

- **Underdo it at the beginning:** If your goal is to walk three miles in forty-five minutes, start with something like three blocks in ten minutes, and work up to it in later sessions. Your tolerance for exercise is considerably less if you are overweight, and you need to sneak up on it. Remember, this is a new lifestyle for you, and there is plenty of time to ease into your new role.

- **The cool-down:** Cooling down after exercise is more important if you are overweight because there is a greater tendency for blood to pool in your legs if you stop suddenly. This can make you either feel faint or actually faint. Gradually diminish your level of activity over five to ten minutes, and let your heart rate return to normal before you become inactive.

- **Temperature awareness:** If you are overweight, you will overheat more readily, especially in the early stages of becoming an exerciser. Avoid hot rooms and, if you exercise outside, the hottest hours of the day. Be sure to drink plenty of fluids before and during your workout. Wear loose-fitting, lightweight clothing. Cotton is best because it wicks moisture away from your body, letting it evaporate and cool you down.

The Head Trip—Think More to Weigh Less

Eating is a means of staying alive, but it's also a behavior that may fulfill a secondary need. Eating can relieve boredom, quiet anxiety, or calm anger. Being conscious of why you are eating can help you go far toward modifying eating habits.

Behavior modification techniques can make an important contribution to your success in losing weight. First, identify your personal eating patterns by keeping a written record of how you eat for a period of two to three weeks. Don't estimate: Most women underestimate their daily food intake. Write down when you ate, what it was, where you ate it (home, restaurant, snack stand, and so on), and how you felt at the time (angry, guilty, frustrated, lonely). Understanding your eating patterns can help you begin to make some positive changes.

For example, if you find that you frequently eat high-calorie snacks while watching TV, try a low-fat substitution, such as fruit. When you feel hungry, it may be that you are only thirsty. Try drinking a glass of water. Go for a brisk walk instead of walking to the refrigerator after a disagreeable confrontation. You can probably think of other substitutes.

Keeping a record of your daily activities for a week or so; it may show you where you can squeeze in some exercise without a lot of fuss. Maybe you can get off the commuter train a mile from work and walk the rest of the way, or park your car a comfortable walk to your destination. Ride a stationary bicycle while you watch the evening news rather than consuming snacks during that time.

Weight control may be a challenge for you in your transition years, but it is a major component of wellness and deserves your attention.

Smoking

There has probably been more said and written about the destructive effects of smoking than about any other human habit. Americans must be listening, because the number who smoke has been declining over the last two decades.

If you are still smoking, you probably would like to quit. Earlier in this book you learned about the relationship of smoking to cardiovascular disease, osteoporosis, lung cancer (the number one cause of cancer death for women), the aging process, skin wrinkles, and earlier menopause. The number of deaths attributable to smoking for all Americans between ages thirty-five and sixty-four is nearly one in five. This exceeds the combined total from suicide, murders, fire, auto accidents, AIDS, alcohol, cocaine, and heroin (Warner 1991). When used as directed, setting fire to tobacco leaves and inhaling the products of combustion is a waste of a perfectly good body. Thirty-five percent of smokers die from a smoking-related disease. As a woman, you currently can expect to outlive your male contemporaries by seven years. If you are a smoking woman, however, this advantage may be lost entirely.

Then there is the issue of passive smoking. Secondhand smoke is estimated to be responsible for 35,000 to 62,000 cardiac deaths each year (Wellness Letter 2000), as well as for 100,000 to 200,000 nonfatal heart attacks and strokes (Glantz 1995). Nonsmoking women exposed to tobacco smoke are 30 percent more likely to develop lung cancer than those who aren't so exposed (Fontham 1994).

Why You May Still Be Smoking

One of the keys to quitting smoking is to be aware of the reasons you smoke. There are a variety of reasons women continue to smoke (Rigotti 1992):

- **Addiction to nicotine:** It's official: Nicotine is addictive. This is a very difficult problem to conquer. Nicotine gum and skin patches may help you.

- **Weight control:** A Surgeon General's report indicated that three-quarters of women gained an average of five to seven pounds after quitting smoking. The American Cancer Society disagrees. They found only about one-third gained weight, and if exercise was combined with an effort to cease smoking, one-third actually lost weight. It may be that you gain weight after quitting because your metabolic rate drops, or it may be simply that you end up using eating as a substitute for the strong oral stimulus of smoking. You may well gain some weight, but estimates are that you would need to gain at least 75 pounds before the risks of obesity begin to outweigh the risks of smoking (Reichman 1996).

- **Pleasant associations with smoking:** After-dinner conversation, coffee breaks, and smoking after sex are three examples.

- **Psychological dependence:** Like overeating, smoking may represent a coping mechanism for dealing with anger, boredom, stress, frustration, and pressure.

- **Coping with stress:** You may use smoking to handle stress; when you stop, you experience more stress, which causes you to light up again.

There are many books and programs available to assist you in your effort to quit smoking. Check the Appendix for the addresses and phone numbers of the American Cancer Society, National Cancer Institute, and American Heart Association

Alcohol

As you sip your evening cocktail after another harrowing day of just being you, you are consuming a very unusual substance. Alcohol is a tiny molecule with no nutrient value, but it is readily absorbed into your bloodstream. Because it is so small and is soluble in water, it is carried to every cell in your body. Other drugs with larger molecules are not as widely distributed, but alcohol, once consumed, is presented with near-endless opportunities to do harm. The array of ill effects on your body and your life from alcohol abuse is astonishing. It is a potent, and sometimes deadly, force in aging. Alcohol can destroy your liver, raise your blood pressure, lower your bone mineral density, enlarge your heart, cause gastrointestinal bleeding, impair your brain function, shatter your sex life, hasten your menopause, decrease your fertility, suppress your immune system, worsen diabetes, increase your cancer risk, sap your energy, increase your stress level, trigger depression, and create social problems, including marital, family, and occupational difficulties.

The Gender Difference

It takes less alcohol over a shorter time span for women to sustain the serious and sometimes fatal outcomes of alcohol consumption (Landau 1994). Part of the reason is that women are generally smaller than men, so they have a smaller volume of blood and other body fluids. If you consume the same amount of alcohol as a man, it will probably not be diluted as much in your body. The effect on your tissues is therefore more intense.

Another important difference is that as a woman, you have less of a stomach enzyme called gastric alcohol dehydrogenase than men do (Frezza 1990). This enzyme's job is to partially break down alcohol in your stomach and reduce the amount of ethanol, an alcoholic drink's active ingredient, that you absorb into your bloodstream. With less enzyme breakdown, your blood alcohol level rises much faster than in men. Your organs and tissues are once again subjected to a more concentrated solution of alcohol.

Alcoholism

Most people who drink overdo it occasionally. The morning after reminds you of it. This doesn't mean you have an alcohol problem. You do have a problem, though, if you fall into either of these two categories:

- **Alcohol abuse:** Drinking impairs your normal life functions, such as your marriage, job, and other relationships.

- **Alcohol dependence:** In spite of the impairments, you have an unrelenting compulsion to continue drinking.

Your genetic background can influence your chances for alcohol dependence. If you have a first-degree relative (parent or sibling) who is an alcoholic, your risk is fourfold. Approximately 5 million American women have serious drinking problems. This may be an underestimate, since women are more introspective about their drinking problems than men and may seek to disguise their overuse of alcohol. Many more women drink alone than men. Although more than twice as many men as women are reported to be serious problem drinkers, this may be largely the result of underreporting of alcohol use by women (Gold 1991).

Health Consequences

For women, heavy drinking is considered to be more than two drinks a day. By now, you are probably already aware that alcohol affects your brain (and therefore your behavior, coordination, and reflexes) and that it can cause cirrhosis of the liver. It is also a significant factor in fatal accidents and in heart disease. How else does alcohol abuse affect you?

- **Skin damage:** Overuse of alcohol can severely damage skin. It has to do with free radicals, which we described in Chapter 9. Collagen and elastin are damaged, which leads to decreased skin tone, sagging, blotching, puffiness, and brown spots. Long-term use may even give you rhynophyma—a red "W. C. Fields" nose. Severe alcoholics in their forties commonly appear to be in their sixties.

- **Effects on sex:** With lowered inhibitions, you are more likely to engage in risky sexual behaviors. These can range from socially risky flirtations to the health risks of sexually transmitted diseases from new or multiple partners. Heavy alcohol use can also suppress orgasms and diminish your sexual desire.

- **Breast cancer:** Women who consume 30 to 60 grams of alcohol daily (two to four bottles of beer, three to five glasses of wine, or two to four shots of liquor) have a 41 percent higher risk of breast cancer than nondrinkers (Smith-Warner 1998). No one knows the reason for the alcohol–breast cancer association, but speculation is that alcohol causes increased estrogen levels, abnormal liver function, immune system suppression, and free radical damage to DNA in breast cells (Ginsburg 1995). If you have risk factors for breast cancer (you have first-degree relatives with breast cancer, are overweight, have never been pregnant, or had your first term pregnancy after age thirty), abstinence from alcohol is your safest course.

- **Obesity:** Alcohol contains seven calories per gram, compared to four calories per gram for carbohydrate and protein and nine calories per gram for fat. There is no nutritional value in alcohol, so any of those calories you do not burn immediately are stored as fat. Since your metabolic rate slowly declines during perimenopause, your need is for fewer calories containing more nutrients. You may not gain weight by drinking alcohol, but you sure won't be better nourished.

- **Fetal damage:** If you are planning a pregnancy, drinking alcohol is a very bad idea. This is true both while you are trying to get pregnant and once you've succeeded. Heavy drinking can cause fetal alcohol syndrome, which causes low birth weight with deformities of the heart, limbs, and face, as well as mental retardation (Autti-Ramo

1992). The specific safe maximum for alcohol in pregnancy is still unknown, so abstinence is safest for your baby.

- **Heart disease:** Heavy drinking can cause high blood pressure, which in turn is linked to an increased workload for your heart and to damaged heart muscle. Alcohol also raises serum triglycerides, which represents a specific risk for heart disease in women. But there's some good news: The Harvard Nurses' Health Study found that moderate alcohol intake (two or fewer drinks a day) can reduce your risk for heart disease (Stampfer 1988). In addition, moderate alcohol use also raises your "good" HDL. Moderate alcohol intake has a positive effect on blood-clotting mechanisms, which decrease your risk for strokes and heart attacks.

- **Osteoporosis:** Low bone mass is common in heavy drinkers, including women who have not reached menopause. The reason is that alcohol interferes with calcium absorption. It also impairs activation of vitamin D by your liver, and this further lowers calcium absorption. In addition, if your diet is nutritionally poor (common for heavy drinkers), your intake of calcium and vitamin D may be deficient. If you have personal risk factors for osteoporosis, limit your consumption of alcohol to fewer than two drinks daily.

- **Immune suppression:** Not much has been published on this subject, but alcohol apparently lowers or alters your immune response to foreign intruders and cancer formation (Reichman 1996). When oncogenes trigger the formation of a cancer cell, your immune system normally resists this abnormal cell and tries to destroy it, but this effect is lessened in heavy drinkers. If your immune system is suppressed, you are more susceptible to infections—everything from the common cold to HIV (the AIDS virus).

There is not much disagreement that drinking alcohol in moderation can do a little good, but it can do a lot of harm if consumption gets out of control. The transition from being a moderate "social" drinker to alcohol abuse and dependence is often a subtle one. The profile of the transitional woman who develops a drinking problem is that of a divorced or separated woman, a woman who lives with an alcoholic partner, a married woman who does not have an outside job, and for a woman whose children no longer live at home. A very common trait of the alcoholic woman is that she is a solitary drinker, and often a secret one (Gold 1991). The good news is that, like quitting smoking, healing begins immediately when you stop drinking.

As we mentioned earlier in this chapter, drinking problems are categorized as either alcohol dependence or alcohol abuse. If your problem is alcohol dependence, and alcohol is literally controlling your life, your best choice for treatment is to enter a detoxification program, either as an inpatient or an outpatient. Inpatient therapy usually requires about a month of treatment. Most cities have such facilities.

If alcohol abuse more accurately describes your situation, a detox program may still be the best plan, but for some, a lesser level of treatment may also work. Alcoholics Anonymous and Women for Sobriety are two effective support groups that can help you. Here are some additional tips:

- **Acknowledge your drinking problem:** The longer you put it off, the more likely you are to suffer permanent damage to your body and to your life.

- **Go public:** Make an announcement of your intention to stop drinking. It's easier for you to quit this way. Tell people important to you (your partner, friends, coworkers) that you are quitting alcohol. The value is twofold. First, you are more likely to stick with your commitment because you have announced it to them. Second, your peers may avoid putting pressure on you to drink when they realize your genuine intention to quit alcohol.

- **Ask your partner to help:** Ask your partner not to drink in your presence. Also, invite your partner to attend counseling and group sessions with you. It may turn out that your partner is enabling (unwittingly encouraging) you to be a drinker and does not realize it. If your partner refuses to participate, you may have to choose between ending your relationship and jeopardizing your recovery.

- **Decline the offer of a drink:** At a party, simply say, "I don't drink." If your hosts insist, leave the party.

- **Avoid drinkers:** Seek out friends who don't drink. One source of new friends is the people you meet in a support group. In the early stages of recovery, when you are most vulnerable to backsliding, it is reasonable to ask friends who do drink not to do so around you. You can't impose that limitation forever, of course, but they may be willing to help you during the early stages. If not, avoid them.

- **Refuse alcohol substitutes:** Avoid nonalcoholic beer and wine. The tastes are similar enough to their alcoholic cousins that they may conjure up the old cravings.

- **Keep busy:** Now may be a good time to invest yourself in volunteer community work, join a theater group, or go back to school. Just make sure it's fun. You may soon realize that being sober is really more rewarding than drinking.

- **Exercise:** Join a health club if you can. Regular exercise relieves stress, improves your body's condition, and puts you in the company of people who enjoy good health.

The overall mortality rate for alcoholic women is four and a half times that of nondrinkers. Your life expectancy is shortened fifteen years by heavy drinking (Reichman 1996). Shortened also are relationships with your partner, children, and friends. Time and human closeness are too precious to throw away on a tiny but deadly molecule like alcohol.

Drug Dependency

Just as you are not immune to alcohol dependence, neither are you immune to dependence on addictive drugs. You may not know a single person who set out to become addicted, but you probably know some addicts. Much has been said and written about inner-city abuse of illegal drugs. As a perimenopausal woman, however, you are more likely to become dependent upon legal than illicit drugs. Drug dependency cuts across all social, cultural, and economic boundaries. One in twenty American women abuses or is dependent on drugs of some type (Gold 1991).

The effects on you of drug dependency can be widespread and devastating. It can turn your body into a toxic waste dump and rapidly age you. You may lose your money, your partner, your children, your job, your friends, and your dignity. You can become malnourished. Neglect of exercise and personal grooming habits contribute to further deterioration. Your intellectual capabilities will become blunted. And the bottom line is that you can die from drug dependence.

How Drug Dependence Can Happen

People take drugs because they make them feel good. If you sprain your ankle, a prescription painkiller makes you feel better. For sinus congestion, an over-the-counter decongestant helps. A line of cocaine may make your brutal daily schedule more tolerable. A tranquilizer gets you some much-needed sleep. That's the start of it. These drugs fill a need in your life. For most people, however, relief is short-lived. Long-term use causes decreased production of endorphins, your own internal opiumlike drug, which, as you know from Chapter 4, you rely upon for relief of pain and other stresses. This encourages greater use of your drug of choice and may eventually result in dependence—you need it just to get by.

What Drugs?

While marijuana, cocaine, methamphetamine, and heroin are the usual suspects, there are many, many more prescription and over-the-counter drugs upon which you may become dependent:

- **Psychotropic drugs:** Medications such as tranquilizers and sleeping pills are common sources of drug abuse in women. Diazepam (Valium), chlorazepate (Tranxene), chlordiazepoxide (Librium), and similar drugs are commonly prescribed for short-term stress control, but these drugs are well known for their addicting capabilities.

- **Amphetamines and other appetite suppressants:** Amphetamines and a whole panoply of similar appetite suppressants, such as phentermine (Fastin) and mazindol (Sanorex) may give you a diminished urge to eat, but the stimulant effect of these "uppers" makes you want to stay with them indefinitely.

- **Painkillers:** These are intended for relief of acute pain, but some pain is chronic and poses the threat of addiction if these drugs are continued for an extended time. They include oxycodone with aspirin (Percodan), propoxyphene (Darvon), codeine-containing drugs, and other analgesics, such as pentazocine (Talwin), hydrocodone (Lortab, Vicodin), and levorphanol (Levo-Dromoran), any of which may become avenues to addiction.

- **Over-the-counter medicines:** These, too, can become addictive. Phenylpropranolamine is the active ingredient in diet pills such as Dexatrim, Acutrim, and Dex-A-Diet. This drug is also found in many other medications, including nasal decongestants (Entex, Ornade), cough medications (Dimetane, Hycomine, Triaminic), and drugs for treating PMS. Phenylpropranolamine has a stimulant effect, and therein lies the trouble—it's another feel-good drug.

- **Alcohol abuse:** A National Institute of Mental Health survey found that women who abuse alcohol are six times more likely to abuse other drugs as well (Gold 1991).

Are You at Risk?

As a woman, you are at greater risk than men for abuse of tranquilizers, stimulants, sedatives, and other prescription drugs (Prochaska 1992). This stems from the fact that women are generally more health-conscious than men and seek care more frequently. Women tend to be more open about their concerns and in touch with their feelings about common disorders such as anxiety, insomnia, weight control, and chronically painful conditions. The drugs warranted for these problems often have a high potential for addiction. Adding to your risk is the fact that women are less likely to come forward with a dependency problem, which results in a more advanced stage of addiction when care is finally sought. The exception to this is in women who work outside the home; if drug abuse is causing trouble at work, help is usually sought earlier.

If you suffer from a mental disorder, such as depression or anxiety states, your risk of drug dependency is raised. Depression quadruples your risk of abuse or dependency. For panic disorder and obsessive-compulsive states, the increase is doubled (Gold 1991).

Another gender-related risk is that women generally have more body fat than men. Sedatives and tranquilizers are deposited in body fat, and they are cleared from women's bodies more slowly than in men. This means that the desired effect lasts longer, and you can get to like it. In addition, the smaller your body, the greater the concentration of the drug, resulting in a more intense response. If the response is a positive one, you may be reluctant to give it up.

Heredity also has a role to play. In his book *The Good News about Drugs and Alcohol*, Dr. Mark Gold writes that drug dependence, like alcoholism, can run in families. His estimate is that one in ten people are genetically predisposed to drug dependency. There is no genetic test for this, so if your family history includes drug or alcohol dependency, be extremely cautious. Avoidance is a whole lot easier to deal with than dependence.

Prevention

There is no question that never getting started on drugs beats trying to stop. Experimentation with illegal drugs, even briefly, can quickly lead to dependency. Addiction is certainly not what you had in mind when, just for a lark, you snorted your first cocaine. But it can be a pretty slippery slope after that. And it's a long way down. Dependency on legal drugs, although it starts with legitimate treatment, can follow the same downward path. Consider these suggestions for steering around a drug problem:

- **Know what you are taking:** When a new medication is prescribed, ask your doctor or the pharmacist about its potential for addiction. This is especially important if you have risk factors that make you prone to dependency—prior drug abuse or mental illness, or a family history of addiction.

- **Use as directed:** Your interests are best served by following the prescription label precisely. Take the medication as frequently and for as long as directed, and then stop. Avoid saving what is left over unless your doctor advises you to do so. Prescription drugs may be even more dangerous than illegal drugs because they are made available to you for a legitimate purpose, and you might worry less about misusing a legal drug than a street drug.

- **Resolve conflicts in your life:** Attempts at using drugs to relieve the stress created by a conflict are only avoidance; it's a temporary measure. Seek out the cause of your frustration, boredom, anxiety, work pressure, or poor relationship and deal with it. Change partners, get a new job, compromise with an adversary, or do whatever is appropriate to deal with the problem. Don't risk having drug dependency on your back along with your conflict.

When to Get Help

There are some very clear signs that your drug use has overstepped normal bounds:

- You can't think of anything except the drugs you are using. Without them you can't start the day, go to work, be happy, be relaxed, go to a party, have sex, get to sleep, or do anything normal.
- You are neglecting your family and friends to obtain and use drugs.
- You are lying to get prescriptions refilled.
- You are missing work because of drug use or drug hangovers.
- You are neglecting your nutritional needs and personal grooming habits.
- You are depleting your savings or selling possessions to buy drugs.

How to Get Help

Drug dependency can happen to you. It doesn't mean that you are of low moral character or unworthy of compassion. For a variety of reasons, some of them not of your choosing or in your control, you may have drifted into dependency. Chronic illness, overwhelming stresses, ignorance of the risks, and many other factors may have played a part in bringing you to this point. You didn't intend to get addicted. You just are. If this is your situation or you think it is, the following suggestions can be helpful (Larson 1993):

- **Ask for help:** Your chances of getting out of this morass alone are not good. Tell someone—your partner, a friend, your doctor, a clergy member—about your problem. This alone will make you feel better. If someone knows about you and cares, you've acquired some support and taken the first step toward recovery.

- **Seriously consider a treatment program:** Drug recovery centers offer both inpatient and outpatient services. As an inpatient, you will be in a nonthreatening environment while your body is detoxified. This setting also provides people skilled in helping you address the underlying causes of your drug dependency. Both are necessary to full recovery. The costs are now covered by many insurance companies and even by some employers.

- **Join a support group:** Support groups can be very helpful. Many twelve-step programs, for example, are conducted by people who have experienced drug dependency. The people you meet will greet your problem with understanding and empathy. Contact Narcotics Anonymous, Alcoholics Anonymous, or Cocaine Anonymous for a chapter near you (see the Appendix).

- **Get back on a healthy diet:** Very few drug-dependent women regard eating well as a priority. The problem can arise from binge eating and obesity in marijuana users to severe undereating and malnutrition in cocaine users. If you are starting a recovery program, a balanced diet will not only supply the needed calories, it can provide the sense of orderliness in your life that you may have lost.

- **Start exercising:** You have probably neglected your body during your drug dependency. If so, starting a regular program of moderate exercise, as we described earlier in this chapter, will make a big difference during your recovery. Your body will feel better, and your spirits will be raised. Depression is common during dependency, and exercise is an excellent mood elevator.

Summary

Destructive behaviors are common human frailties. For some, they result from an unfortunate shuffling of the genetic deck. For others, these behaviors arise from bad choices. Fortunately, the latter is the most common cause of destructive behavior (Prochaska 1992). If you chose it to begin with, you can also "unchoose" it. It isn't easy to change long-standing habits and behaviors, but as a perimenopausal woman, you have years ahead of you in which to benefit from discontinuing destructive behaviors that can endanger your wellness.

O O O O

11

Relax for a Change: Management of Stress and Depression

As a perimenopausal woman, you may encounter some new stresses (hot flashes, sleep disruption, mood shifts, short-term memory changes), but your stress response will likely be similar to your past experiences with stress. Like most people, you probably don't have a perfect handle on coping with stress. The first half of this chapter explains what stress is, how to recognize it, how it can affect your health, and how to cope with it. The second half covers the relationship of stress to the development of depression—both minor and major forms—and bipolar disorder.

What Is Stress?

Stress can be described as the sum of your biological reactions to any adverse stimulus that tends to disrupt your homeostasis, or balanced state. (Homeostasis is a constantly changing balance in the physiological, psychological, and social spheres of your life.) Stress throws you off-kilter. The adverse stimulus can be physical, such as threat of an impending injury; it can be mental, as when you worry about paying your bills; or it can be emotional, like anger. A stressor is any change arising internally or externally, whether real or imagined, that requires you to react or adapt to it. Each individual reacts differently to stress. If your compensating reaction to stress is inadequate or inappropriate, it can lead to additional problems.

Stress control is an important part of your wellness program. By understanding the relationship between stress and your health, you can better control it.

What Link Does Stress Have to Other Disorders?

Sixty to ninety percent of office visit complaints are rooted in lifestyle habits and stress (Notelovitz 1993). In addition, while infections of various sorts have historically been the predominant cause of death and disease, stress-induced disease has now assumed this mantle in industrialized cultures. Stress is linked to cardiovascular disease, respiratory disease, arthritis, insomnia, infertility, chronic pain, depression and even cancer. Negative emotions, anxiety, loneliness, grief, and depression will suppress your immune system (Kiecolt-Glaser 1991; Kiecolt-Glaser 1996). This puts you at risk for a variety of illnesses, including common colds and failure to respond to vaccines.

How Does Stress Do It to You?

Stress upsets your body's homeostasis. Even though events frequently disturb that balance, a series of ongoing minor adjustments will usually bring you back into balance. This fine-tuning occurs at many levels: biochemical, cellular, organ-system, psychological, interpersonal, and social.

For example, let's say your stressor is that you are very cold. Your homeostatic responses might be:

- **Biochemical:** Your stress hormones, epinephrine (adrenaline), norepinephrine, and cortisol, are increased. These prepare you to take whatever action might be necessary to combat the cold. This is your "fight-or-flight" capability.

- **Cellular:** Your declining body temperature causes certain cellular metabolic functions (like digestion) to slow, in an effort to conserve energy for more important tasks.

- **Organ-system:** The heat-regulating mechanism in your brain signals your skin capillaries to constrict and keep more blood located centrally in your body, where it is warmer. Your brain triggers shivering to generate heat from your muscles.

- **Psychological:** You worry that you might be freezing to death.

- **Interpersonal:** You ask, "May I borrow your coat?"

- **Social:** You say, "Let's get off this frozen lake and go home."

Voila! Your homeostasis is regained by your appropriate responses to stress.

Each time you are confronted by a stressful or threatening situation, your brain instructs your sympathetic nervous system to rapidly release stress hormones into your bloodstream, readying you to fight or flee. This served our distant ancestors very well when they were being charged by a woolly mammoth and it still works for us in emergencies. But most of the stresses we face don't actually require such extreme coping techniques. The fight-or-flight reaction is hard on your body and your health, which is why it's important to find ways to control your responses to stress, matching them to the actual magnitude of the threat.

Stress responses have more significance for women than for men because stress hormones stay in your bloodstream longer than in a man's (Harvard Women's Health Watch 1999). Stress hormones suppress your immune system; this means you are more at risk for infectious diseases and other illnesses if such episodes are frequent or chronic. Controlling the damage caused by these responses centers around first recognizing stress and then coping with it.

Recognizing Stress

It is often easier to recognize the symptoms of stress than its source. The symptoms may be emotional, physical, behavioral, or cognitive, and you may sometimes have symptoms in all of these categories. Take a look at Table 11.1 for a listing of some typical symptoms. The source of stress that generates these symptoms is sometimes obvious, such as loss of a family member, divorce, a job change, or moving to a new town. Some aren't so obvious. For example, biological changes due to estrogen decline can be sources of stress.

Table 11.1. Symptoms of Stress			
Emotional	**Physical**	**Behavioral**	**Cognitive**
Anxiety	Rapid heart rate	Critical of others	Forgetfulness
Nervousness	Restlessness	Can't get things done	Can't make decisions
Anger, acute or chronic	Headaches	Bossy with others	Fuzzy thinking
Irritability	Stomachaches	Overeating	Diminished creativity
Loneliness	Insomnia	Excess smoking	Lost sense of humor
Boredom with life	Sweaty palms	Overuse of alcohol	Constant worrying
Feeling pressured	Fatigue	Neglect of personal habits	Trouble concentrating
Fearfulness	Breathlessness	Decreased sexual desire	
Crying	Tension, neck and shoulders		
Unexplained sadness			

Adapted from: Benson and Stuart 1993

If you are also experiencing other biological changes (unrelated to hormones), such as graying of your hair, the need for glasses, and wrinkles, you might not recognize any one of them as a stressor. You may nevertheless feel stressed without other apparent causes. In this case, it could be that the aging process itself is unacceptable to you.

Whatever the cause of your stress, once you recognize it, you are in a much better position to effectively deal with it.

Tolerating Stress

Some people adapt to stress more naturally than others. One investigator (Kobasa 1982) refers to such people as having "stress-hardy" personalities. These individuals are able to experience stress without undergoing the typical physical or mental stress responses. People with stress-hardiness are characterized by three important attitudes : acceptance of life's challenges, a sense of control over its vagaries, and a commitment to their families, their work, and their life in general. They tend to take control of their lives instead of passively accepting their lot, and are more likely to regard challenges as opportunities for personal growth than as threats to be avoided or escaped. People who react to stress with an attitude of helplessness represent the opposite number of the stress-hardy. Most of us fall somewhere between these extremes.

Closeness is a fourth characteristic of the stress-hardy personality (Benson 1993). This refers to the ability to establish relationships in which a person can both provide and receive social support. This type of person appears to be much more stress-resistant than someone who feels isolated from personal contact.

As you may have begun to suspect, the larger view of stress is that it is not always bad for you. Your reaction to stress is what governs its effect on your life and your health. It makes sense to reduce heavily stressful influences in your life as much as you can and to learn strategies for coping with stress. But adopting a strategy of avoiding all stress may not make sense. Instead of regarding all stress in largely negative terms, you can try to perceive it as an exciting challenge—a stimulus to achievement. Actively coping with hardship (stress) challenges your intellect and engages your emotions. Indeed, you may obtain a more desirable result by changing your reaction to a stressful situation than by changing the situation itself.

Performance and efficiency increase as levels of anxiety and stress increase, but then, as stress continues to increase, performance and efficiency decline (Yerkes 1989). (Ever notice how a slightly messy office is the most productive one, or how happy seemingly disorganized families are?) The point is that total stress avoidance can be unhealthy. You do, however, need to know how to handle the heavy stuff.

Strategies for Coping with Stress

Effective coping is dependent on a number of factors, some of which we've already talked about in this book: a healthy diet, adequate exercise, relaxation techniques, and psychological adjustments that produce a positive attitude. Not all kinds of coping are equal, though. Eating a balanced diet is a good way of coping with stress; a food binge is not. Regular exercise is a good coping mechanism, but being a couch potato is a bad one.

Restoring homeostasis (balance) by psychological means involves what are called defense mechanisms. These relatively automatic mental maneuvers modulate the intensity of your emotional reaction to a stressful situation so that your behavior in dealing with it is appropriate. Good coping utilizes mature defenses, and poor coping uses immature defenses. Over the long term, poor coping can lead to a number of social maladjustments, such as chronic anger and estrangement. It also may lead to true psychological illnesses, such as depression and anxiety states.

Your built-in defense mechanisms help you counteract the everyday stresses of life: when you've misplaced your car keys, your child's soccer team just lost, or you have incinerated the family dinner. You may handle these stresses without even noticing how you did it. When the stresses are extreme (as when a spouse dies) or long lasting (you lose your job), they can overwhelm homeostasis, and their effects can become harmful to your health. There are several ways you can reduce the negative impact of stress.

Prioritize the Tasks That Face You

Sometimes your stressor is not a major one, but an accumulation of little things that are annoying. They may have taken months or years to pile up on you, or maybe the list just started yesterday morning. Try ranking these tasks into categories according to their relative priority: (1) essential, (2) important, and (3) trivial. A good way to assign rank is to ask yourself: "What is the worst that could happen if I don't get this done?" You'll find that many things you first thought were crucial, just aren't. Concentrate on the essential items, delegate to others as many of the important tasks as possible, and ignore the trivial stuff altogether (Landau 1994). When assigning priorities to your list, be sure to include "time for myself" near the top of your "essential" column. Even if it is for only a few minutes, plan something that pleases you and is just for you—perhaps luxuriating in a warm bath.

Eat a Healthful Diet

If you are under stress, you may be too distracted to focus on your nutritional needs. Nevertheless, good nutrition is more important than ever; stress raises your metabolic rate and increases your energy needs. A diet emphasizing complex carbohydrates that are high in fiber diminishes PMS because of the calming effect from increased serotonin. It works for stress control as well.

Get Regular Exercise

Aerobic exercise provides a useful outlet for your fight-or-flight energy. Endorphins released during vigorous exercise elevate your mood, leaving you in a state of natural relaxation at the end of your workout. Your blood pressure declines, your pulse rate decreases, your muscles become relaxed, and tension is released. You will sleep better, and your mind will also participate in the general relaxation. Exercising for stress relief is most beneficial if you do it twice daily for about thirty minutes: A brisk walk will do nicely, and it can also qualify as time for yourself. Remember that exercising just before bedtime can prevent sleep.

Get Plenty of Rest

Insomnia is a common accompaniment to stress. Insomnia causes chronic fatigue, which can be an additional stressor. Prescription sleeping pills can provide relief in acute situations, but many are addicting and they become less effective over time. You can also become dependent on over-the-counter sleeping aids. For problems with early awakening, two new nonaddicting sleeping medications may help. Zaleplon (Sonata) and zolpidem (Ambien) provide continued sleep with no daytime sedative effect or rebound insomnia. Regular exercise can contribute to your sleeping well. In addition, consider the following recommendations for helping you sleep (Benson 1993):

- **Spend less time in bed:** The average adult needs only seven to seven and a half hours (Hauri 1990). Spending too much time in bed is a mistake if you have problems with insomnia.

- **Eat a light carbohydrate snack an hour or two before bed:** A snack such as cookies or cereal may help to increase your production of serotonin, which promotes sleep.

- **Control your sleeping room:** It should be dark, quiet, and reasonably cool. Pull the shades, wear eye covers, and use ear plugs if necessary to manage your sleeping environment.

- **Maintain a sleeping schedule:** Go to bed and get up at the same time every day. Your body will accommodate to your schedule.

- **Avoid caffeine late in the day:** Coffee, tea, and colalike soft drinks are the chief suppliers of this sleep-robbing stimulant.

- **Use your bed exclusively for sleep:** Except for having sex, of course. Don't eat, watch TV, talk on the phone, or work in bed.

Look for Social Support

The transitional years can be accompanied by some major life stresses: divorce, infidelity, work dislocation, children leaving home, financial problems, or single parenthood. Joining a group of women who are facing similar problems can reduce your stress significantly. Support groups for various health concerns abound in most communities. Find them through newspaper listings, community hospitals, religious organizations, mental health clinics, and the ever-reliable word of mouth.

Learn Some Relaxation Techniques

There are a number of relaxation techniques from which to choose. Deep breathing is simple, yet effective. Other methods include meditation, self-hypnosis, biofeedback, yoga, t'ai chi, massage, visualization and guided imagery, acupuncture, and acupressure. Find out what works for you. The goal of all of them is to elicit what Benson (1993) calls the "relaxation response": You diminish your oxygen consumption and decrease your breathing rate, heart rate, and blood pressure. This is the opposite of what happens during a fight-or-flight stress response.

Deep Breathing

Deep breathing is one of the most widely used methods to relax. (It helps hot flashes too.) It is often the starting point for other relaxation techniques, such as meditation, visualization, and yoga. To elicit the relaxation response, try this:

- Seat yourself comfortably in a quiet room and close your eyes.

- Relax all of your muscle groups by consciously thinking of them one at a time. (See the next section.)

- Breathe in and out slowly through your nose, and concentrate on the air you are moving both into and out of your body.

- Repeat a neutral word or phrase silently. This repetition tends to keep extraneous thoughts out of your mind.

- Allow about ten to twenty minutes to complete this routine.

- At the end, sit quietly for another minute or two before slowly opening your eyes.

Progressive Muscle Relaxation

Progressive muscle relaxation is a great way to relieve muscle tension. Alternately tense and relax all muscle groups in your body, starting with your toes and feet and progressing through your calves, thighs, buttocks, back, hands, arms, neck, and face. It is most effective if you start with slow breathing. This routine takes ten or fifteen minutes to complete, so be sure to allow for enough solitude to do it. Try this technique a couple of times a day.

Meditation

Meditation is a well-known alternative in relieving a wide variety of ailments, and stress relief is not the least of them. Meditation uses the breathing techniques we have already covered. It often involves repeating a mantra (word or phrase) and incorporates various other relaxation methods.

Meditation helps you learn to have a quiet inner self and to live more actively in the moment. You may become both more alert and energetic and more serene. You can meditate sitting or lying down, while enjoying a peaceful walk, or even during other forms of exercise. It takes some training to get started, so look for a beginner's class at your community center, church, or local mental health clinic.

If you decide to try meditation, make a commitment of several months. It can take this long before you appreciate the positive effects it can have on your life.

Visualization and Guided Imagery

Visualization is a way of filling your mind with a relaxing image. You close your eyes, doing the deep breathing exercise we've already described, and focus on an image of utter serenity or profound joy—perhaps a past event in your life that made you feel that way. Think about every detail of the event: the time of day it happened, the surroundings, who was there, what was said, what you were wearing, how it felt, how it smelled, what you were feeling. If focusing on an actual event doesn't work for you, guided imagery can help. This involves listening to a voice, either in person or on tape, that helps you create an image of serenity in your mind.

Hypnosis can also be used as a form of guided imagery. It is a safe and effective means of relaxing, but it requires the help of someone specifically trained. You can also learn to relax using self-hypnosis.

Laughter

Humor is a proven stress reliever, both psychologically and physiologically. A good laugh relaxes muscles, oxygenates your system, lowers blood pressure, and has a unique ability to defuse a confrontation. As Victor Borge observed: "Humor is the shortest distance between two people." Look for the humor in seemingly sober moments; there usually is a thread of it somewhere. Start remembering jokes people tell you, then retell them with your own embellishments. Keep a scrapbook of really great jokes or cartoons you see in newspapers and magazines and look through it when you need a grin. Make a point of seeing funny movies—the laughter of an audience is infectious.

A good sense of humor is available at a moment's notice to improve your mood, defuse a confrontation, lower your blood pressure, and relieve your anxiety. Here is a five-point plan for improving your health and your life with laughter (Wilde 1997):

- **Laugh out loud:** Physically laughing increases your oxygenation, improves your circulation, lowers your blood pressure, and even has a positive influence on your immune system. Laughter and longevity apparently go hand-in-hand: George Burns made it to 100, Lucille Ball to her late seventies, and Bob Hope, Milton Berle, and Red Skelton all survived to advanced ages.

- **Laugh at yourself:** At its roots, laughter is an expression of love. If you can laugh at your own shortcomings, you basically like yourself. Abraham Lincoln, never known as a handsome man, said when he was accused of being two-faced: "If I had two faces, would I be showing you this one?" Abe was comfortable with himself.

- **Maintain a lighthearted attitude:** Attitude is a choice you make, so why not make it upbeat? A joyful spirit makes you more productive, helps control stress, and defuses resentment. When things are tense, open a joke book or listen to a tape; and then see how smoothly things go afterward.

- **Find something funny every day:** Some days you may have to dig pretty deep to find something funny; life is like that. Maybe it will be only a cartoon in the newspaper, but find something.

- **Find the funny side of life even when you are up to your neck in alligators:** You might as well laugh instead of cry. A famous humorist wrote that just as life does not cease to be funny when we have a serious problem, life does not cease to be serious when we laugh.

Laughter is good for you. It doesn't cost a dime, is tax-free, fat-free, cholesterol-free, and nontoxic. Humorist Josh Billings said: "There ain't much fun in medicine, but there's a heck of a lot of medicine in fun."

Religion

Many people benefit from a commitment to a formal religion and a deeply felt set of values and beliefs. By this time in life, you may be starting to become aware of your own mortality. Religious traditions and beliefs can provide a sense of depth and meaning at a time in life when you have acquired the wisdom to appreciate them. A commitment to religion can help you develop an awareness of a larger reality and promote your understanding of life's meaning (Moyers 1993). The peace you derive from this kind of awareness is a good antidote for stress.

Yoga

Yoga is a system of physical exercises, postures, and stretching combined with deep breathing that requires you to focus on your body. You may discover that yoga is not just a wonderful way to relax, but is also a way to improve flexibility in your body. Look for yoga classes at your local community college or on videotape. (It is probably a good idea to start with a class to learn the basics.)

T'ai Chi

T'ai chi ("tie-chee") is a discipline of exercise and breathing that originated in China. It means "Salute to the Sun" and is the exercise of choice for aging Asians to greet the new day. T'ai chi emphasizes breathing, body alignment, and flexibility, which makes it similar to yoga. The difference is that the techniques of t'ai chi are designed to stimulate your body as well as to relax it, which is why it is an effective way to start your day. It is becoming increasingly popular in the U.S., so look for announcements and ads for local classes.

Acupuncture

Acupuncture is an ancient Chinese technique wherein tiny needles are inserted at specific locations to positively alter the flow of energy, called qi ("chee"). It works for many people to advance healing, promote overall well-being, and induce relaxation. The benefit you receive is dependent upon the skill of the practitioner, so be sure you see a licensed acupuncturist. Acupressure, a similar technique, applies pressure, but not needles, to the appropriate locations.

Massage

Massage can be an extremely pleasurable and relaxing experience. You can learn many of the various techniques yourself using a book or video, but it is probably better to start with a professional. You can often find massage therapists at beauty salons and health clubs. Mutual massage is a good option; in addition to its relaxing benefits, it can provide an affectionate and romantic interlude for you and your partner. Many women also find it relaxing to have a facial performed by an experienced and sensitive esthetician.

Hot Tubs and Saunas

Hot tubs and saunas feel great after a workout, or even if you just want to relax before going to bed. Usually, about fifteen minutes in water or air around a hundred degrees is all it takes.

CAUTION! After exercising, avoid water or a sauna that is too hot; it can divert too much blood from your central circulation into your skin and cause you to faint. If you have not cooled down after exercise or you have just consumed a large meal (which concentrates blood in your abdomen for digestion), entering a hot tub or sauna can lower your blood pressure sufficiently to cause fainting. So tubbing or taking a sauna alone is not always a good idea.

Biofeedback

Biofeedback is a method of inducing relaxation that uses various recording devices to monitor heart rate, blood pressure, and skin responses. When you are tense, the recordings are dramatically different from when you are relaxed. Biofeedback teaches you to identify tension in your body. Then, using visualization, guided imagery, and other relaxation techniques, you can monitor whether, and how much, your tension is being relieved. In this fashion you are taught how to do it for yourself.

Psychotherapy

Short-term therapy with a psychologist (rather than a psychiatrist, whose training is in mental illness) is less structured and more personalized than most of the above techniques. A major goal of stress management is to first identify the stressor; you may need some counseling to help identify it.

Many health-care professionals and their patients rely on prescription drugs for managing stress. Use of tranquilizers and antidepressants for stress management may be regarded by some as "avoidance," but these drugs may be useful in acute and chronic situations.

Beyond Stress—Psychiatric Illnesses

If a healthful diet, exercise, relaxation techniques, and other psychological adjustments are not successful in controlling your stress, it may be that you are suffering from a more serious mental illness, such as major depression, one of a variety of anxiety states, or panic attacks. If the causes of your stress have long passed but the symptoms of stress persist and are causing serious disruptions in your life—perhaps making it impossible for you to work or threatening the functioning of your family—you may have a significant problem that requires professional intervention. Let's examine two of these illnesses so you'll know what to look for—or better yet, what you probably don't have to worry about.

Major Depression

"Depression" is one of the most hard working words in our culture. We use it to describe everything from economic hard times to weather conditions to a bad hair day. Like most people, you probably have occasional bouts of the blues, short-lived episodes of moodiness, discouragement, sadness, or loneliness. These are a normal part of life, and they are referred to as minor depression. For the most part, minor depression is self-limiting and does not pose a health threat. We can cope with it.

Serious depression that just doesn't go away is major depression, a true psychiatric illness requiring psychotherapy and antidepressant medication. Depressive disorders are characterized by a persisting disturbance of mood, a loss of sense of control, and intense mental, emotional, and physical anguish, and they disrupt relationships, family, job, and social functioning (Depression Guideline Panel 1993). The American Psychiatric Association categorizes severe depression in two ways: major depression, also known as unipolar depression, and manic-depressive illness, now known as bipolar depression. We'll look at bipolar depression in the next section.

The lifetime chances of your dying during a major depression are greater than your lifetime risk for dying from breast cancer, due to to the 15 percent suicide rate among untreated depressives. It's a serious disorder (Gise 1996).

Diagnosis of Major Depression

The *Diagnostic and Statistical Manual of Mental Disorders* outlines some markers for major depression. Two factors are (1) feeling depressed most of the day, nearly every day and (2) taking markedly diminished (or no) interest or pleasure in most or all activities, most of the day, nearly every day. If you have either of these symptoms together with at least three of the following, you may have a major depression:

- Significant weight loss or gain (about 5 percent in a month) even when you are not dieting, or increased or decreased appetite nearly every day.

- Insomnia or hypersomnia (sleeping too much) nearly every day.

- Psychomotor (mental and physical) agitation or retardation nearly every day.

- Fatigue or loss of energy nearly every day.

- Feelings of worthlessness; excessive or inappropriate guilt nearly every day.

- Diminished ability to think or concentrate, or indecisiveness nearly every day.

- Recurrent thoughts of death (not just fear of dying); recurrent suicidal thoughts without a specific plan; a suicide attempt; or a plan for suicide.

(Note: Hypothyroidism, unrecognized diabetes, adrenal disorders and other metabolic illnesses can mimic depression, and they must be considered before a diagnosis of depression is reached.)

CAUTION! If the above describes you, or comes even close, you may be suffering from major depression. Since only 20 to 25 percent of those who meet the above criteria receive appropriate treatment (McGrath 1990), we urge you to avoid inadequate treatment and seek immediate help from a physician experienced in diagnosing and treating depression.

Causes and Risk Factors

A number of factors may predispose you to depression (McGrath 1990):

- A childhood loss, such as death or prolonged illness of a parent, or divorced parents.

- Physical or sexual abuse by a parent, spouse, or partner. Twenty-five percent of depressed women were sexually abused as children.

- Low self-esteem.

- Socioeconomic deprivation. Inadequate education plays a major role.

- Family history of depression. In some families it occurs generation after generation.

- Stress from multiple lifestyle roles, such as spouse, mother, homemaker, occupation outside the home, community responsibilities.

- Unhappy marriage or unhappy divorce.

- Young children at home.

- Recent childbirth. Up to 8 to 10 percent of mothers with new babies suffer major depressive symptoms (O'Hara 1991).

- Bodily disfigurement from trauma or surgery.

Depression was considered solely a psychiatric illness until abnormalities in serotonin were revealed in the 1990s. Depression is now believed to be caused by an imbalance in brain chemicals: Too many serotonin receptor sites on brain cells remain empty. In women with such an imbalance, the predisposing factors mentioned above influence the likelihood and severity of depression (ACOG 1993).

Hormonal change may influence major depression. Perimenopausal symptoms such as hot flashes, which disturb sleep, can contribute to depression (Sherwin 1993). Symptoms of major depression are much more pervasive, severe, and disruptive than those of perimenopause; do not confuse the two. There appears to be a slight increase of the rate of depression in transitional women. The stress induced by perimenopausal changes may trigger a major depression in a woman who is already teetering on the brink of it, but it is rare for perimenopausal symptoms to be a solitary cause.

Hypoglycemia, or a low glucose level in the blood, is a common cause of depressionlike symptoms. Brain function is hampered by low glucose levels, creating such symptoms as irritability, fatigue, anxiety, headaches, and depression. Removing refined carbohydrates from the diet is often enough to solve this problem (Notelovitz 1993). Food allergies can play a major role for people suffering from depression (Ojeda 1995). If your therapist can't get a handle on why you are depressed, this would be a reasonable avenue to explore.

About 5 to 10 percent of all women experience major depression at some time, regardless of age (McKinley 1987). There is a slight increase in the rate of depression during the perimenopausal transition, but women over age forty-five have less depression than younger women. The profile of a women at risk for depression is someone who has children under age five at home, is divorced or has a poor relationship, has less than a high school education, and is undergoing economic hardship—any of which might be true of any contemporary transitional women.

There appears to be a gender difference in the incidence of major depression. A study of major depression in North America, Europe, the Middle East, Asia, and the Pacific Rim (Weissman 1996) found that women are more likely to experience major depression than men. In North America, the incidence in women is twice as high as in men. The gender difference for women begins at puberty and ends at menopause. Around the age when women go through menopause, rates of depression become higher in men.

The differing ways women and men define themselves may help explain the gender difference. Psychologically, women tend to define themselves primarily through their relationships with other people: partners, children, family members, friends, coworkers (Kaplan 1986). Relationship problems are common sources of depression for women. Women may turn inward and examine their responsibility for a relationship gone awry (Nolen-Hoeksema 1987). This tendency to analyze relationships, if combined with little power to create a positive change, can lead to feelings of helplessness, despair, and depression. On the other hand, men tend to define themselves on the basis of physical ability, sexual prowess, occupational success, and societal impact. When stressful problems arise in these areas, men tend to turn outward, becoming involved with hobbies, sports, other women, more work, and other distracting pursuits. This difference may in part explain why men have a lower rate of depression than women before midlife.

To summarize, there are multiple bio-psycho-sociological factors that put you at risk for major depression. You and your health-care adviser must take all of them into account if you are experiencing major depression.

Treatment of Major Depression

People suffering from depression are often embarrassed by their perceived "weakness." In addition, far too many depression sufferers and their physicians erroneously believe that a pep talk about keeping your chin up is all you need. Unfortunately, failure to get proper treatment usually results in prolonged suffering, lost productivity, and a severely diminished quality of life. The good news is that major depression is treatable.

Treatment is successful for 70 percent who use antidepressant medications, and the success rate is higher still if psychotherapy is used in addition (Gise 1996). Major advances in the understanding of the neurobiology of depression have led to the development of newer and safer antidepressant medications. The serotonin-booster medications prescribed for major depression, such as Prozac, Zoloft, Paxil, and Serzone have been especially helpful for women whose depression has been aggravated by the serotonin-lowering effect of diminished estrogen.

Make sure your physician or therapist knows of any relationship problems you are having; strong relationships are a core constituent of your well-being. It is also important to disclose any history of depression in your biological family, and your use of alcohol, prescription drugs (including HRT and high blood pressure medications, which can influence depression), and over-the-counter and street drugs.

What You Can Do to Diminish Your Symptoms

In addition to treatment by a nonphysician therapist or psychiatrist, there are steps you can take on your own to alleviate the symptoms of a major depression. Here are some suggestions:

- **Incorporate healthy habits:** As in treatment for stress, a healthy diet, regular exercise, relaxation techniques, and support groups are important parts of the mix in dealing with major depression.

- **Avoid isolation:** A family member, your physician, a member of the clergy, or a trusted friend can all serve the need you have for a close and intimate human contact.

- **Avoid self-treatment:** Persistent fatigue from lack of sleep may tempt you to power up during the day with caffeine or sweets. At night a couple of cocktails or some wine may seem to be the way to relax. Tranquilizers or sleeping pills at bedtime might help you get to sleep. All these are only avoidance techniques, and they do not help depression.

Major depression is a highly treatable, biologically based disorder. If you are aware of the symptoms and knowledgeable about the availability of treatment, you can get help early if you need it.

CAUTION! SAMe (S-adenosylmethionine) is one of the hottest nonprescription supplements on the market for depression. It is not an herb, hormone, vitamin, or any sort of nutrient. SAMe is a chemical produced naturally in all animals, and known to be essential to many biochemical processes including substances vital to transmission of nerve impulses and influencing emotions and moods (Wellness Letter 2000). In the U.S., an unregulated supplement; it's strictly a prescription product in Europe. It is being promoted here as a nearly magical treatment for depression, arthritis, and liver disease. Though more than forty studies have shown SAMe to be effective for depression, almost all have used intravenous administration. In the oral form, it is poorly absorbed and less than 1 percent becomes bioavailable (Gaster 1999). SAMe is transformed into homocysteine in the body, which raises a concern because homocysteine is implicated in the development of atherosclerosis and coronary heart disease (Eikelboom 1999). It may harm people with bipolar disorder by inducing mania. SAMe is also expensive, averaging $240 for a thirty-day supply. For these reasons oral SAMe cannot currently be recommended for treatment of depression.

Bipolar Depression (Manic-Depressive Disorder)

Bipolar depression, which affects women and men equally, is characterized by cycles of alternating depression and elation. Changing from the trough to the peak is usually gradual, but occasionally it can be dramatic and rapid. Symptoms of the manic phase include hyperactivity, decreased sleep, decreased appetite, racing thoughts, and psychotic behavior, as well as inordinate elation, grandiose notions, disconnected thoughts, inappropriate social behavior, poor judgment, nonstop talking, irritability, and a startling increase in sexual desire. During the depressive cycle, you may experience all the symptoms of major depression.

Bipolar depression, like major depression, is related to chemical imbalances in the brain's neurotransmitters. There are also emotional and situational factors, such as an upsetting life experience, substance abuse, lack of sleep, or other situations resulting in excessive stimulation. When these factors are present in a person with bipolar disorder, the normal brain mechanisms for restoring calm functioning don't always work properly. It is therefore not surprising that treatment involves a combination of medication (Tegretol, Depakote, lithium), psychotherapy, and support groups.

On average, people with bipolar disorder see three to four doctors and spend over eight years seeking treatment before a correct diagnosis is made (Consensus Treatment Guidelines for Bipolar Disorder 1996). Earlier diagnosis and proper treatment can help prevent the following:

- Suicide—the rate is highest in the initial years of illness

- Alcohol/substance abuse—which occurs in over 50 percent

- Marital problems and work problems

- More difficult treatment if the illness has been of long standing

- Incorrect, inappropriate, or partial treatment if bipolar disorder is mistaken as depression alone. Antidepressants without antimanic medication make the overall illness worse.

The National Depressive and Manic-Depressive Association (NDMDA) has chapters throughout the country that sponsor support groups and provide lending libraries, as well as medical advisors and facilitators. To find out if there is an NDMDA chapter near you, refer to the Appendix.

Summary

Stress is an unavoidable fact of living. In some ways, stress plays a positive role in your life, requiring you to evolve with changing circumstances. However, when stressors start to threaten your equanimity, it is crucial to recognize and take steps to cope with them; your physical and emotional health may be on the line. You can use a variety of coping techniques to bolster your ability to handle stress positively.

Sometimes, though, you may be overwhelmed by events to the point where major depression or other mental illnesses result. Fortunately, a number of treatments are available if mental illness does strike.

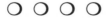

Section III

Making Change Easy

12

Sexuality: Good Sex Doesn't Need to Change

Sexuality is more than the biological urge to reproduce. It involves the time-less desire for emotional and physical intimacy. Sex can be one of the most gratifying experiences that life has to offer at any age. With maturity, sexuality can be expressed in a variety of ways, including shared interests, companionship, and holding hands at the movies as well as by sexual intercourse. Sex, like your body, changes as you progress through life, but the desire to be sexual is never extinguished for most people.

This chapter begins with a discussion of the all-important role of psychological factors in your sex life. Emotions such as attitude and self-image are crucial to your sexual enjoyment. Then we take a look at certain biological factors that may have a negative impact on your sexual pleasure, and how to deal with these changes in ways that protect your sexuality. Armed with this information, you can proceed with confidence toward (and beyond) menopause with your sexuality intact.

Sexual Desire

Sexual desire, or libido, is a blending of several diverse influences:

- Hormone production, which accelerates at puberty, causing sexual organ development and body growth

- Testosterone production, resulting in fantasies in both genders

- Psychological development, which contributes to knowledge and attitudes about sexuality

- The social influences of cultural, religious, and family perceptions of sexuality

- Physical development and general health

Libido is the net effect of these influences, resulting in sexual fantasies, sexual arousal, and the motivation to have sex.

Psychological Influences on Sexual Desire

Your brain is the most important and sensitive sexual organ throughout your life. Many women lose their sexual desire solely because of psychological influences. They are often so pervasive, you may not even recognize their presence, let alone their influences on your sexuality.

Psychiatrists and sex therapists believe that the most influential factors by far are psychological. Attitude is the keystone of a healthy libido, so let's talk about some things that influence your attitude toward sex.

Past Experience

If sex has been an enjoyable and integral part of your life, your sexual desire should persist in spite of the biological changes that perimenopause and menopause bring.

Some women at midlife no longer want sex. This may be due to past experiences such as cultural and religious influences, trauma, and relationship problems. If your desire for sex has diminished or if sex has never been enjoyable or fulfilling for you, the biological changes of late perimenopause and menopause may provide a convenient reason to opt out of being sexually active.

TIP! One-quarter to one-third of adult women endured childhood sexual abuse (Lechner 1993; Russell 1986). Many women who had such childhood experiences often do not remember them until they are over forty. If you are a victim, you may just now be finding out about or remembering it.

The complicated emotions such as guilt and anger that result from childhood sexual abuse and adult memory can interfere with your sex life in some very specific ways. Women who were sexually abused often have a difficult time trusting their sexual partners, even though they love them, because love was associated with pain when they were children.

There may be physical symptoms as well. You may have pain or insufficient lubrication of your vagina when you try to have sex. You may experience vaginal muscle spasm called vaginismus; vaginal penetration during vaginismus is extremely painful or simply impossible. More than 35 percent of women who experience abdominal and pelvic pain with sex were the victims of sexual abuse as children (Lechner 1993). Nevertheless, these symptoms can be from a variety of causes other than childhood abuse, so be cautious in reaching this conclusion.

If you believe you have a history of childhood sexual abuse, get professional help. The complicated problems arising from childhood sexual abuse often take years of therapy and hard work to resolve.

Stress

If you are worried about a serious illness, a family crisis, or a financial problem, having sex may be very low on your agenda of important things to do. Solving the problem usually restores your sexual desire.

Depression

Depression may have a dampening effect on sexual desire. In addition depression is associated with changes in the adrenal hormone cortisol. This in turn can diminish pituitary production of FSH and LH, causing an adverse effect on ovarian secretion of your sex hormones. Bingo—depressed sexual desire. Effective treatment of depression restores desire for most women.

Physical Vitality

You already know, from earlier chapters, many good reasons to remain physically active and in good physical health. Here is one more: Sexual desire can remain high if you feel physically fit.

Routinized Sex

If you are in a long-term relationship, sex may get boring. If romance, sensuality, and intimacy are left out, sexual desire may wither. You may start blaming your slumping sexual desire on PMS or on perimenopause and diminishing hormone levels. You may blame your partner for your dampened desire.

To escape this situation, some women (and men) seek a new sex partner or turn more to self-stimulation. These methods of dealing with decreased sexual desire can lead to misgivings and feelings of guilt. Instead, try using differing positions, lubricants, sexy lighting and music, and more verbalizing. Heed your fantasies and allow them to lead you. Make a date for having sex, and be sure to keep it. After one or two such encounters, you may rediscover the magic.

Self-Image

Another psychological challenge for women in the perimenopausal years is to resist the cultural stereotype of what constitutes a sexy woman. Worry about physical attractiveness quickly translates to worry about sexual attractiveness, and dampens desire. Your body is not like it was two decades ago. This is true of men, too, of course, but it is culturally more acceptable to be a man whose hair is graying and whose middle is growing than to be a woman with physical characteristics of midlife. Your healthy sexual desire is intimately involved with your understanding that good sex does not require a perfect body.

Culturally imposed distortion of self-image commonly results in eating disorders (anorexia, bulimia, fad dieting). Weight loss from these disorders can adversely affect hormones throughout the body. A weight level as little as 10 percent below ideal body weight can be enough to shut down ovarian function, with cessation of menstrual periods and lessened production of estrogen and testosterone (Reichman 1998), curbing sexual desire.

Partner Availability

Sexually inactive women report their sexual desire progressively recedes (Bachman 1991). The same appears to be true for women who have partners but have infrequent sex. Sexual desire, multifaceted though it may be, is dramatically influenced by your partner's demonstrations of sexual interest in you. For example, if your partner is having erection problems, he may be profoundly embarrassed by and reluctant to display his incapacity. Though his interest in you sexually may be undiminished, you may interpret this behavior as a symptom of disinterest. Your self-esteem may be damaged, causing sexual desire to plummet. A number of other issues can be at the root of infrequent sex; good communication between you and your partner is essential for dealing with them.

Biological Influences on Sexual Desire

Along with the significant psychological factors we have described, a broad range of biological factors influence sexual desire. While these factors can have a potent effect on your desire, they are not nearly as influential as your sexual attitude.

What Is Sexual Response?

According to the landmark work of Masters and Johnson (1966) female response to sexual stimulation falls into four stages:

- **Sexual excitement:** Sexual excitement can begin in any number of ways—with fantasies, hugs, stroking, whispered endearments. Your pelvic blood vessels dilate and congest the region with blood. Vaginal lubrication results, as very slick secretions pour out through your vaginal walls. Muscles throughout your body begin to tense.

- **Plateau:** In the plateau phase, your sexual arousal increases dramatically. Your clitoris, becomes enlarged from blood engorgement and exquisitely sensitive to being touched. The folds at the entrance of your vagina (labia) become swollen from blood engorgement. Your heart rate and rate of breathing increase, and you may be perspiring. Your upper vagina becomes dilated and lengthened, while the muscles surrounding your lower vagina tense.

- **Orgasm:** This is the climactic moment, or moments, of sexual response. The physical and emotional excitement generated is maximized and you may feel compelled to relinquish your sense of control. Rhythmic contractions occur in your uterus and lower vagina. There may be multiple orgasmic peaks or a single intense one.

- **Resolution:** During resolution, pelvic vascular congestion promptly subsides. You are engulfed in a feeling of profound relaxation during which peace and warmth and closeness may be maximal. A few moments of hypersensitivity may occur occasionally in your vaginal lips, and particularly your clitoris, during which you are too sensitive to be further stimulated. Once this passes, repeat arousal and additional orgasms are possible.

This four-stage pattern of sexual response remains generally unchanged throughout life, although individual components may vary as time passes. What excited you sexually at twenty may be very different from what works a couple of decades later. Lubrication may take longer. Reaching an orgasm may also take longer, be less intense, and occur less reliably, and the intensity may change from rocketlike to Roman-candlesque. The number of orgasmic contractions may diminish. During your perimenopausal years, none of these may be an issue. If they are, there are many steps you can take to manage them. As for those postmenopausal years down the road, take comfort in knowing that women at any age can enjoy sex.

Better Sex Through Chemistry

Sexual desire is an urge that motivates women (and men) to seek out, initiate, and engage in sexual activity. But sexual desire is not merely a subjective sensation or simply a cognitive event. It is modified by social behavior, as well as by neurotransmitters and hormones. For example, women generally have a higher level of sexual interest at the midpoint of their cycle, when production of sex hormones is at their peak. Let's look at the role of hormones, and some nonhormonal drugs and other products in sexual desire.

The Role of Male Hormone

A landmark 1985 study on sex hormones divided women whose ovaries had been removed into four groups. Each one of four types of medication: estrogen, testosterone, a combination, or a placebo (Sherwin). The groups on testosterone or estrogen plus testosterone reported an increased level of desire, arousal, and sexual fantasizing, while those on estrogen or a placebo did not.

Testosterone, according to this study and others since (North American Menopause Society 1998), is the hormone behind sexual desire. By contrast, estrogen's role is more closely connected to physical aspects of sexuality, such as vaginal lubrication, other arousal responses, and orgasm (Sarrel 1990). Estrogen mediates these responses through receptor sites on the nerves that supply your vagina, clitoris, and other pelvic structures. By contrast, testosterone mediates its effects directly on receptor sites in your brain. These studies and others have resulted in the increasingly common use of testosterone to boost female sexual interest and fantasizing. Acknowledged criteria for use of testosterone replacement therapy (TRT) are (Beck 1995):

• Significant loss of libido—no motivation, fantasies, or arousal

• Global libido loss—nothing and nobody is a turn-on

• Diminished sense of well-being

• Inability to become aroused, no matter what

• Significant loss of nipple and/or clitoral sensitivity

• Inability to have orgasm, or severely diminished orgasm quality

• Loss of pubic hair

• Fatigue, depression, irritability, nervousness, insomnia, or poor concentration

When TRT is appropriately used, you can expect improvement in most of the above areas.

DHEA (dehydroepiandrosterone) is a weak male hormone that has been the subject of much hype and promotion in the food supplement industry as a fountain-of-youth additive. While small studies to date have shown an improved sense of well-being with DHEA, most have not shown a direct effect on sexual motivation and fantasies (Morales 1994). One recent study did find improved sexual desire with DHEA (Arlt 1999).

Sexual problems from lowered hormone levels are not common during perimenopause, but there are exceptions: If your ovaries have been removed or if you are taking low-dose birth-control pills, you may need a testosterone supplement to maintain normal levels of sexual desire. The Pill lowers free testosterone levels.

The Role of Estrogen

The functioning of your clitoris, vulva, vagina, and uterus depends upon estrogen support. When estrogen is withdrawn, there is a 60 percent decrease in the blood supply to the genital area and these structures undergo atrophic changes. Such changes can have an adverse impact on sexual arousal and pleasure.

Your vagina may be the first to complain of estrogen decline. Diminished blood supply causes thinning of your vaginal lining and a reduction in mucus production. Long before your doctor can see any evidence of thinning, you may notice a reduction in moisture. After menopause, if you take no preventive measures, these changes can become more extreme. Your vagina can eventually lose up to 90 percent of its thickness, as well as most of its elasticity (Sachs 1991) making sex very painful.

Vulvar changes from estrogen deficiency are slow and subtle also, and mainly postmenopausal. The skin covering labia becomes thin and inelastic. Fatty tissue is lost and the labia appear shrunken. There is less pubic hair. Vulvar dryness may cause an itchy condition, called pruritis.

With estrogen depletion, your uterus, including your cervix, also shrinks over time. In rare cases, painful uterine contractions occur during orgasm. Your clitoris will also have fewer functioning nerve fibers, so it will be less sensitive to stimulation.

Other estrogen-related changes can also interfere with your sex life. For example, if hot flashes are depriving you of sleep, you may be too tired to enjoy sex. Or your sensory perceptions may be altered since an adequate estrogen level is a factor in the sensitivity of skin nerves.

Don't panic over all this information—the changes we've described are slow to develop; and may not become bothersome until after menopause. Even if you are taking oral estrogen though, you may need topical estrogen to prevent or reverse these atrophic changes.

Nonhormonal Drugs

Sildenafil (Viagra) has been successful in treating erectile dysfunction in men, so it is being studied in women as well. As expected from its chemical makeup, Viagra increases blood flow to female genitals, resulting in better vaginal lubrication and clitoral engorgement, although improved orgasms were not observed (Meston 1996). In a small study of women whose libido was suppressed by antidepressant drugs, Viagra improved libido, vaginal lubrication, and orgasmic response (Nurnberg 1999).

Herbs

Ginseng was reported to improve erections and libido in men, but women were not studied (Reichman 1996). The exclusion of women may stem from the fact that the word ginseng means "man root." Studies of women should obviously be done.

Black cohosh has been shown to improve hot flashes, sleep disruption, and vaginal dryness, all of which can cause decreased sexual desire. Elimination of these estrogen-deficiency symptoms can lead to improved sex.

Other herbs believed to be aphrodisiac are myrtle, sarsparilla, kava kava, echinacea, licorice, damiana, and dong quai. Thus far there has been no scientific evidence that they improve libido or sexual response.

Pheromones

Animals are attracted and aroused by scents they exude, called pheromones. The assumption that humans also have this capability has resulted in an array of products claiming to cause female arousal. Some manufacturers include DHEA, a weak male hormone, in their "pheromone" products, but so far there is no good science backing its effectiveness. On the other hand, researchers have tested a variety of scents and found that a combination of black licorice, cucumber, baby powder, lavender, and pumpkin pie caused increased female sexual arousal. Of these, black licorice with cucumber had the greatest effect, while cherry inhibited arousal. Men's cologne actually reduced female arousal (Azar 1998; Hirsch 1995).

In the future many other nonhormonal drugs and products may be found to be effective for improving sexual arousal and desire.

Medical Illness and Your Sex Life

A major physical illness at any age can affect both your interest in having sex and your physical ability to do so. If the illness is temporary, desire usually returns when you start feeling better. However, some chronic diseases may have long-term effects:

- **Arthritis and orthopedic problems:** Joint pain and reduced range of motion from arthritis and other orthopedic problems can interfere with the mechanics of having sex. Experiment with different positions, strategic use of pillows, and sensuous hot baths to accommodate your disability. (That might be interesting even if there are no orthopedic problems.)

- **Chronic heart or lung disease:** If you have severe heart or lung disease, you may be fearful that having sex can be dangerous to your health. In fact, this concern can come up in terms of any disease that makes you physically unfit. It may be helpful to know that the energy required to have sex is about the same as climbing two flights of stairs. Sex, of course, is generally a lot more fun.

- **Diabetes:** If poorly controlled, diabetes causes loss of orgasmic ability in about one-third of women within four to six years after diagnosis of the disease (Reichman 1996). It pays off sexually to take care of yourself if this disease is diagnosed. Diabetes in a man can also cause erectile dysfunction, which can drastically reduce sexual encounters for you.

- **Hypothyroidism:** Because hypothyroidism (which we talked about in Chapter 5) can cause profound fatigue and depression, it can also seriously dampen sexual interest and your ability to reach an orgasm. Low thyroid hormone levels depress your male hormone production, resulting in lessened sexual desire. Too much thyroid hormone may suppress ovulation and ovarian hormones. So one of the first tests to get if your libido has declined is a thyroid stimulating hormone (TSH) blood level.

- **Sexually transmitted disease (STD):** The effect of STDs on sexuality is uniformly negative. This can be from either the adverse symptoms an STD can cause (irritation, vaginal discharge, pain), or because of the fear of giving it to, or getting it from, a sex partner. Therefore, safe sex turns out to be the best sex.

- **Pain with sex:** Pain with sex, called dyspareunia, is the most common sexual complaint reported to gynecologists, occurring in 10 to 15 percent of women (Meana 1997). In 76 percent, the pain results from physical conditions such as vaginal infection, chronic inflammation of glands at the vaginal opening (vestibulitis), vaginal dryness or thinning from estrogen loss, vaginal muscle spasm (vaginismus), bladder or urethral infection, pelvic inflammatory disease (PID), endometriosis, and other forms of pelvic abnormalities. If pain with sex is your problem, you deserve a careful evaluation to determine the cause and appropriate treatment.

- **Erectile dysfunction (ED):** Few would dispute that ED can potentially curtail your opportunities for sexual encounters. There are other men, of course, but if your partner is a valued companion, his problem with ED is partly yours as well. Many factors can be involved in ED (Harvard Women's Health Watch 2000):
    - **Psychological.** Depression, anxiety, stress, and relationship problems account for 20 percent of ED.
    - **Medical.** Impaired blood flow to the penis from vascular disease, or nerve damage to the penis account for the other 80 percent of ED.
    - **Surgical.** Prostate surgery for benign enlargement results in ED for about 20 percent of men who have this procedure.

- **Drug side effects.** Antidepressants, tranquilizers, blood pressure drugs, alcohol, steroid abuse for muscle building, smoking, recreational drugs: Of the 80 percent of ED with a medical cause, one-quarter is related to drug side effects.

A wide variety of effective treatment modalities are available, up to and including Viagra, depending upon the underlying cause. Your understanding and support will be necessary adjuncts to his dealing successfully with ED.

Medications and Recreational Drugs

A variety of prescription and over-the-counter medicines, while helping one health problem, may be detrimental to your sexual health. Selective serotonin reuptake inhibitors (SSRIs—see Chapter 3), such as Prozac, Zoloft, and Paxil, may improve depression, but they cause a decreased sexual desire in up to 75 percent of users of either gender (Labbate 1994). Tranquilizers (Valium, Tranxene, Xanax) can relieve your stress in some ways, but they may create another stressful problem by blunting your sexual responsiveness. Beta-blockers (Lopressor, Inderal, Tenorman) are effective for lowering high blood pressure, but up to 50 percent of women and men who use beta-blockers in high doses experience lower sexual desire and lessened ability for arousal and orgasm (Medical Letter 1992).

Antihistamines do a good job of drying up a drippy nose or congested sinuses, but they may also cause vaginal dryness and decreased sexual lubrication. A variety of adverse effects on sexual functioning may occur with antacids (Tagamet, Pepcid, Zantac), the antialcohol drug disulfuram (Antabuse), the seizure control drug phenytoin (Dilantin), gemfibrozal (Lopid) for high cholesterol, and the anti-inflammatory drug naproxen (Anaprox, Naprosyn).

Alcohol can also cause sexual problems. It is well known to lower inhibitions, which may make you feel like you are about to be a sexual Olympian. However, arousal levels are actually lowered in about 40 percent of intoxicated people of both genders in spite of their feeling sexually uninhibited (Reichman 1996).

Marijuana, cocaine, heroin, and LSD may all produce a temporary increase in sexual desire and functioning ability, but chronic use and abuse can lead to significant sexual dysfunction.

Sex after Surgery

The major problems in the area of sex posed by major surgery are generally not that you will lose sexual capability through surgery; that seldom happens. The problems lie in what that surgery may do to your body image and self-esteem. For example, after a hysterectomy some women feel that they are no longer whole because they can no longer reproduce, and their partners may feel the same way.

If you have a hysterectomy, it may temporarily dampen desire because of postsurgical tenderness in your vagina. If this surgery results in shortening of your vagina (unlikely unless it is radical surgery for cancer), this may make sex feel different for a few weeks, until the vagina stretches. Some investigators feel that the cervix functions as a trigger for orgasm in about 10 percent of women and that uterine contractions are an integral part of orgasmic pleasure (Helstrom 1994). In spite of uterine loss, however, women who had good sex preoperatively still had it postoperatively. One study of 1,300 women who had hysterectomies for benign (noncancerous) conditions found that frequency of sex, vaginal lubrication, and orgasms all increased after recovery from the operation (Rhodes 1999). On the other hand, surgical removal of both ovaries (oophorectomy) eliminates your major source of estrogen and testosterone; sexual desire may plummet if estrogen and testosterone are not replaced.

Disfiguring surgery, such as a mastectomy or a colectomy followed by colostomy (removal of the colon and diversion of fecal material through the abdominal wall into a collecting receptacle) can have potent negative effects on self-image and desire. Surgical reconstruction of a new breast often helps in diminishing post-mastectomy emotional turmoil. Fortunately, most breast cancers are being treated by lumpectomy (removal of a cancerous lump with conservation of the breast), a less drastic measure.

Later in this chapter you'll find some suggestions for dealing with issues like these.

Some Keys to Good Sex

The perimenopausal years, and the entire process of aging, do not preclude your need for intimacy and sexual pleasure; these are lifelong. But unless you make the effort to understand and cope with the changes in your body, your sex life may suffer. Let's look at some things that can help you cope.

Communication

Communication is more than mere talking; it involves being understood and understanding in return. But communicating about sexual issues is often not easy. You may talk about it, read about it, see references to it on TV, and watch it on videotape. But that exposure does not necessarily make you able to communicate about the more important sexual issues, such as caring, sharing, intimacy, and personal sexual preferences. However, partners who do discuss sexual issues (what feels good, what doesn't, erection difficulties, lubrication) can do a great deal to resolve sexual problems.

In *Making Sense of Menopause*, author Faye Kitchner Cone presents guidelines for improving your ability to communicate. She calls this "getting your verbal juices flowing." To effectively communicate about a problem, you must be patient, caring, and open, and avoid a self-centered approach. The principles are as follows:

- **Enlist your partner as a fellow problem-solver.** Agree in advance that your goals are to improve mutual satisfaction and harmony. This gives you a common goal, the pursuit of which will promote a sense of intimacy.

- **Find out more about your partner's sexual needs and preferences.** It may be true that your unsatisfied needs and preferences are the reason you have convened this committee of two. Nevertheless, if you have shown an interest in your partner's needs, this unself-centered approach can result in your partner's becoming more sensitive to, and inquisitive about, your needs. In addition, you may learn some things about your partner's preferences that vary considerably from your previous impressions.

- **Don't be confrontational.** The last thing you want is to turn this into an argument, so don't ambush your partner with your pet grievance: "I fake orgasm because you fake foreplay." Drawing a line in the sand does not serve your purposes. Instead, make your partner feel safe in talking to you by explaining that you are interested in making your sex life satisfying for you both. Keep in mind that this needs to be a dialog, not a lecture.

- **Regard this as a process, as opposed to an event.** Your committee of two may need to be convened several times to accomplish your mutual goal. This attitude of a process is especially important if your first attempt at communication stumbles a bit. You have too much riding on resolving your differences to gamble on a single all-or-nothing conversation. If you need to table the discussion for a better time or a more appropriate setting, decide on a time to resume. In the meantime, both of you will have time to think. Total agreement may not be a realistic possibility, but compromise is a wonderful way to come together.

- **Nonverbal communication works, too.** The primary goal of this communication process is not mere talking, valuable as it might be, but rather that you and your partner are meeting each other's needs. If either or both of you are aware that a positive change is needed, you may be able to communicate this by altering your approach to having sex. For example, buy a new teddy, burn scented candles, take a warm bath together, introduce lubricants, or try new verbal expressions during sex. Then depend upon positive or negative feedback to decide whether or not to keep your innovations on the menu.

In communicating with your partner, the obligation you both have is to be receptive to new thinking and suggestions, sensitive to personal preferences, and nonjudgmental. Avoid canned speeches; communicate from your heart.

Maintaining Vaginal Moistness

As we've pointed out, after age forty you may notice slightly less abundant secretions in your vagina. Penetration during sex may become uncomfortable. By your mid- to late forties, this may have progressed to a sense of dryness, with painful sex. After menopause, if your vaginal lining has thinned, the dryness can be even more accentuated.

Regular Sexual Activity (Vaginal Conditioning)

As a transitional women, you may be confronted with a sexual dilemma. On one hand, your capacity for having sex may be robust, your ability for arousal undiminished, and emotional maturity may have given you confidence in initiating sex. On the other hand, in spite of this, your frequency of having sex may be diminishing. Studies show that the rates of having sex gradually decline for women and men from age twenty to forty. After forty, the decline accelerates. It is common for women in their late thirties to have sex about sixty times per year, but a decade later, the frequency is halved (Cone 1993).

The change from frequent to infrequent sex can sometimes create problems with loss of lubrication. Masters and Johnson (1970) noted that women who experience sexual stimulation on a regular basis, about twice weekly, do not lose their vaginal secretions or sexual lubrication. This was true for women well into their sixties.

The key word here is stimulation. It doesn't have to be intercourse; other techniques, such as self-stimulation and nonvaginal sex with your partner, can work just as well. Using a vibrator can also stimulate secretions. Sexual excitement, regardless of its origin, stimulates blood flow to your pelvic organs, including your vagina. This keeps your ability to produce normal secretions intact. Because you utilize the same muscles whether sex consists of intercourse or an alternative technique, they benefit as well. The bottom line is that like other parts of your body, your vagina needs regular workouts to stay in shape; but you don't have to go to the health club to do it. Masters and Johnson coined the phrase "Use it or lose it," which has since been used for advice on everything from athletic prowess to government funding.

Kegel exercises are a good addition to your vaginal workout. These exercises were introduced in the early 1950s by Dr. Arnold Kegel, a urologist (Kegel 1951). The original purpose was to help control a type of involuntary urine loss called stress incontinence. Sex therapists soon discovered that it is also beneficial in improving sexual sensitivity and vaginal muscular control. Kegel exercises improve the strength of the pubococcygeus (PC) muscle which forms the floor of your pelvis and surrounds your urethra, vagina, and anus. You can teach yourself how to contract your PC muscle by stopping the flow during urination, or by placing two fingers in your vagina and contracting around them. To do the exercise squeeze your PC for five to ten seconds, then slowly relax it, wait ten seconds, and repeat. Do a set of about ten to fifteen repetitions and work up to three to five sets per day. Sexual improvement derives from doing "flutter" Kegels. Here you just squeeze, squeeze, squeeze as fast as you can during each set. You don't need to be passing urine or have your fingers in your vagina to do these exercises, of course, so you can do them any time.

Lubricants

Lubricants, even if you are on hormone supplements, are often helpful. Some women are reluctant to use sexual lubricants because they feel somehow defeated by having to admit the need for them. They can make a big difference in your sexual enjoyment, and in your partner's. Try introducing a lubricant as part of your sex play, and use it on your partner as well. There are many water-based commercial products available (such as Astroglide, H-R Jelly, Today Personal Lubricant, and K-Y Jelly). Good old reliable saliva (not sold in stores) also works. One drawback of the above water-soluble lubricants is that they dry quickly; you may need more than one application. Pure vegetable oils (right out of your kitchen) last longer and work well as lubricants.

CAUTION! Avoid lubricating with petroleum-based products like Vaseline. They weaken latex condoms and may mask the signs of vaginal infections.

A longer-lasting lubricant alternative is a vaginal suppository (Lubrin) that melts in your vagina and lasts about three hours, simulating natural secretions. A better method is to restore the secretions themselves. In estrogen deficiency, your vagina produces fewer secretions, which reduces its normal acidity. You can restore normal acidity by using a vaginal moisturizer (Replens, Gyne-Moistrin), which stimulates production of natural secretions. These products are about the same consistency as hand lotion and have bioadhesive qualities that make them last about three days.

Hormones If You Need Them

Hormone production fluctuates and gradually declines during perimenopause, and perimenopausal women often wait to use HRT until late in the transition. Still, if you are plagued with perimenopausal symptoms that are blunting your sexual desire, supplementing your flagging estrogen levels now may be helpful. To do this, you can use low-dose birth control pills, patches, and hormonal creams.

If you are using the Pill, you may also need to take a testosterone supplement to enhance your sexual desire. Increased hair growth, acne, and

deepening of the voice are common worries for women who consider testosterone supplements, but this occurs in less than 5 percent if low doses are
used (Sherwin 1996).

Female Sex Device

The FDA has approved a new method of improving clitoral
engorgement (Mitchell 2000). Called Eros-CTD (clitoral therapy device), it is a
soft suction cup with a tube attached to a handheld vacuum device. After
clitoral engorgement is achieved, the cup is removed. The system is
FDA-approved for sale by prescription only for treatment of the female
equivalent of male impotence.

Partner Availability

We all have lifelong needs for caring, sharing, and intimacy. These factors contribute to our normal desire for sex with a partner. Life circumstances,
such as divorce, separation, disabilities associated with aging or illness, relationship problems, or death may result in your being without a suitable partner or with sharply reduced opportunities to have sex. These situations may
not diminish your interest in sexual gratification. There are a number of
methods to deal with this problem:

- **Masturbation:** Masturbation is a way to experience pleasure and discharge sexual tension if you do not have a partner or are not sexually
  active with your partner. You may have been brought up to feel guilty
  about self-arousal, but there are significant benefits to this healthy and
  harmless sexual practice. In addition to stimulating vaginal secretions,
  sexual release is well known to dissipate the harmful effects of stress.
  Self-stimulation can also increase your understanding of your sensuality and promote better sex with a partner.

- **A change in partners:** In the transitional stage of life, many women
  experience a loss of their partner, often as a result of death or divorce.
  Some women choose a new partner after events like these, perhaps
  simply someone whose company they enjoy and with whom they
  have pleasurable sex. A new partner can be a potent source of re-
  newed sexual energy.

- **Nonvaginal sex:** If you and your partner are looking for alternatives
  to vaginal sex because of pain or discomfort, oral sex is a pleasurable
  method to both give and receive satisfaction. Mutual masturbation is
  another option that satisfies the need for closeness and relief of sexual
  tension.

Touching

We all need to hug and be hugged, to caress and be caressed, from infancy to advanced old age. Touching is thought to have a critical influence on mental health and our sense of well-being. Some researchers believe that this is mediated through the endorphins (Kaverne 1989). So warm hugs (lots of them) are important to your health, and they say volumes about how you feel toward your partner. Tactile stimulation can certainly lead to great sex, but this does not need to be the goal or inevitable end point of the activity. Touching is satisfying on its own.

Timing Is Everything

Make time for sex. You may have children at home, a household to manage, a job to look after, a busy social schedule, community and political obligations. . . . Not only may you lack the energy for sex, you may not have the time for it. Just remember that when the frequency of sex declines, so does your desire for it. Try making an appointment—well, call it a date—with your partner. You may find yourselves "dating" a lot more after the first one or two. It also might be worth reexamining the responsibilities that keep you too busy for sex, and possibly rearranging your priorities.

Another useful technique is to try sex in the morning or midday. A good night's sleep will do a world of good for your fatigue, so you may have a lot more energy for sex in the early part of the day.

Sex Therapy

A frequent comment of sex therapists is, "When sex goes well, it accounts for 15 percent of a marriage; but when sex is bad, it's 85 percent." The common human trait of difficulty in discussing sexual matters has contributed to making sex therapy a growth industry in the U.S. If you have tried communicating, lubricating, masturbating, dating, hormones, and more, but nothing is working, now is the time to bring in some third-party help. A sex therapist can give you a whole new perspective. Most sex therapists are licensed psychologists, social workers, or psychiatrists. Being a sex therapist requires specialized education and licensure, so be sure to see someone who is properly credentialed. Many are not.

Before you decide on a sex therapist, take an honest look at the root of your problems as a couple. If bad sex seems to be resulting from poor communication and disagreements about nonsexual issues, a marriage counselor may be a better choice for resolving your differences. If you still can't agree or are unable to decide upon the major source of your difficulties, a psychologist might be a better choice to help you sort it out. (You may even find a psychologist who is also a sex therapist!)

Summary

Aging and sexuality are not at opposite ends of a spectrum. Sexual activity and sexual pleasure are experiences for which you have a lifelong capability. It is an inescapable fact that living your life will bring change to your anatomy and physiology, which can also bring change to your sexuality. It is also true that the major controlling factor in sexual enjoyment is your brain. (Your body may be the orchestra, but your brain is the conductor.) With the cooperation of your brain, you can take advantage of a number of well-proven techniques that favorably influence the anatomic and physiologic changes that time imposes on your body and lead to enjoyable sex. With a healthy attitude, you can express this vital core of your emotions and your humanity for as long as you live. You may experience your sexuality as an expression of love, as a fountain of erotic pleasure, as a means of communicating your desire for caring and intimacy, as a private island where problems cease and pleasure is maximal, or as a time of total acceptance. Regardless of how you experience it, there is no reason your sexuality cannot flourish as the years pass.

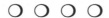

13

Looking Good While Changing: Skin Care, Hair Care, and Cosmetic Surgery

Cultural demands often hold women to an unrealistic standard of youth and beauty. But don't worry—this is not one of those "how-to-stay-young-forever-no-matter-what" chapters. It simply offers suggestions for helping you present your best image—the one that makes you feel good—so you can move on to other matters in your life. If you're happy to let the natural signs of aging progress without interference (and many women are), feel free to skip this chapter.

Change has been the topic of this book, and that theme continues here, as we address changes in your appearance during perimenopause. The passage of time is unstoppable, of course, but there are ways of coping with it. Let's look at the causes and prevention of appearance changes that occur over time, as well as some treatment suggestions.

Skin

The earliest visible signs of aging come in your body's largest and most public organ: your skin. You may not have known your skin is an organ, but it is, and it serves many important functions. First and foremost, though, it covers you up. Your intact skin is a barrier to invasion by microorganisms; it

Alphabet Soup	
AHA	Alpha hydroxy acids
MED	Minimal erythema dose
SPF	Sun protective factor
UV	Ultraviolet

transmits sensations, both pleasurable and painful; and it is vital to regulating your body temperature. It also functions as part of your immune system. Like other bodily organs, your skin changes with the years, but some of the adverse changes are avoidable and treatable. Let's start by considering its components.

A Bit of Biology

Normal skin is a biological marvel. Figure 13.1 is a schematic of your skin's normal architecture. On the right side you will notice there are three layers bracketed: epidermis, dermis, and subcutaneous tissue. Skin consists of those first two layers. The third layer is made up mostly of fat. The epidermis is the layer you can see, and the dermis is the infrastructure. The dermis is the life support system for the visible part of your skin. Distributed through the dermis are blood vessels, nerves, oil (sebaceous) glands, sweat glands, and hair follicles, which are all supported by connective tissue fibers called collagen and elastin. The dermis transports nutrients to the epidermis; whatever happens in the dermis has an effect on your skin's surface appearance.

Your epidermis is made up of the five sublayers (each called a stratum or layer) noted on the upper-left side of Figure 13.1. These are the layers from which you get a continuous resupply of new skin cells. The new cells are generated by the germinal layer (also called the basal layer), and gradually work their way to the surface, where they die and are sloughed off. Transit time from the germinal layer to the stratum corneum takes on average about four weeks in adults. In children it only takes about two weeks. So you get a new skin about once per month.

Although the appearance of your skin is influenced by both internal and external factors, sunlight is responsible for 75 to 90 percent of the changes we associate with aging skin (Takeuchi 1998). Internal influences include good nutrition and a well-functioning microcirculation of blood to deliver those dietary nutrients to your skin. Externally, your skin is subject to various environmental influences such as ultraviolet damage from sunlight, weather conditions (hot, cold, humid, dry, windy), and pollutants. Fortunately, normal, healthy skin has many defenses for the hazards to which it may be exposed. It is constantly guarded by specialized cells that alert the general immune system to an invasion by bacteria, viruses, and other intruders. Your skin can also produce antioxidant molecules, which neutralize free radicals and prevent them from damaging skin cells and the collagen support matrix. In addition, your skin is a semipermeable structure that regulates the flow of water out of your body and helps prevent dehydration. In spite of these defenses,

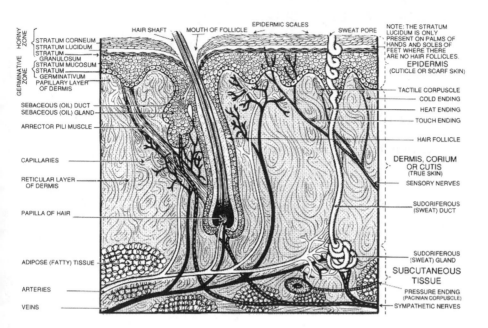

Source: Joel Gerson. 1992. *Milady's Standard Textbook for Professional Estheticians.* rev. ed. ; Milady Publishing Co.

Figure 13.1.   Normal Skin Architecture

your skin is still a fragile organ and susceptible to major changes from the inevitable processes of aging.

The Aging Process

Aging in cells throughout your body appears to be genetically programmed at birth. Each of your trillions of cells has DNA strands in its nucleus on which genes are located. The genes control a variety of cellular metabolic activities, including how frequently the cell will reproduce itself and how long it will live. For skin cells, as we mentioned, that's about one month. As aging occurs, genes are altered and the genetic messages are gradually changed. Cells throughout your body slow down the process of division into new cells. Cells throughout the body also diminish hormone production and production of the nearly three dozen growth factors necessary for new cell formation. (We discuss growth factors in a moment.) Although genes are partly responsible for aging skin, we can't emphasize enough that sun exposure is the major player. You can't change your genes, but you can certainly diminish future sun damage.

What Causes These Changes?

There are several theories about what causes our bodies, including our skin, to age:

Genetic Programming

Planned obsolescence seems to be part of the grand plan of nature. Plants and animals start from seeds, grow to maturity, reproduce, and then decline. Your skin is a reflection of this process.

Hormone and Growth Factor Depletion

Over time, diminished production of hormones and other growth stimulators, called *growth factors*, slows cellular metabolism. Hormones, as you know, are biologically active chemical messengers. Growth factors are also biologically active intercellular messengers. They are produced by cells and attach to receptor sites on cell surfaces, where they direct the cell to perform certain functions, such as reproducing itself or changing its metabolism. Aging cells have fewer receptor sites to which growth factors can attach, so the cells slow their metabolic activities. Slower metabolism changes the appearance and function of all tissues, including the skin. The greatest drop in growth factor production is after age forty, and the most visible sign is in your skin (Notelovitz 1993). As a result of diminished cellular activity, as well as the accumulation of sun damage, both of which diminish collagen and elastin, lines and wrinkles appear.

Photoaging from Ultraviolet (UV) Sunlight

UV light has two wavelengths: UVA, or long waves (320 to 400 nanometers), and UVB, or shortwaves (280 to 320 nanometers). UVB causes sunburn and subsunburn exposures (called suberythema dosage), which damage the epidermal layer of your skin. Research has linked both basal cell and squamous cell cancers to UVB exposure (Wikonkal 1999; Mitchell 1999). UVB not only contributes to photoaging, but there is increasing evidence that it is also responsible for the alarming increase in melanoma, the most dangerous form of skin cancer (Atillasoy 1998). UVB damages DNA in genes, which explains the increase in all forms of skin cancer from sun exposure. As few as two bad sunburns before age twenty may predispose you to skin cancer when you get older (Paige 2000). This is a very good reason to put a sunscreen on your children whenever they are exposed to the sun.

UVA's long waves penetrate the deeper layers of your skin, and cause damage to the infrastructure: the collagen, elastin, and blood vessels. It is responsible for most photoaging, and some skin cancer as well. Most sunscreens do not protect against UVA (Leenutaphong 1992).

DNA damage to the cellular genes from UV light is caused by free radicals, which are released as a result of the inflammatory response (sunburn). (Chapter 9 discussed free radicals.) The DNA-damaged cells produce

DNA-damaged daughter cells and, over time, this leads to aging, cellular malfunction, and possibly skin cancer.

Actual Skin Changes

Visible skin changes actually begin slowly in your twenties, but the process speeds up and tends to be more noticeable in your mid-thirties (the start of your transitional years). UVA radiation damages elastin, which gradually results in accumulation of massive amounts of abnormal elastic material and results in a condition called solar elastosis. The result is individual patches of skin thickening, and loss of smoothness. Damaged elastin doesn't allow your skin to bounce back as well when stretched.

UVA radiation also reduces your skin's collagen network, making your skin thinner. With less collagen, there is less space for your skin to hold water, and it loses its plumpness. So, the overall effect of UVA radiation on your epidermis is thinning, the creation of fine, dry lines, and the development of solar elastosis. As the damage continues, fine lines eventually become deep wrinkles.

UVB rays cause immunosuppression (a suppressed immune system) in your skin. In such an unprotected state, the free radicals released by the inflammation of sun exposure are unchecked in their attack on collagen, elastin, cell membranes, and the vital DNA elements of the cell nucleus. A suppressed immune system in the skin is associated with 90 percent of basal cell and squamous cell cancer, and in 50 percent of melanoma (Wikonkal 1999; Mitchell 1999; Atillasoy 1998).

So, now you know chronic sun exposure causes a breakdown of the collagen fibers in your skin, which results in thinning of the epidermis. Here's what happens as skin ages:

- **Skin cells:** The number of cells in the basal layer of your epidermis decreases, and those still left are slower to divide; regeneration slows. It takes more time for cells to migrate from the basal layer of your epidermis to the surface. Sun damage reduces the overall thickness of your epidermis, but the number of dead cells in the outermost sublayer (stratum corneum) increases. These dead cells are therefore present for a longer period of time, which can dull your skin's appearance. More pigmentation accumulates, giving the skin a discolored look.

- **Oil and sweat glands:** These glands become less effective, so your skin becomes drier. It may get scaly or develop cracks.

- **Collagen and elastin:** The amount of collagen and elastin in your skin decreases. These connective tissues in the dermis comprise more than 90 percent of your skin's bulk between the ages of twenty and forty (Reichman 1996). Collagen gives your skin plumpness, and elastin gives it (you guessed it) elasticity. You can get a good idea of how these elements are working in your skin with a simple test: On the back of your hand, pinch some skin and raise it up. If your skin is young, when you release it, it springs back into position almost more quickly than you can see it. Older skin, with diminished collagen and elastin, takes much longer to bounce back. In addition, the loss of collagen and elastin contributes to thinner skin and one of the hallmarks of older skin: wrinkles.

- **Fatty tissue:** Fatty tissue under the dermis breaks down. This further reduces the thickness of your skin and may change the angles and contours of your face. Loss of fatty tissue combined with thinner skin can make your bony structures more prominent, in contrast to the rounder face of your youth, and make veins appear more prominent as well.

- **Microcirculation:** As microcirculation decreases, the blood supply to your skin is reduced. Skin can become less glowing and look less healthy. Your skin gets cold more easily because of the diminished circulation—unless you're having a hot flash, of course.

As these deteriorating conditions progress, the initial change is usually some fine smile lines about the eyes. Eventually, radial wrinkles, called lip stitches, form around the mouth. You've got about twenty-five years between smile lines and radial wrinkles, so there is plenty of time to take preventive measures.

Skin Abuse

In addition to the normal results of aging, there are many ways you can unintentionally abuse your skin. Pinching pimples may be a longtime habit, but it can leave scars. Scrubbing your face roughly or removing your makeup with wild abandon can also damage your skin; the same is true of tugging the skin around your eyes when you use eye pencils. Most facial tissues are made from wood pulp, which is abrasive. A better plan is to use a dry washcloth or cotton balls to remove your makeup. It treats your skin gently and still removes surface skin debris.

Neglecting your skin falls in the category of abuse. Failure to use a sunblock is a good example. Moisturizers are a must if you are to avoid drying and premature aging. (You'll find out more on these products later in the chapter.) Neglecting to remove makeup at night will cause clogged pores, skin eruptions, and unhealthy looking skin.

Habitual squinting and frowning can also cause wrinkles—the ones that make you look like you're squinting and frowning! You're going to get some wrinkles no matter what, so why not make them smile lines?

Skin Care from the Inside

The condition of your skin is a fair barometer of how well you are treating your body. If you have been neglecting your overall health, your skin may tell the tale.

Diet

You probably already know what we're going to say. Your diet should be balanced, which means rich in fruits, vegetables, whole grains, and complex carbohydrates, as we described in Chapter 9. A high animal-fat intake is bad for your cardiovascular system; but contrary to popular belief, dermatologic research has shown that it has no negative effect on your skin. Neither a high-fat nor a low-fat diet in acne patients makes a difference in their acne (Fulton 1996). The same is true of a diet rich in sweets. On the other hand, chronic dieters who are not getting adequate fat or protein commonly experience dry skin and dull hair; your skin likes your diet balanced.

Fluids

Good hydration is essential for smooth, healthy skin. Fluids are stored in the spaces between collagen fibers in the dermis. This aids in maintaining the plumpness of your skin. It takes about two quarts of water consumption daily to meet your skin's needs (Eskin 1995). You can buy commercial skin moisturizers, but you'll achieve the same effect just by drinking water.

Alcohol

Alcohol dehydrates your body, which you now know is bad for your skin. Chronic alcohol abuse causes dilation of skin capillaries, particularly on the face and nose. Alcohol also interferes with your ability to absorb B vitamins, which are important to your skin's ability to heal itself.

Smoking and Drug Abuse

Nicotine causes blood vessel constriction, resulting in diminished oxygen and transportation of nutrients to your skin. That encourages wrinkles; cigarette smokers often have wrinkles equivalent to those of people more than a decade older, typically around the mouth and on the outer part of the eyes. Smoking causes an earlier decline in estrogen production, which has a deleterious effect on collagen formation in the skin, leading to more wrinkles. Smokers also have poor healing of injured skin, and this contributes to the appearance of aging.

Drug abuse is one of the worst skin abusers because of the dietary and personal grooming neglect that may accompany such a lifestyle. It not only ages you faster, but you will look drawn and haggard while you age.

Skin Vitamins

Several vitamins have been studied for their beneficial effects on skin:

- **Vitamin A:** This vitamin keeps your skin soft and prevents scaling and drying. It also is an antioxidant, so it protects your skin cells and collagen from free radical damage.

- **Vitamin C:** Because oral vitamin C is an antioxidant, it may have a role in prevention of photoaging.

- **Vitamin E:** Although dietary and supplemental vitamin E is an important and useful antioxidant, research has failed to find any benefit from topical use. Indeed, there is a high incidence of allergic responses to its use on the skin (Paige 2000). This is the main antioxidant vitamin for collagen protection.

- **B-complex vitamins:** The B-complex vitamins assist in tissue repair and prevent skin scaling and cracking.

Regular Exercise

Regular exercise is a major stimulant to blood flow, which contributes to vibrant-looking skin. Some experts believe that a vigorous workout does more to enhance blood flow and transport nutrients to your skin than the various creams, masks, and facials now available for these same purposes. It is less expensive, too.

Skin Care from the Outside

There are some effective external techniques for improving your skin's health and for treating damage you may have already sustained. Some techniques involve making simple behavioral changes. There are also some new products on the market that do more than just cover up your skin problems cosmetically. These products stem from research in the late 1980s and early 1990s into the fundamental reasons skin deteriorates, and from a more pharmaceutical approach to dealing with these underlying causes (Leverette 1991). The goal of many skin-care products is to prevent damage and to heal it. External skin care doesn't have to be time consuming, expensive, or complicated, but it should be consistent.

Protecting Against Sun Damage

Since skin damage from sun exposure occurs over the long term and is generally irreversible, sun protection is vital to preventing photoaging. There are several steps you can take.

One of the simplest techniques is simply to avoid the midday sun. The most intense rays are from 10 A.M. to 4 P.M., from March to October. You can even get indirect exposure while sitting in the shade or riding in a car, or on a cloudy day. Reflections of the sun on snow and water cause intense UV exposure. Another commonsense technique is to wear protective clothing. A broad-brimmed hat, long sleeves, and wide sunglasses offer good protection.

Using a sunscreen or sunblock is another important preventive measure. Sunscreens have been shown to reduce the incidence of squamous cell skin cancer, a very dangerous form, by 39 percent, but they don't change the frequency of the less worrisome basal cell skin cancer (Green 1999). Sunscreens absorb UV light and sunblocks reflect it. The only two sunblock types are those containing titanium dioxide or micronized zinc oxide (Paige 2000). The zinc oxide favored by lifeguards for years has been refined. It still works, but it is no longer a thick white paste.

Sun protective agents are rated by a system called minimal erythema dose (MED). This refers to the length of time it takes for your skin to turn pink when exposed to the sun. Sun protective factor (SPF) indicates how much longer it takes to reach your MED. The higher the SPF, the longer it takes to reach your MED.

Apply a sunscreen or sunblock about half an hour before you go out, or you will not achieve full protection. For everyday protection, a SPF of 15 is adequate, as long as you reapply it every two hours during sun exposure, no matter what it says on the label. Even heavily pigmented skin burns if exposed to sun for long periods of time. If you are near the water, at a high altitude, or close to the equator, double the strength of your sunscreen.

Products stating they are "waterproof" will continue to protect your skin for eighty minutes in the water, but "water-resistant" products work for only forty minutes.

Most sunscreens do not screen out UVA radiation, the type most responsible for photoaging. Newer sunscreens containing a chemical called avobenzone or Parsol 1789 do absorb some, but not all, UVA and protect your skin significantly better than older products.

The FDA is implementing new regulations for sunscreen products. There will be three categories: minimum (SPF 2 to 12), moderate (SPF 12 to 30), and high (SPF over 30) (Women's HealthSource 2000).

Bottom line: If you are in the sun, protect your skin with adequate clothing, a hat, and sunglasses.

Are Sunscreens Harmful or Helpful?

The incidence of melanoma has been steadily rising as the use of sunscreen has increased. Researchers have become concerned that the sunscreen, which has not screened out UVA radiation, has allowed people to stay in the sun longer without burning, thereby increasing their risk of skin cancer (Autier 1997). While this is a compelling argument, it is not true.

There are several reasons for the increase in melanoma unrelated to sunscreen use. Since World War II, more and more people have moved to sunshine states (California, Florida, Arizona). This alone can account for the increased incidence of melanoma. In Australia, where the incidence is of epidemic proportions, the government has conducted a successful campaign to educate people as to the dangers of sun exposure. Australians are using significantly more sunscreen and there has finally been a plateau in the incidence of melanoma.

In the past, several sunscreen products have been "Ames test" positive. This means the product caused DNA damage when applied to the skin. In all instances, the substances that caused a positive test were contaminants (Paige 2000).

Skin-Care Products

Your skin is rather resistant to chemical penetration, but it is not impervious. Applying certain products to the skin can achieve internal effects. The estrogen skin patch, which we described in Chapter 7, is a good example. This bit of information has spawned a huge industry in skin-care products. When you select a product, read the label carefully. The first ingredients listed are the ones that will do you the most good. The further down the list an ingredient appears, the less likely that the product supplies a significant amount of it. In general, the fewer ingredients the better. Try to avoid products that contain fragrances, artificial colorings, and especially alcohol. Some of the claims made by manufacturers of skin products are simply hype, but many can be effective. Let's examine some of the choices.

Acnegenic

In the past, some products caused acne and blackheads because they blocked pores. Today, reputable cosmetics are subjected to the "rabbit ear test." Before marketing, each cosmetic is rubbed into a rabbit's ear. If it doesn't cause blackheads, it is nonacnegenic or noncomedogenic and will say so on the label.

Cleansers

Mild soap and water may be the only cleanser your skin needs. Some manufacturers of skin products would like you to believe that you need a cleanser, but you probably don't. If you have a condition such as eczema, that results in dry, flaky skin, a cleanser can help remove the excess skin debris. Manufactured cleansers in liquid, cream, bar, and gel form commonly contain varying combinations of water, allantoin, propylene glycol, urea, aloe vera, and other products to remove dirt, grease, and makeup. Some cleansers contain alpha-hydroxy acids in varying strengths to assist in removal of dead skin debris. (You can find inexpensive nonsoap cleansers in pharmacies and department stores.)

Toners

A number of different toners are on the market, but you probably don't need to use a toner at all. Most of them are mildly astringent and recommended for use on oily skin, especially around the "T" zone of the nose. Toners can actually irritate your skin, and they cause a rash in some women with sensitive skin. Soap and water works just as well as a toner to degrease your skin, and is a lot cheaper.

Moisturizers

Moisturizers can be very helpful for perimenopausal skin that has become somewhat thinned from collagen loss and therefore holds less moisture. Moisturizers are made up of two components: humectants, which are substances that attract and hold water (glycerin, glycol, sorbitol, gelatin), and occlusives (also known as emollients), which seal water in your skin (mineral oil, lanolin, petrolatum). Moisturizers have their effect on the epidermis, but their molecules are too large to penetrate the dermis, so no benefit is derived at that level except for helping to prevent water loss. The available products vary in texture from light (slightly watery feel), to medium (lotion feel), to heavy (butterlike). The grade that works for you depends, among other things, on the oiliness of your skin, the climate, and the season of the year. Cleanse your skin before applying a moisturizer. An ideal time for a moisturizer is after your bath or shower when your skin is still damp (McCallion 1993). Moisturizers can also be the base for your makeup since they last most of the day (Hayman 1996).

The existence of alpha-hydroxy acids (AHA) has been known for many years, but in the late 1980s, skin researchers demonstrated their benefits to skin (Leverette 1991). AHAs are derived from fruit and animal products: tartaric acid from grapes, malic acid from apples, citric acid from citrus fruits, and lactic acid from sour milk. A widely used AHA called glycolic acid comes from sugar cane. Most AHA products contain between 5 and 15 percent glycolic acid. If you use much higher concentrations, do so only under the direction of a dermatologist.

AHA products work by resurfacing your skin (Stiller 1996). Glycolic acid and other AHAs penetrate the stratum corneum of your skin and break up the buildup of dead skin cells that make your skin look dull and unhealthy. As your skin sheds these cells, areas of irregular pigmentation are also often eliminated or reduced, as are irregularities in your skin contour, such as the depth of fine lines. This leaves a fresher looking skin.

Glycolic acid also allows for more rapid regeneration of new cells, and it helps empty your pores of skin debris, which is an aid in acne control. When combined with sun protection, skin resurfacing with glycolic acid can aid in reversing some of the damage aging skin has suffered and in preventing further deterioration. Your interests are best served if you start a glycolic acid regimen under the supervision of a dermatologist or an experienced esthetician. Maintaining the improvements may require long-term use; you can implement a home treatment plan of glycolic acid in the strength your skin specialist recommends.

It may take three to six months to achieve maximum benefits with home use. When used in lower concentrations (5 to 20 percent), as in products for salon or home use, a longer period of use is necessary for improvement. The effect appears to be cumulative, though, so slow progress is okay. Dermatologists use higher glycolic acid strengths of 50 to 70 percent to deal with deeper wrinkles and to allow the acid to penetrate into the dermis, where collagen formation is stimulated (Moy 1995). Deep chemical peels, which we talk about a little later in the chapter, are one way to administer higher-strength glycolic acid. The results are more rapidly accomplished than with home use, but skin irritation is more severe.

Tretinoin

Tretinoin (Retin-A, Renova) is a vitamin A derivative applied in a lotion, cream, or gel directly to the skin to remove dead cells from the stratum corneum. Its primary use has been for treatment of acne, but it also speeds up the turnover of dead surface cells, so it can also be helpful for perimenopausal skin (Eskin 1995). Tretinoin reverses some of the effects of photoaging, lightens your skin, and improves blood flow to the skin. Progress is slow, but it does provide cosmetic improvement after a few months. Renova is a milder product than Retin-A, so is less likely to cause skin irritation. Both products increase sun sensitivity, which means you have to minimize exposure to sunlight by using sunscreens and protective clothing.

CAUTION! Do not take tretinoin during pregnancy. It has caused delayed fetal bone mineralization in laboratory animals. Studies on humans have not been conducted.

Topical Vitamins

Interest in using vitamins on the skin has been widespread, and many products have been marketed with glowing claims. But researchers have not been able to show they are beneficial. In some instances, as with vitamin E, topical vitamins are actually harmful. Vitamin A is necessary for healthy skin, but dietary sources are considered adequate. Topical vitamins C and E have not been shown to be beneficial to skin health in spite of claims that they are. So at this time, vitamin skin products are not considered useful.

A Routine for Daily Care

You can incorporate a few simple practices into your daily schedule to ensure that your skin stays healthy over time.

Daily Facial Care

Good facial skin care can be achieved in only a few minutes each day. In the morning there may be no necessity for cleansing your face if you have done it before retiring. Just stimulate your skin with a cold washcloth and pat dry. Then apply a moisturizer if you have dry skin and put on any makeup you wear. During the rest of the day, you don't need to do anything except perhaps touch up your makeup. Remember to use a sunblock before putting on your makeup if you will be out of doors. In the evening, use a cleanser (a makeup-removing one if necessary) and apply a moisturizer before going to bed. Some skin experts recommend using a moisturizer with AHA for your bedtime application.

Daily Hand Care

Even if you have a young-looking face, your hands can tell a lot of tales. If you wash them frequently or they are often wet during the day, the consequence can be dry skin. Wash with a mild cleanser. Apply a hand cream every time you wash your hands. (Lotions and oils are not as effective as hand creams.) Just keep some cream handy at all your sinks. Using a cream only takes a few seconds, and you should notice improvement in days. At night, apply a moisturizer before you climb into bed. You can use the same one you use for your face, but cheaper ones will also work quite well.

When doing wet household chores using harsh detergents and cleansers, wear white cotton gloves under heavy vinyl work gloves. The white gloves absorb the perspiration and the vinyl protects your hands from household irritants. Wear cotton gloves when you dust as well. In cold weather, wear leather gloves when you go out, to protect your hands from weather effects. Make sure you have a sunscreen on your hands when you are out in the sunlight and reapply it every two hours in the sun. Between 10 A.M. and 4 P.M., wear protective gloves if you must be in direct sunlight.

If you have liver spots, those irregular brown pigmented areas, glycolic acid–laced moisturizers will help them fade, as long as you also use a sunscreen when you are outside (Leverette 1991). As discussed earlier, UV exposure is the primary cause of these discolored skin areas.

Daily Body Care

Taking a bath, especially a long hot soak, can dry your skin. Try to keep those luxurious soaks to a minimum; save them for when you especially need to relax or as a treat. If you have dry skin, try adding a half-cup of pure sesame or almond oil or a capful of neutral, mild bath oil. Some women become allergic to bath oils, so use with caution. Use a mild cleanser that is nonalkaline (meaning it contains no mineral salts, such as sodium bicarbonate). During your shower, try rubbing a loofah sponge vigorously over your skin from the neck down to help remove dry and dead cells from the surface of your skin. Using a loofah also increases blood circulation and tones your skin. After your bath, pat your body dry and use a moisturizer, all over your body, including your feet, while you are still slightly damp. This helps retain the moisture in your skin.

We tend to overwash in the U.S. (Hayman 1996). In the winter, when the weather is cold and blustery and you've turned up your heating system, your skin can become much drier than during the other seasons. Showering or bathing only adds to the problem. Try taking a shower every other day, with a sponge bath in between to minimize the drying effects of washing away your skin oils.

Hair

In your perimenopausal years, you can expect your hair to become thinner, drier, more brittle, and less shiny. To top it off, white and gray hair becomes coarse and doesn't reflect light the same as pigmented hair, so it can look dull. Why do these things happen?

Each of your hairs is made up of a number of plates, which are composed of a hard keratin that is also the primary constituent of nails. (Soft keratin is the main component of the dead surface cells of your skin.) The keratin plates are situated close to each other and give a hair shaft its strength. As you get older, the number of plates deposited in each growing hair declines, as cells in the hair follicle become less active. The plates don't adhere as well to each other, which makes your hair more brittle and inclined toward split ends.

Hormone changes also influence the condition of your hair. Normal estrogen levels make your hair lustrous by promoting oil production from skin glands, and androgens promote hair growth. As estrogen declines, you secrete less oil in your scalp, resulting in drier hair that appears dull. During estrogen decline late in the perimenopausal years or after menopause, androgen production does not decrease at the same rate, so there is relatively more male hormone influence. This is the cause of increased facial hair. Hair loss at this time of your life, however, is the result of loss of hair follicles due to aging.

Another adverse influence is the cumulative effect of many years of perms, straightening, blow-drying, and coloring if peroxide is used as part of the coloring process. This contributes to a dry, brittle appearance. Fortunately, since you grow six inches of hair every year, this kind of damage can be reversed with time.

To reverse or control these changes, estrogen replacement can be helpful if you are deficient in that hormone. Experts also recommend the following principles of routine hair care:

- **Use a mild shampoo.** Choose a shampoo with no alcohol, and with emollients such as panthenol, that won't dry out your hair. Concentrate on using the shampoo on your scalp and the roots. If you avoid washing the ends, there is less drying. They will be adequately cleansed when you rinse.

- **Use a conditioner or a cream rinse every time you shampoo.** Conditioners penetrate the hair shaft, which softens your hair while adding nutrients and shine. Protein cream rinses add body to your hair. Cream rinses are not as penetrating, but they provide a light conditioning, detangle your hair, and still give it shine.

- **Dry your hair carefully.** Use a wide-toothed, hard rubber or plastic comb (metal breaks the hair) to gently detangle your hair. Ideally, you should allow your hair to dry at least partially on its own. Gently towel-dry your hair before blow-drying. Hold your hair dryer at least six inches away from your head to minimize heat damage.

Gray Hair

As time passes, the pigment-producing cells in your hair follicles begin to falter, and graying gradually results. It's an immutable fact of living. If you decide to go gray, be aware that your hair will be coarser and more brittle, so be sure to use moisturizing and protein conditioners. To prevent yellowing, a violet-toned shampoo is ideal. On the other hand, if you decide to defer having gray hair, a couple of options exist. A process called low-lighting (the opposite of highlighting) can accentuate the natural coloring of your hair. Low-lighting involves selective coloring of your natural hair in a deeper shade. With salt-and-pepper hair, low-lighting enhances the pepper aspect while improving texture (Hayman 1996). Ask about it at your salon.

The other option is total coloring. There are two types of coloring available: permanent and semipermanent—the so-called rinse that washes out after a few shampoos. Before you decide to color your hair, it's a good idea to use a rinse to see whether you like the color. Coloring your gray hair changes its texture, making it more manageable.

If you choose to color your hair, try not to perm it as well. For coloring to work, the cuticle (outer coating) of the hair shaft is broken down to allow the coloring agent to penetrate into the center of the hair shaft. This weakens hair. A perm works much the same way, and combining these two procedures can result in significantly weakened hair, which can break off at the scalp and leave you temporarily very short of hair—as in mainly bald. Some people develop allergies to the coal tar pigment in some dyes, especially black dye, which seems to be much more allergenic than other colors (Fisher 1995). Color rinses, which are not as penetrating as total coloring, do not jeopardize your hair strength.

For years there was concern that hair tints were carcinogenic, and to some extent they are. Your increased risk of developing cancer when you tint your hair is the same as if you smoke one cigarette a month; that's not much risk.

Unwanted Hair

As estrogen decline progresses and your androgen influence increases, you may notice more hair on your upper lip, chin, nipples, and abdomen below your navel. This occurs very gradually and is not harmful, but you may find it objectionable from a cosmetic standpoint. Estrogen replacement will help prevent this if you are deficient in that hormone, but there are other methods for dealing with it too:

- **Shaving:** The most basic way to remove hair. The problem is that you may need to shave every three or four days.

- **Bleaching:** Using over-the-counter preparations to bleach the hair can camouflage it.

- **Plucking:** Plucking out the unwanted hairs by their roots lasts longer than shaving.

- **Waxing:** Waxing also pulls hairs out by the roots. Like plucking, it is somewhat painful, but it gets the job done faster than plucking one hair at a time.

- **Depilatories:** These are chemical creams for removing hair. They do a good job, but occasional skin allergies occur. It's best to test the cream on a small patch of skin before widespread use. For dealing with facial hair, a prescription product called Vaniqa is available, which inhibits an enzyme necessary for hair growth. It is applied twice daily as a moisturizer, but it must be used continuously to prevent regrowth.

- **Electrolysis:** This process uses electrical current to destroy hair follicles. It is a tedious and painful process, but it lasts longer than other methods. If the unwanted hair is being caused by hormonal shifts, electrolysis is not a permanent solution, and you may need to repeat the procedure every few weeks or months.

- **Antiandrogens:** Flutamide (Eulexin) and finasteride (Proscar) are two antiandrogen drugs that have been shown to reduce hirsutism (excess hair growth) by 40 percent in six months and up to 58 percent in a year of use (Fruzzetti 1999).

- **Laser removal:** Lasers have surpassed prior methods of hair removal. They destroy specific colored objects such as dark hair and tattoos, but they cannot identify blond hair. Electrolysis is still needed for that. Compared to electrolysis, six-month hair counts with laser treatment decreased an average of 74 percent as opposed to 35 percent with electrolysis. In addition, it is sixty times faster than electrolysis, and less painful (Gorgu 2000). Laser treatment is more expensive, but its efficacy and speed outweigh the cost difference.

Veins

Spider veins and varicose veins are common in transitional women. Spider veins are those bluish-reddish veins that appear just below the skin's surface. They are flat and harmless. Either laser therapy or sclerotherapy can eliminate them. In sclerotherapy, a concentrated solution of salt water or another irritant is injected into the vein, causing scarring, which stops the blood flow. Dermatologists, general surgeons, and plastic surgeons usually perform sclerotherapy. It leaves a whitish blemish less noticeable than the original veins. New spider veins can still form, so you may need more than one treatment.

Varicose veins result from the failure of small one-way valves in the vein. These valves prevent backflow of blood between heartbeats and ensure that blood flow continues back to the heart. When the vein loses its elasticity and dilates, these valves stop preventing backflow, and blood tends to pool by gravity in dependent parts of your body such as your legs and vaginal labia. Varicose veins are raised, bulging, and serpentine-shaped, with a bluish hue. In addition to a dull ache, they cause decreased blood flow and increased clotting. When a clot (thrombus) forms, the vein becomes inflamed, resulting in a painful condition called thrombophlebitis. In a superficial (surface) vein, thrombophlebitis is not a serious threat. In deep veins however, a portion of the clot may dislodge and be carried to your lungs, resulting in a life-threatening emergency called a pulmonary embolism. Treatment for superficial thrombophlebitis consists of heat, rest, and elevation of the leg, but for deep vein thrombophlebitis an anticoagulant (anticlotting) medication is used to prevent pulmonary embolism.

The tendency to develop varicose veins runs in some families. They also occur during pregnancy, with prolonged standing, in overweight people, and in those with sedentary lifestyles. Once varicose veins develop, surgical removal may be necessary. Surgery does not prevent new varicose veins from forming. Prevention is the best game in town, and you can achieve it by following these guidelines:

- Exercise regularly

- Elevate your legs

- Avoid prolonged sitting, standing, and crossing your legs

- Avoid becoming overweight

Keep Smiling

Coffee or tea drinking or smoking cause stains on your teeth. Tooth-brightening toothpaste may help remove stains, but can damage your tooth enamel. Cosmetic bonding of new material over your teeth works well to hide the stains, but it is expensive. A less expensive technique involves the use of a whitening gel, which bleaches your teeth. Long-term use of whitening products can cause brittle teeth.

Periodontal disease is the most common cause of tooth loss during perimenopause (Eskin 1995). The problem is created by the buildup of plaque—a colorless film—on your teeth. If you don't remove plaque by flossing, using tiny brushes (called proximate brushes) between your teeth, and/or visiting the dentist twice a year, the plaque hardens into tartar (calculus). Bacteria in your mouth become incorporated into the hardened plaque, irritating your gums. This results in loss of gum tissue and the supporting structures of your teeth. Pockets of infected tartar eventually develop below the gum lines and start destroying the bone tissue. With less and less support, your teeth start loosening and can eventually fall out.

During perimenopause, make sure your calcium intake is sufficient to prevent osteoporosis in your jaw.

Cosmetic Surgery

More and more American women are opting for the "last resort" procedure of plastic surgery. Women with smile lines, frown lines, wrinkled necks, protruding tummies, and broad hips are hearing the siren call of the quick fix. Record numbers of Americans are undergoing facelifts, eyelid revisions, facial resurfacing, tummy tucks, breast implants, and body contouring with liposuction. These procedures often work, but they are expensive and not without risk. The cost can be very dear both financially and in terms of the effects of potential complications. The overall complication rate is low, in the range of 2 percent, but this is just an average. As with any other surgery, when you have cosmetic surgery you are at risk for complications from anesthesia, infection, bleeding, allergic reactions, and scarring; these operations are not a simple, quick fix. In addition, most cosmetic surgery is not covered by health insurance, so check with your insurance carrier or HMO before you decide to have any procedure.

If you are considering having a doctor perform plastic surgery on you, be sure to get answers to these questions:

- **Are you board-certified in plastic surgery?** You can get this information by examining the doctor's diploma on the wall or by asking. You can also call the American Board of Medical Specialties at 800-776-2378. Certification requires special training and completion of a rigorous examination by peers who are qualified in the specialty.

- **What are the possible complications?** This information should be laid out to you explicitly and in terms you understand.

- **How many operations such as mine have you done?** Experience with the proposed procedure is some assurance that you will obtain the desired result.

- **Is it likely I will need more surgery?** Touch-ups and redoing an undesirable outcome are common. Find out if there is a charge for it.

- **Do you have before-and-after pictures?** The results on other patients may be important to you in making your decision. Just remember that good results on someone else are no guarantee for your own outcome.

- **Will you be doing my surgery?** Don't settle for a conference with an associate or an office nurse. In teaching hospitals, resident doctors in training may be scheduled to do your surgery under the supervision of your doctor. If this is objectionable to you, say so.

- **Where do you have hospital privileges?** The answer to this question not only tells you what type of hospital, it tells you that this doctor has been reviewed by peers on the hospital staff. Such reviews look at a doctor's record of competence and proper indications for the surgery performed.

- **Will this be an office operation?** If so, find out whether the office operating suite has been accredited for ambulatory surgery. Ask your doctor, or call the American Association for Accreditation of Ambulatory Surgery Facilities at 847-949-6058.

The following are a few of the nonsurgical (no cutting involved) procedures in current use.

Chemical Peels

The purpose of a chemical peel is to remove the outer layers of skin from the face, neck, chest, hands, arms, and legs with acids (ASDS 1994). In the process, fine wrinkles are also removed. Estheticians do peels with mild concentrations of glycolic acid, which we talked about earlier in this chapter. A series of treatments is usually required. For severe acne- or sun-damaged skin, up to 70 percent concentrations of glycolic acid may be necessary. Deep wrinkles require stronger acids, such as phenol, salicylic acid, or trichloracetic acid. Dermatologists and plastic surgeons perform these peels. It takes three to five days to recover from the skin redness of a superficial peel with low concentration acids, and up to a month from a deeper peel because of swelling, blistering, and crusting that occur with stronger concentrations of acid. Your face will be reddened after deeper peels, and this may take three months or more to fade. A chemical peel makes your skin very sensitive to the sun until your skin returns to normal. Stronger peels occasionally result in permanent lightening of the skin and can lead to irregular pigmentation.

Chemical peels do not remove loose or sagging skin. (That's what a face lift does.) They also do not remove deep scars and may not change pore size in skin.

Dermabrasion

Dermabrasion, done under general anesthesia, removes the scarred and weathered outer skin layers using high-speed rotary brushes. It can also remove fine wrinkles and soften acne scars (Epps 1995). Recovery takes about two weeks, and redness fades in three months. You must observe strict sun avoidance for several months, until the pigment has returned to your skin. The effect is permanent—until new wrinkles form. Complications include scarring, infection, irregular pigmentation, and grooving of the skin. Plastic surgeons and dermatologists perform dermabrasion.

Laser Resurfacing

Laser resurfacing is an alternative to the chemical peel or dermabrasion. It uses a carbon dioxide pulsed laser beam to selectively destroy the sun-damaged outer and middle layers of skin, which are replaced when new skin grows (Brumberg 1997). Laser resurfacing is effective in removing fine lines and smoothing out deeper wrinkles (Alster 1996). It is also used to remove stretch marks, birthmarks, acne scars, and tattoos. Long-term follow-up has shown continued improvement in the reduction of solar elastosis (discussed earlier in this chapter) for two years after the initial laser treatment. When laser resurfacing is combined with topical tretinoin, the effects of laser therapy are even further enhanced. Like peels and dermabrasion, laser resurfacing cannot regenerate sagging muscles. Following treatment, your skin will be swollen and reddened for up to a month, and three months may be necessary for a complete return to normal. Complications include scarring and irregular skin pigmentation. While loss of pigmentation is the most common complication, it appears related to the contrast between the healing new skin and the extent of the preexisting photo-damaged skin.

For a referral to a board-certified laser surgeon, call the American Society for Dermatologic Surgery at 800-441-2737. You can also write to the American Society for Laser Medicine and Surgery at 2404 Stewart Square, Wausau, Wisconsin 54401.

Summary

This chapter has dealt extensively with the cosmetic effects that aging and lifestyle may have on your body. It has given you suggestions and tools to modify or modulate the changes to which you may be subjected. You can pick and choose among them or ignore them entirely; just make sure your choice makes you feel good about yourself.

O   O   O   O

14

Gynecologic Surgery and Medical Treatment: When the Unexpected Happens

You're ready. You've had every lesson you could take. You can finally ski down the fall line (that's "straight down the hill," for you nonskiers) with your skis parallel. You can shift your weight to the downhill ski without thinking about it. You can take the bumps with your legs, without moving your body. You're good! But suddenly, out of nowhere, a snow snake appears and grabs your skis, and down you go. (A snow snake is what causes you to fall just when everything is going well.) This is similar to what happens to you when things start to go wrong in perimenopause: bleeding through your clothes without warning; wetting your pants when you cough or sneeze or even think about having to go to the bathroom. Whatever it is, you're flat on your face—a snow snake got you.

Unexpected changes like these often require surgery or a major lifestyle change. When symptoms occur, you may be reluctant to take time out for such bodily "inconveniences." This chapter is about the unplanned changes that can occur during perimenopause, and describes a variety of surgical and nonsurgical strategies that are available to manage these problems.

Abnormal Uterine Bleeding

During perimenopause, irregular menstrual bleeding is a common accompaniment to the decline of ovarian hormone production. For the most part, these changes are not serious. They can usually be managed with hormone supplements or even weathered without any treatment at all. Sometimes uterine bleeding gets out of control, however, and becomes truly abnormal. The medical term for this condition is dysfunctional uterine bleeding (DUB).

What Causes Dysfunctional Uterine Bleeding?

The first half of your normal menstrual cycle is dominated by the production of estrogen. Estrogen causes your endometrium to regenerate after you have shed it in a menstrual period. During this regeneration, your growing endometrium is supported by blood vessels arranged in fairly straight lines. At midcycle, ovulation takes place and you begin to produce progesterone in large quantities. Progesterone thickens your endometrium, preparing it to receive a fertilized egg. (Your body wants to get pregnant, even if you don't!) Progesterone changes those straight blood vessels to corkscrew shapes. When you shed this lining at your next menstrual period, uterine contractions (cramps) squeeze these corkscrew vessels closed to limit the amount of blood loss.

If you don't ovulate, you don't produce progesterone. If progesterone is not available to convert your straight vessels to the corkscrew type, your vessels don't close completely, so your bleeding is heavier when you menstruate. This is called dysfunctional uterine bleeding,

Most of the time dysfunctional uterine bleeding begins when your period is due; but it can also occur earlier or later in your cycle. It often begins without warning. You may be at a meeting, walking through the mall, or teaching a class when you feel warmth between your legs. You look down and, to your great embarrassment, see a patch of bright red blood.

During perimenopause you may begin to ovulate less frequently. As you get closer to menopause, you usually stop ovulating, so dysfunctional bleeding may occur monthly. The embarrassment is bad enough, but you may also become anemic from blood loss. Menstrual bleeding is the main source of iron loss in women, and the most common cause of iron-deficiency anemia in the developed nations (Fairbanks 1995). Chronic anemia can impair your body's immunity, increase the frequency of serious infection, and even cause you to bleed even more heavily. It's time to see your doctor.

Tell Me What's Wrong—Diagnosis

Dysfunctional uterine bleeding is caused by hormonal changes, but abnormal bleeding may be caused by other factors. You and your doctor need to know the cause of your abnormal bleeding so it can be treated effectively.

To determine the cause of your bleeding, your doctor will perform an office procedure called an endometrial biopsy. A small amount of tissue is removed from the uterine cavity and evaluated microscopically. Almost all biopsies will confirm the diagnosis of dysfunctional uterine bleeding. Occasionally, the biopsy reveals polyps or fibroids (described later in this chapter). The biopsy also screens for uterine cancer, which is rare in perimenopause (Brill 1995).

In the past, an operation called a dilation and curettage (D&C) was the principle technique for obtaining endometrial tissue. In recent years, endometrial biopsy has largely supplanted the D&C. In a 1982 study, Grimes established the advantages of an endometrial biopsy over a D&C based on several factors: convenience, adequacy of tissue sample, complications, diagnostic accuracy, and cost. The D&C is now used chiefly for certain therapeutic treatments rather than diagnosis.

CAUTION! Make sure your health-care provider has a microscopic diagnosis before treating your abnormal bleeding. Although uterine cancer is rare in your age group, it is cured 93 percent of the time when a timely biopsy is done at the onset of abnormal uterine bleeding (Cramer 1994).

Medical Treatment of Dysfunctional Uterine Bleeding

A variety of medications are helpful in controlling DUB. These medications make up for the progesterone you lost when you didn't ovulate; they include both male and female hormones, as well as nonhormonal treatments. Herbal products and creams can be used to replace progesterone (discussed in Chapters 7 and 8), but they don't work consistently to control this bleeding problem.

Female Hormones

Progesterone therapy is used in women who are not ovulating and who are bleeding heavily. Both natural progesterone and synthetic progestins can be used (see Chapter 7 for more about these drugs). Oral progestins such as medroxyprogesterone (Provera, Cycrin), norethindrone (Micronor, Nor-QD), and norethindrone acetate (Aygestin) simulate ovulation when given in large enough doses. The progestins cause the blood vessels in the lining of your uterus to corkscrew. When you stop the progestin, the vessels constrict, returning your menstrual bleeding to normal.

After several months of progestin therapy, your blood loss can be reduced by as much as 20 percent (Cameron 1990). Women who have progestin intolerance can use micronized progesterone vaginal gel. This gel prevents the development of an abnormal uterine lining without increasing your blood levels of progesterone.

Birth control pill therapy is targeted at women who are still ovulating but experiencing heavy bleeding, and whose endometrial biopsy is normal. The Pill contains both estrogen and progesterone. This combination of hormones prevents the uterine lining from thickening, which decreases menstrual bleeding by as much as 50 percent (Brill 1995). Birth control pills are contraindicated in certain perimenopausal women. If you smoke or have migraine headaches, high blood pressure, a history of blood clots in your legs, or fibroid tumors, you can't take the Pill. It is also contraindicated for women who don't tolerate progestins (Leventhal 1996).

The progesterone-impregnated IUD can be used in all women who bleed heavily—those who ovulate and those who don't. With this IUD in your uterus, bleeding will be reduced by 65 percent over a twelve-month period (Brill 1995). Your uterine lining is affected by direct contact with the progesterone in the IUD, and progesterone levels within your uterus are much higher than can be achieved by taking progestin by mouth. The endometrial lining becomes very thin, so you bleed very little during your menstrual period. The greatest reduction in bleeding from any nonsurgical method is seen with the use of the progesterone-impregnated IUD (Brill 1995; Coleman 1997; Barrington 1997). The blood level of progesterone isn't increased with this IUD, so you can use it even if you have a progestin intolerance. It must be replaced every year.

The levonorgestrel-releasing IUD contains a very powerful synthetic progestin. It has shown an even greater benefit, reducing bleeding by 86 percent after three months of use and by 97 percent after twelve months (Coleman 1997; Barrington 1997). Some women have irregular light bleeding after the placement of this IUD, but the bleeding stops after three months of use in all but 3 percent of women (Wang 1998). It does increase progesterone levels slightly, so another 3 percent discontinue its use because of systemic side effects (Coleman 1997). It must be replaced every seven years. FDA approval of this IUD is expected in late 2000.

Nonhormonal Treatment of DUB

Nonsteroidal anti-inflammatory drugs (NSAIDs) also work to control dysfunctional uterine bleeding. Mefenamic acid (Meclomen) has been shown to reduce abnormal bleeding by 50 percent (Brill 1995; Cameron 1990). It also decreases menstrual cramps, which is a bonus. Mefenamic acid even reduces bleeding in some women with known fibroids (Brill 1995).

Ibuprofen (Motrin, Advil) and naproxen (Anaprox, Naprosyn, Aleve) are also NSAIDs; they reduce bleeding but are not as effective as mefenamic acid. In addition, there's a downside to taking these medications. If you have a history of ulcer disease, are allergic to aspirin, or bruise easily, you won't like what the NSAIDs do to you. You may have an upset stomach, reactivate your ulcers, and increase your bruising. If you have diabetes, asthma, kidney, or liver disease, NSAIDs should not be used because they may increase the complications associated with these diseases.

Male Hormone

Danazol, a derivative of the male hormone testosterone, dramatically reduces your menstrual blood loss when taken daily in doses of 200 to 800 milligrams (Brill 1995). Taking danazol also reduces menstrual cramps. Lower dosages are associated with irregular bleeding, and higher dosages have bothersome side effects. Since the drug is a derivative of testosterone, it may lower your voice, so don't use danazol if you use your voice professionally. The medication may also decrease your breast size, increase your weight, and cause acne.

Surgical Treatment of Dysfunctional Uterine Bleeding: Endometrial Ablation

Surgery may be needed to stop abnormal uterine bleeding. Until 1981, a hysterectomy was usually performed when medical management was unsuccessful in controlling such bleeding.

When you have abnormal bleeding and progesterone intolerance, severe cramps, migraine headaches, premenstrual syndrome, prolapsed (fallen) uterus, or involuntary urine loss, a hysterectomy is still your first choice to stop heavy menstrual bleeding. However, your only problem is abnormal bleeding and you don't plan any future pregnancies, an alternative treatment can be used: endometrial ablation (Goldrath 1981). This surgical procedure destroys your uterine lining (endometrium) and stops the bleeding. Your doctor may pretreat you with danazol, depo-medroxyprogesterone, or a GnRH agonist, which stunts your endometrium so its deepest layers can be destroyed, thus achieving a higher success rate (Goldrath 1990; Amso 1998). Once the endometrium is destroyed, it can't regenerate, and your problems are solved.

An endometrial ablation is an operating room procedure under general or spinal anesthesia. Because it is an outpatient procedure, most women can return to normal activities within a week. There may be some minor bleeding for about six weeks, but from then on bleeding is either minimal or stops altogether for 50 to 80 percent of women (Brill 1995). Approximately 10 percent of women have no change in their bleeding patterns whatsoever. These women will still need a hysterectomy or the levonorgestrel IUD to control their bleeding (Fedele 1997).

As with any surgical procedure, there are certain risks associated with an endometrial ablation. The procedure destroys most of the endometrial lining, forming a scar, which prevents remaining cells from bleeding but not from developing into cancer cells after menopause. Therefore women who have had an endometrial ablation must take progesterone along with estrogen for hormone replacement to prevent remaining cells from becoming cancerous. If you cannot tolerate progesterone, you shouldn't have an endometrial ablation.

Your menstrual period may return two to three years following an ablation because your endometrial lining has grown back. Occasionally, scar tissue may block the cervical canal (the channel between the endometrium and vagina). Trapped menstrual blood may cause severe pain, requiring a hysterectomy for pain control (Magos 1991).

The complication rates for endometrial ablations are very low: less than 3 percent for rollerball ablations (Lefler 1991) and less than 1 percent for thermal balloon ablations (Amso 1998). Thermal ablations are only performed when there are no uterine abnormalities such as fibroids, which may explain the lower complication rate.

Researchers are continuing to develop newer methods to destroy the endometrium. One freezes the endometrium (cryosurgery); one burns the cavity using a metallic membrane; another uses an expanding wire mesh that coagulates the endometrium in two minutes. These advanced instruments may improve success rates over methods now available (Oliver 2000).

Let's turn now to some physical causes of abnormal bleeding: polyps and fibroids.

Polyps and Fibroids

Polyps and fibroids are the two most common nonhormonal causes of dysfunctional uterine bleeding. Often the doctor detects fibroids during an initial pelvic examination. Polyps are more difficult to diagnose. Let's start by looking at the diagnosis and treatment of polyps and then at the somewhat more complicated issues involved in the treatment of fibroids.

Polyps: Diagnosis and Treatment

Endometrial polyps are teardrop-shaped glandular growths of the endometrium. They hang into the uterine cavity and are not sloughed off during menstruation. Instead, they remain attached to the uterus, which causes prolonged and sometimes heavy bleeding. Polyps do not have abnormal cells and are not considered to be tumors.

Since polyps do not respond to hormonal drug therapy, they must be removed. When abnormal bleeding is cause by a polyp, endometrial biopsy can easily miss the polyp and the laboratory report will be normal. For this reason, if polyps are suspected, they can be more reliably detected by inserting a fiber-optic device, called a hysteroscope, to visualize the interior of the uterus for easy identification and removal.

What Are Fibroids?

Except for the thin glandular endometrium, your uterus is composed exclusively of muscle. Most women are aware of this because of the two "big Cs"—cramps that come with your periods, and contractions when you deliver your babies. A fibroid (the medical term is leiomyoma) is a benign muscle tumor of the uterine wall. Fibroids are hereditary. They usually begin to grow when a woman is in her early forties. Estrogen is the catalyst that makes them grow. Thirty percent of all women have fibroids sometime during their lifetime, but only one-fifth of these women have symptoms and need to be treated (Parker 1995. Myomectomy).

Fibroids can occur at various places in your uterus. The only ones that will cause you trouble are those that grow on the inside wall of the uterus and push their way into the uterine cavity (endometrial cavity). They cause abnormal bleeding in two ways. First, they interfere with the corkscrewing of the blood vessels in the endometrium during the second half of the menstrual cycle, simulating dysfunctional uterine bleeding. Second, they push into the cavity, causing pressure on the opposite wall, making the endometrium abnormal there also. Fibroids that grow into the uterine cavity are called submucous fibroids. Some submucous fibroids hang down into the cavity itself. These pedunculated fibroids cause abnormal bleeding, and lots of it. Unfortunately, progestins do not stop the bleeding caused by submucous fibroids. In some women, mefenamic acid or ibuprofen can decrease the bleeding by constricting the blood vessels. The levonorgestrel IUD reduces this bleeding for some women, but most women will eventually need surgery.

Fibroids rarely cause infertility unless they are located inside the uterine cavity (Brill 1995). Pregnancy is unaffected by the presence of fibroids, except for a slightly higher rate of cesarean section births (Parker 1995. Myomectomy).

Fortunately, fibroids are never cancerous. (There is a rare cancer that resembles a fibroid in the early stages, but it's extremely uncommon in perimenopausal women.)

Treating Symptomatic Fibroids with Medication

Fibroids can't be cured with medications, but a medication called gonadotropin-releasing hormone agonists (GnRH-a) works nicely to shrink them and stop them from bleeding.

GnRH is the hormone your hypothalamus sends to the pituitary gland. It tells your pituitary to release FSH (follicle stimulating hormone) and LH (luteinizing hormone), and they in turn stimulate your ovaries to make estrogen and progesterone. A GnRH agonist is a drug that blocks GnRH, interrupting your ovarian hormonal cycle. You stop producing estrogen and progesterone. Sounds like menopause, doesn't it? That's right; a GnRH agonist causes a temporary menopause and stops uterine bleeding. Not surprisingly, then, side effects of GnRH agonists include hot flashes, vaginal dryness, skin aging, and possibly osteoporosis if the medication is used for too long.

Treating fibroids with GnRH agonists (by injection or with a nasal spray) is only a short-term measure to control bleeding, clear up anemia, and shrink fibroids. The next step in treatment is either a hysterectomy, the surgical removal of individual fibroids (myomectomy, discussed below), or uterine embolization (also discussed below). You can reduce the side effects of a GnRH agonist by taking low-dose estrogen and progesterone—called add-back therapy. Add-back therapy does not negate the benefits of the GnRH agonist, but it controls hot flashes, usually stops your menstrual period, menstrual cramps, and PMS. GnRH agonists are not prescribed for longer than six months because of risks of osteoporosis.

The levonorgestrel IUD was used to treat five women with heavy bleeding due to fibroids. The bleeding was controlled and their fibroids reduced in size (Singer 1994). Several other studies have shown women using the levonorgestrel IUD have a lower incidence of fibroids than women using the copper IUD (Silvin 1994; Coleman 1997; Fong 1999), suggesting the levonorgestrel IUD has an inhibitory effect on both the development and growth of fibroids.

Surgical Treatment of Symptomatic Fibroids

There are two surgical approaches to dealing with symptomatic fibroids: hysterectomy and myomectomy. In a hysterectomy, your uterus is removed, as well as all your fibroids. Hysterectomies are performed for other reasons besides fibroid removal, as you'll find out later in this chapter. In a myomectomy, individual fibroids are removed, but not the uterus.

The appropriate operation for removing fibroids is based on your fertility status, your desire for future pregnancies, your age, and surgical feasibility. You and your doctor will make these choices together. Let's start with a look at the types of myomectomy.

Intrauterine Myomectomy

An intrauterine myomectomy is the removal of fibroids located inside the uterus. The operation is nearly identical to an endometrial ablation. When you have only one or two intrauterine fibroids, you are highly unlikely to need a hysterectomy later on.

Surgical risks for this procedure increase when the uterus is enlarged because of the fibroids. These risks include fluid overload (extra fluid in your blood stream), the chance of incomplete removal of the fibroids (which could require additional surgery), and uterine perforation. For a woman with a large number of fibroids, the safest surgery is a hysterectomy, an embolization (described later on), or a myomectomy through an abdominal incision (described next).

Extrauterine Myomectomy

An extrauterine myomectomy involves the removal of the cauliflower-shaped fibroids on the outside of the uterus either by an open abdominal operation, through a laparoscope, or using a combination of these techniques.

The open abdomen method is used for very large fibroids because the empty space in the uterus created by the removal can be closed with sutures. This makes subsequent childbearing safer. For small fibroids and in women for whom future childbearing is not an issue, fibroids can be destroyed or removed using a laparoscope inserted through a small incision. A third technique, called a laparoscopically assisted myomectomy, combines the use of a laparoscope and a small open abdominal incision to remove small fibroids. With this method, the empty space can be sutured closed to safely allow childbirth (C. H. Nezhat 1996; F. Nezhat 1996; Dubuisson 1996).

The following complications are associated with an abdominal myomectomy (and less frequently with a laparoscopic myomectomy):

- **Adhesions:** Following an abdominal myomectomy, 92 percent developed adhesions between the uterus and bowel (Tulandi 1993), but only 46 percent had adhesions following a laparoscopic myomectomy (Parker 1995. Myomectomy). Adhesions are pieces of scar tissue that bridge the gap between the uterus and the bowel, fallopian tubes, and ovaries. They can obstruct the tubes, causing infertility, block the intestines, and cause chronic pelvic pain. Adhesions are caused by the heavy blood loss during this operation.

- **Blood loss:** Fibroids have an abundant blood supply. When they are removed, the typically heavy blood loss can be reduced by injecting a drug called vasopressin directly into the fibroid (before removal) or by placing a tourniquet or clamps around the uterine vessels. In spite of these efforts, however, postoperative bleeding can be a complication. Blood transfusions or reopening the abdomen to stop the bleeding may be necessary. Sometimes a hysterectomy is the only option at this point. There is less blood loss with a laparoscopic myomectomy because the fibroids are smaller. Indeed, it is uncommon to need either a blood transfusion or a hysterectomy following laparoscopic myomectomy for small fibroids (Parker 1995. Myomectomy).

- **Infertility:** You may become infertile because of adhesions following an abdominal myomectomy. Adhesions form between your ovaries and fallopian tubes 56 to 93 percent of the time following an abdominal myomectomy (Tulandi 1993). These adhesions may prevent the egg from reaching the fallopian tube or the sperm from reaching the egg. The myomectomy may also cause scar tissue within the uterus, making the endometrial lining inhospitable to the fetus and compromising your ability to successfully complete a pregnancy.

- **Recurrence:** Even if you have surgery to remove fibroids, you have a one in four chance of growing more and needing a repeat operation at a later date (Malone 1969). Due to the risks involved, physicians typically recommend a hysterectomy instead of a multiple myomectomy if you have completed your childbearing. For smaller fibroids, though, the laparoscopic myomectomy is a less invasive operation because fiberoptic technology is used instead of an open incision. You have less pain and usually go home the same day.

- **Pregnancy:** When pregnancy is still part of your plans, another aspect of the laparoscopic procedure must be considered. Surgery weakens the uterine wall. When a woman does get pregnant following a myomectomy, she has a small risk that her uterus will rupture (Harris 1992; Garnet 1964). The risk of uterine rupture is greater when a woman has had a laparoscopic myomectomy than when she has had the traditional abdominal procedure (Harris 1992). As a result, doctors are reluctant to remove fibroids with a laparoscope in women desiring pregnancy. However, if you don't want more children and have only one or two small fibroids, a laparoscopic myomectomy may be your best choice.

Fibroid Embolization

In 1995, J. H. Ravina and other French radiologists used an X-ray technique called embolization to successfully stop massive bleeding from fibroids in sixteen French women who were too weak to withstand a hysterectomy. Radiologists frequently use an embolization technique to stop bleeding, but this was the first time embolization was used for women with bleeding fibroids. Using artery catheters and X-ray dye as a visual aid, small (500-micron) poly-vinyl-alcohol particles were injected into the uterine arteries. These particles traveled to the bleeding vessels, clotted them, and stopped the bleeding. The fibroids supplied by these small vessels then died. Because two other arteries supply blood to the uterus, the uterus didn't die.

Following the embolization, 85 percent of these patients didn't need a hysterectomy; their fibroids shrank in size and their heavy bleeding stopped. Since the 1995 report, these doctors have embolized over 400 French women, with similar results. The same procedure is now being used in radiology centers around the United States (Goodwin 2000).

We see the advantages of this new technique as follows:

- No general anesthetic: the procedure is done under sedation.
- No surgery: this is an X-ray procedure done with the aid of an X-ray machine.
- No adhesions or other postsurgical risks.
- A 40 to 70 percent decrease in fibroid size: the bigger they are, the smaller they get.
- All fibroids die, not just the ones the doctor can see or feel.
- No regrowth of treated fibroids. Fibroids often recur following a myomectomy.

- High cure rate: only 10 to 12 percent of the patients needed a hysterectomy because the procedure failed to stop the bleeding (Goodwin 2000).

Unfortunately, fibroid embolization does create some problems:

- The sudden decrease in the fibroid's blood supply causes pain equivalent to the pain of a mild heart attack. The pain continues until the whole fibroid dies off.

- The bigger the fibroid, the more it hurts.

- Flulike symptoms result from the inflammatory reaction to the dying fibroid.

- A smelly and profuse discharge develops as the fibroids inside the uterus die and are discharged through the vagina. You just have to wait it out.

- You may need hospitalization because of the pain and fever.

- There are no statistics on pregnancy complications, but doctors worry that there will be a decrease in the blood supply to a fetus because of the embolization. Although several centers have reported successful pregnancies following an embolization (Dieden 2000), this procedure is still not recommended for women who wish future pregnancies.

- You may need an emergency hysterectomy if you develop an infection due to necrosis of extremely large fibroids (Goodwin 1999; Vashisht 1999).

- A small risk of pulmonary emboli or stroke is associated with any arterial catheterization procedure.

As with any procedure, embolization doesn't work every time. One patient out of five failed to respond and needed a hysterectomy or myomectomy anyway.

Hysterectomy

We've already mentioned two valid indications for doing a hysterectomy: uncontrollable bleeding and symptomatic fibroids. Other indications for a hysterectomy include cancer and precancerous conditions, infection, severe endometriosis, pelvic pain, and uterine prolapse. First, though, it will be helpful to know more about the operation itself, the various ways it can be carried out, and the reasoning behind choosing one technique over another.

According to the National Center for Health Statistics over 600,000 hysterectomies are performed each year in the United States. By age sixty, one-third of American women will have had a hysterectomy (Carlson 1993). Hysterectomies are the second most common major female operation after cesarean sections. The $5 billion annual cost to our health-care system for hysterectomies has stimulated efforts to find alternatives. The newer medical and surgical technologies discussed earlier in this chapter have reduced the number of hysterectomies by 20 percent.

If your doctor recommends a hysterectomy, making your decision will be easier if you understand some of the terminology surrounding this procedure. The following list of definitions will help. In addition, Figure 14.1 illustrates normal pelvic anatomy; and Figure 14.2 illustrates the structures removed in the various operations.

- **Total hysterectomy:** Removal of the entire uterus, including the cervix (the opening into the vagina), but not the ovaries or the fallopian tubes.

- **Total abdominal hysterectomy and bilateral salpingo-oophorectomy (TAH & BSO):** An abdominal operation that removes the entire uterus, fallopian tubes, and both ovaries.

- **Subtotal abdominal hysterectomy:** Removal of the main body of the uterus but not the cervix.

- **Vaginal hysterectomy:** Removal of the entire uterus through the vagina, with no abdominal incision.

- **Laparoscopically assisted vaginal hysterectomy (LAVH):** The laparoscope and other necessary instruments are inserted through several small abdominal incisions to help the surgeon remove the uterus vaginally.

- **Laparoscopic subtotal hysterectomy (LSH):** Removal of the main body of the uterus but not the cervix through the laparoscope.

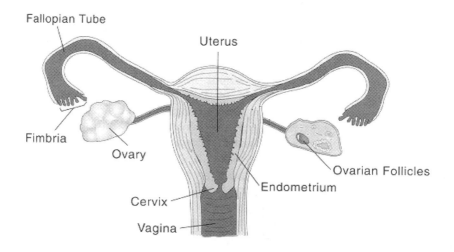

Figure 14.1.   Normal Pelvic Anatomy

Dark outline = structures removed

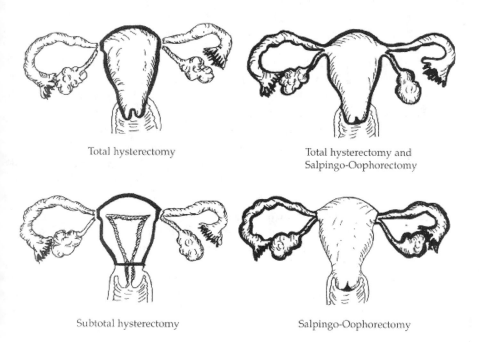

Total hysterectomy

Total hysterectomy and
Salpingo-Oophorectomy

Subtotal hysterectomy

Salpingo-Oophorectomy

Figure 14.2. Pelvic Operations

- **Oophorectomy:** An abdominal or laparoscopic operation to remove one or both ovaries. Immediate menopause occurs only if both ovaries are removed.

- **Salpingectomy:** An abdominal or laparoscopic operation to remove one or both fallopian tubes.

Why Should You Have a Hysterectomy?

Hysterectomies generally fall into two categories: nonelective and elective. A nonelective hysterectomy is required when you have invasive cancer of the endometrium, ovary, or cervix, life-threatening uterine hemorrhage, or uncontrollable life-threatening infection. In these cases, there are alternatives to hysterectomy in only two conditions: Invasive cervical cancer is sometimes treated with radiation instead of surgery; and uterine hemorrhage due to fibroids can be treated with embolization. But don't delay your operation if you have any of these problems. Time has run out to try alternative therapies.

Elective hysterectomies are performed when the indications are less urgent. You have more time to plan for your surgery or to try alternative therapies. Indications for an elective hysterectomy include persistent abnormal uterine bleeding and symptomatic fibroids, both of which we've already discussed. Other indications are:

- **Endometriosis:** This may be caused by your menstrual blood flowing backward through the fallopian tubes into your abdomen. Most women's bodies destroy this blood and tissue, but some do not. In these women, the endometrial tissue becomes implanted in sites outside the uterus, commonly on the ovaries, fallopian tubes, peritoneum (abdominal lining), and intestines. Every time you have a menstrual period, the endometriosis implants bleed also. This results in painful adhesions, menstrual cramps, and painful intercourse. Your doctor may treat your endometriosis with a GnRH agonist, danazol, or birth control pills, but the treatment is effective only as long as the medication is taken. Hysterectomy with removal of the ovaries cures this disease, but it is a last-ditch therapy after medical treatment fails.

- **Precancerous conditions of the uterus:** Cryosurgery, LEEP, and a cervical conization (described in Chapter 6) can be used to treat precancerous lesions of the cervix. Progestin therapy can often treat precancerous lesions of the endometrium. But a hysterectomy always cures both precancerous conditions.

- **Chronic pelvic pain:** This condition is often difficult to diagnose and treat. Causes range from nerve damage, endometriosis, and adhesions from sexually transmitted diseases or previous surgery, to psychological sexual trauma. A hysterectomy is an absolute last-ditch treatment for chronic pelvic pain.

- **Prolapse of the uterus:** Prolapse (sagging) of the uterus is more commonly found in postmenopausal women; the uterus sometimes protrudes outside of the vagina. As an alternative to hysterectomy, methods such as pessaries (a plastic or soft rubber device placed in your vagina to keep the uterus in place) can help. Prolapse is a nuisance, so many women opt for a hysterectomy.

Half of all hysterectomies are done for abnormal uterine bleeding, and half of these uterine specimens are reported to be free of disease (Brill 1995). The fact that the tissue was "free of disease" does not mean these operations were unnecessary. Nevertheless, this has generated so much negative press about unnecessary hysterectomies that many women feel they have somehow failed if they agree to have this operation (West 1994). Many women opt for a hysterectomy because the alternative therapies are not well tolerated or are simply not working.

Study after study has shown that women who opted for hysterectomy were more satisfied with the outcome than women choosing other forms of therapy (Alexander 1996, Dwyer 1993). This is true even though the other treatments are less invasive, have fewer complications, and involve quicker recovery.

Now let's take a closer look at the various types of hysterectomies.

Types of Hysterectomy

All hysterectomies involve detachment of the five ligaments that support the uterus, tying off the blood vessels, and pulling the ligaments together to prevent a later vaginal prolapse. This can be done with an abdominal, vaginal, or laparoscopically assisted vaginal (LAVH) procedure.

Abdominal Hysterectomy

Currently, 70 percent of all 600,000 hysterectomies done in North America each year are done through an abdominal incision (Munro 1995). Prior to 1950, the majority of hysterectomies done in North America were subtotal abdominal hysterectomies, leaving the cervix in place. Antibiotics of that era were not as effective as they are now. Removal of the cervix required opening the vagina, resulting in a higher incidence of postoperative infection from the vaginal bacteria. Since 1950, physicians have favored removal of the cervix along with the uterus (a total hysterectomy) to prevent cervical cancer. (Cervical cancer is discussed in Chapter 6).

Today, the thinking on this subject is changing again. An intact cervix can preserve bladder function, maintain sexual pleasure, and prevent vaginal prolapse after a hysterectomy (Lyons 1996). Cervical cancer is caused by human papilloma virus (HPV), which also causes genital warts. If you don't have HPV, you may be able to keep your cervix with minimal risk. One study found that less than 0.3 percent of 1,104 women who underwent subtotal hysterectomies subsequently developed cervical cancer (Storm 1992). Most subtotal hysterectomies (removal of the body of the uterus but leaving the cervix behind) are performed abdominally rather than vaginally, but subtotal laparoscopic hysterectomies are becoming more common every year (Simon 1999). We discuss this operation later on.

What are the disadvantages of abdominal hysterectomy? For one thing, a large abdominal incision is necessary. The recovery period is longer and more painful than for either a vaginal hysterectomy or LAVH. The incision may become infected, and blood may collect under the skin. For these reasons, only the most difficult hysterectomies are done abdominally. Women with invasive cancer of the female organs (with the exception of some very early cervical or endometrial cancers) have abdominal hysterectomies because the surgeon needs to remove diseased tissue other than the uterus (Montz 1995). Other reasons for an abdominal hysterectomy include large fibroids, severe endometriosis, and severe adhesions from multiple prior operations and multiple cesarean births.

Abdominal hysterectomies usually require a three- to four-day hospitalization and then six weeks of recuperation. This compares with a one- to two-day hospitalization and a two-week recuperation for a vaginal hysterectomy or LAVH.

Vaginal Hysterectomy

A vaginal hysterectomy is an option for women who have a relatively small uterus, some relaxation of uterine supporting structures, and a large-enough vagina to allow the instruments in and the uterus out. Typically, candidates for vaginal hysterectomy have had at least one vaginal birth and have none of the problems requiring an abdominal hysterectomy. There are no external incisions, so postoperative pain is strikingly less than with an abdominal hysterectomy. This translates to a shorter hospital stay and full recovery in two to three weeks (Van Den Eeden 1998).

One common complication with vaginal hysterectomy (and LAVH) is an inadvertent incision in the bladder during the surgical removal of the uterus. This incision is easily recognized and easily repaired; but if it happens to you, you'll need to wear a catheter for seven to ten days while your bladder heals. The chance of this complication is much lower with abdominal surgery.

Laparoscopically Assisted Vaginal Hysterectomy (LAVH)

This operation combines abdominal surgery through a laparoscope with vaginal surgery. By operating through a laparoscope, the surgeon can cut scar tissue that would otherwise prevent the uterus from being removed vaginally. The uterus is freed from its attachments with instruments inserted through three or four small incisions in the abdomen. Once it is detached, the uterus is removed through the vagina.

The advantage of an LAVH is the conversion of an abdominal hysterectomy to a vaginal one. Your length of hospital stay and recovery time for an LAVH is about the same as for a vaginal hysterectomy. An LAVH takes a little longer to perform than either a vaginal or abdominal hysterectomy, but it is worth the effort. Removing the entire uterus and cervix by the laparoscope, however, involves prolonged surgical time and a significant increase in the complication rate over an LAVH (Nezhat 1996). For those reasons a total laparoscopic hysterectomy is believed to be an unacceptable alternative to the LAVH (Nezhat 1999).

Many critics, who are not concerned with pain and the timely return to normal activities, say that the greater operating room expenses associated with an LAVH more than offset the savings of an extra two or three days in the hospital. These expenses include a longer operation and costly disposable instruments. Van Den Eeden (1998) disagrees. He found the LAVH to be less costly than an abdominal hysterectomy. There is no denying, however, even by the critics, that you feel better and return to your normal lifestyle much more quickly—in about three weeks—if you have an LAVH instead of an abdominal hysterectomy.

Laparoscopic Subtotal Hysterectomy (LSH)

As surgeons have developed greater confidence and skill using the laparoscope, more and more operations have been converted from open procedures to laparoscopic surgery. This is true in general surgery and orthopedic surgery as well as gynecological surgery. The laparoscopic subtotal hysterectomy (LSH) has fewer complications, shorter hospitalization, a quicker recovery time, and a faster return to normal activities than is found with an abdominal subtotal hysterectomy. LSH converts the otherwise painful and prolonged recovery from an abdominal incision to the relative ease of laparoscopic surgery. Patients undergoing an LSH have fewer complications and less postoperative pain (Liu 1992). Many women who have an LSH go home in less than 24 hours (Simon 1999). Because of technical difficulties, women electing an LSH must be of normal weight, have a small uterus, and have a normal Pap smear.

Hysterectomy Complications

Minor complications of hysterectomies include bladder and incision infections, skin edge separations, anemia, and in rare cases, a drug reaction (usually a rash and itching).

Most studies show major complication rates to be low. Major complications from abdominal hysterectomies occur in less than 1 percent of surgeries (Munro 1995). Major complications occurred in 4.5 percent of vaginal hysterectomies and 2.5 percent of LAVHs.

The more serious complications from abdominal hysterectomy include injury to the bladder, intestine, and ureter (the tube from the kidney to the bladder). Major postoperative complications include significant bleeding, infection with abscess formation, total wound separation, and adhesions. For vaginal hysterectomies, LSH, and LAVH, major complications include injury to the bladder (as mentioned for the abdominal procedure), but also significant bleeding and abscess formation. Numerous studies in the past two decades show that most complications of hysterectomy are minor ones. Major complications do occur, however, and they deserve a closer look.

Heavy Bleeding

All patients lose blood during any surgery, but you can take iron pills for three or four weeks to correct the minor blood loss from a hysterectomy. When heavy bleeding does occur, your own blood can be saved and returned to you with a cell saver. This is a machine that collects and filters the blood you lose during surgery. It often avoids the need for a blood-bank transfusion. When there is a possibility of a blood-bank transfusion, you can give one or more units of your own blood prior to surgery, which can then be given back to you during or after the operation.

Adhesions

Adhesions rarely cause problems. Infrequently, however, they can be dense and cause tissues and organs to stick together. When organs are immobilized by adhesions, normal body movement may cause pain. Future surgery may be complicated by the presence of adhesions, and the organs themselves (most commonly the bladder and intestines) may be damaged in the process of surgical separation.

If you have had several cesarean sections, you may have dense adhesions between your bladder and uterus. It may be difficult surgically separating the two during a hysterectomy, and it's possible the bladder may be injured. The injury can be easily repaired, but you will have to wear a catheter for the seven- to ten-day healing period.

Ureteral Injury

The ureters—the two tubes that carry urine from your kidneys to your bladder—pass within a quarter-inch of your uterus. This close proximity puts the ureters in harm's way during a hysterectomy. In rare cases, a ureter may be damaged, requiring corrective surgery to restore normal function.

Serious Infection

You have a significant risk of serious infection after a hysterectomy because the surgery enters the vagina, which is teeming with bacteria. Your vagina exists in perfect harmony with its normal bacterial flora, but when these same organisms are transported into the abdominal cavity during a hysterectomy, serious infections may result. Preoperative prophylactic antibiotics reduce your risk of serious infection by 50 percent for all types of hysterectomies (Reggiori 1996; Tanos 1994). Although there is some debate over the use of antibiotics to prevent disease, especially with the emergence of "superbugs," there is no disagreement at all about the use of these drugs in hysterectomies. Without antibiotics, there is a high risk of infection (Medical Letter 1995).

Damage to a Major Blood Vessel

In an LAVH, instruments are inserted through the abdomen, in an area close to major blood vessels. The vessels may be inadvertently torn during the operation, causing heavy bleeding that can be stopped by pressure and several stitches. Occasionally, a larger incision is needed to see the vessels and stop the bleeding.

Long-Term Complications

Some problems resulting from a hysterectomy occur months to years after the surgery. You may develop bladder dysfunction, a hernia of the intestines into the vagina, vaginal prolapse, bowel obstruction, and sexual dysfunction (Lyons 1996). When they are feasible alternatives, an endometrial ablation, fibroid embolization, or subtotal hysterectomy are all procedures that decrease the risk of long-term complications.

Elective Removal of Ovaries as Part of the Hysterectomy

Should you have your ovaries removed when you have your hysterectomy? There is no easy answer to this question. Your ovaries produce the hormones that keep things running smoothly, and if they're removed you experience instant menopause. Why not leave them alone to do their job? On the other hand, removal of your ovaries at the time of your hysterectomy prevents ovarian cancer. That's a compelling reason to have them removed. Let's take a closer look at this debate.

What about Cancer?

Ovarian cancer (discussed in Chapter 6), while rare in perimenopause, remains the leading cause of death from gynecologic malignancy, and the fourth most frequent cause of death from cancer for women in the United States (Maiman 1995; Cramer 1994).

Approximately three-quarters of malignant ovarian tumors are detected only after the disease has spread throughout the abdominal cavity (Maiman 1995). The continued high risk for ovarian cancer is the main reason ovarian removal is recommended when a hysterectomy is being performed.

When Gilda Radner died in 1989 from ovarian cancer following extensive infertility treatment, the foundation that bears her name publicized the existence of a blood test, CA-125, that could detect ovarian cancer. Unfortunately, CA-125 is not specific for ovarian cancer in perimenopausal women unless levels are extremely high—and by then it's too late. Women who have fibroids, endometriosis, ovarian cysts, cirrhosis of the liver, other cancers, or are pregnant or having their menstrual periods produce high levels of CA-125 (Parker 1995. The case for laparoscopie). Most elevated CA-125 levels will be false positives in perimenopausal women (Maiman 1995). Twenty-five percent of women with ovarian cancers will have a normal CA-125 value (Creasman 1997).

Two genes, BRCA-1 and BRCA-2, appear to be responsible for the majority of familial breast cancer occurring before menopause. 60 to 80 percent of women carrying these genes will develop breast cancer and 30 to 60 percent will develop ovarian cancer. The rate may reach 85 percent when there is a strong family history (Mann 1998). Women at significant risk for carrying these genes have three first- or second-degree relatives who have developed breast cancer before menopause, or are of Ashkenazi Jewish descent with two relatives with premenopausal breast cancer. Women carrying these genes need to discuss prophylactic removal of their ovaries with their physicians.

A tumor-suppressor gene (named gene p53) responsible for two-thirds of all ovarian cancer has been discovered (Schildkraut 1997). Uninterrupted ovulation of many years' duration causes mutations of this gene, which results in ovarian cancer. Women who have had fewer than three children are known to be at higher risk for ovarian cancer. A tubal ligation may reduce the risk of ovarian cancer by as much as 70 percent (Harvard Women's Health Watch 2000). Women who have taken the Pill for ten years or longer cut their risk for ovarian cancer in half (Schildkraut 1997). To date, though, there is no reliable method to detect ovarian cancer early, which is the only time when it matters. Even when the genetic test for the altered p53 gene is available, it will only detect in two-thirds of women at risk. A biomarker called lysophosphatidic acid (LPA) may soon be available as a more reliable screening test.

Contributing Factors

Now let's look at some specific factors to consider in terms of whether you should have your ovaries removed (oophorectomy):

- **Hereditary ovarian cancer:** For certain familial cancers, doctors recommend an oophorectomy when a woman has finished her family. When you need a hysterectomy for other reasons, having your ovaries removed at the same time may prevent ovarian cancer.

- **Limited remaining ovarian function:** If you are close to menopause, your ovarian function will soon be dramatically reduced. Based on your individual risk factors, you may consider your risk of developing ovarian cancer too great to justify keeping your ovaries for the few years they will continue to function.

- **Shortened ovarian life:** If your uterus is removed, some of the blood supply to your ovaries is lost. Studies have shown that many perimenopausal women who retain their ovaries after a hysterectomy will be menopausal within a few years—a significant factor in making your decision (Cooper 1999).

- **Ovarian cysts:** Ten percent of women who have a hysterectomy will develop painful recurrent ovarian cysts during the remaining years before menopause (Mancuso 1991). These cysts are not cancer, but they hurt and often need to be removed, which means a second operation. Ovaries can usually be removed using a laparoscope, but cysts may be hidden in scar tissue after a hysterectomy and impossible to remove without a large abdominal incision.

The removal of normal ovaries at the time of a hysterectomy is not foolproof; however, it does reduce your chance of developing ovarian cancer by 90 percent. Cancer of the ovary can develop in ovarian cells that exist outside the ovary. These cells are too few in number to be visible at the time of a hysterectomy, but they can later develop into ovarian cancer even if your ovaries have been removed.

The primary reason to keep your ovaries is their continued production of hormones in just the right amount and at just the right time.

The Bottom Line

When you need a hysterectomy, most gynecologists recommend that you keep your ovaries if you are less than forty years old. Between age forty and forty-five, if you have severe PMS symptoms, menstrual migraines, or significant endometriosis and you are having a hysterectomy, your symptoms will decrease or disappear with the removal of your ovaries (Casper 1990). If you are close to menopause or postmenopausal, your doctor will usually recommend that you have your ovaries removed.

When you are pondering the question of ovarian conservation or removal, ask and get answers to these three questions:

- Are my ovaries still functioning? How long can I expect that to continue?

- If I choose to keep my ovaries, how likely is it that I will need future ovarian surgery?

- Do I have familial cancer risk factors that may shorten my life if I keep my ovaries?

Elective Hysterectomy Accompanying Removal of the Ovaries

Should you have a hysterectomy when you have your ovaries removed? If you choose to have your ovaries removed because of a strong family history of hereditary ovarian cancer, or if you have ovarian cysts or tumors, should you have your uterus out as well? The answer is maybe. Let's consider the factors involved.

Once your ovaries are removed, you will need hormone replacement (HRT). If your uterus is removed at the same time, you won't need to take progesterone to prevent endometrial cancer and you won't ever have another menstrual period—which means no more PMS, menstrual migraines, or anything else associated with your periods.

On the other hand, there is a much higher complication rate from a hysterectomy than from an oophorectomy. In a study of 200 women who had their ovaries removed, 100 women kept their uterus and 100 did not. Twenty-three of the 100 women who had hysterectomies also had serious complications (Gambone 1992). The only complication in the 100 women who did not have hysterectomies was a wound infection. If you can take progesterone without adverse side effects, the removal of your ovaries without the removal of your uterus lowers your risk of complications.

You Needed That Hysterectomy and You Don't Miss Your Uterus—So Why Are You So Sad?

Posthysterectomy sadness is common; 25 percent experience it (Alexander 1996). It is also a short-lived effect of the operation.

An element of that sadness may have to do with a woman's loss of childbearing capability or her relationship to her sexual partner. Women who regard menstrual periods as a monthly affirmation of their femininity, believe them to be a time of cleansing, or have other strongly held beliefs about them may find their absence unsettling. The importance of childbearing is implanted early. Most young girls play with dolls and plan to have children. The loss of this ability can and does have a psychological impact on most women.

In 1996, Alexander and others studied 204 women who needed treatment for abnormal bleeding. Ninety-nine had had a hysterectomy, and the rest an endometrial ablation. The researchers found no lasting psychiatric illness in either group. In addition, both groups experienced the same degree of sexual interest and intensity of orgasm as they had prior to surgery. During the first six postoperative months, the women who had undergone the hysterectomy had significantly more anxiety and depression, but this was gone by twelve months.

The degree of sadness following a hysterectomy is negligible for women who have had a prior tubal sterilization. We believe this may be because they have already come to terms with the loss of their ability to have children. Women with a strong family history of depression and those who have a hysterectomy following unsuccessful treatment of infertility are more often depressed postoperatively (Hendricks-Matthews 1991). Typically, though, the sadness following a hysterectomy passes quickly. Your new sexual freedom and liberty from the pain and embarrassment of out-of-control periods more than make up for any sadness you feel.

Summary of Treatment for Abnormal Uterine Bleeding

When you have abnormal uterine bleeding, the cause must be determined before treatment is undertaken. If a hormonal imbalance is diagnosed, it can be treated by various medications, or by endometrial ablation. When the bleeding is due to a structural change such as polyps or cancer, surgery is necessary to correct the abnormal bleeding. Fibroids can be treated by various operations, including the removal or destruction of the fibroids themselves, or by a hysterectomy, or by fibroid embolization. Hysterectomies do save lives and remain the most common treatment for dysfunctional uterine bleeding as well as genital cancer. Whether to have your ovaries removed while having a hysterectomy or keep them is a difficult decision and must be based on your assessment of the risk of ovarian cysts or cancer, as well as your desire for continued natural hormonal production.

Loss of your uterus is rightly regarded as a significant event and a major life change. You and your doctor must address many complex issues before deciding on this or any other operation. You are a valuable and necessary part of the decision-making process. Being informed is a good way to begin.

Ovarian Cysts

A cyst is any closed cavity lined with cells that contains liquid or semisolid material. Cysts are painful, often during sex, but rarely malignant (Maiman 1995). An enlarged ovary can be detected during a pelvic examination, but the examination can't distinguish a fluid-filled cyst from a solid tumor. An ultrasound examination provides more information; it differentiates between a clear fluid cyst, a cyst with particles in the fluid, and a solid tumor. If a solid tumor is found, your doctor will usually advise its immediate removal. When you have an ovarian cyst, the ultrasound can help you and your doctor decide on the correct treatment.

Several types of ovarian cysts are common to perimenopausal women.

Functional Ovarian Cysts

Functional cysts occur as the result of everyday activity in your ovaries. Perimenopausal women's cysts are almost always functional cysts: smaller than a golf ball, filled with clear fluid, occurring in one ovary at a time, and almost never cancerous. These cysts are painful, but they usually disappear over two to three months without any therapy except watchful waiting.

There are various types of functional ovarian cysts. In general, only when a cyst is larger than a golf ball does it require drainage or surgical removal. In this case, it may not be a functional cyst and won't go away without treatment. When they are purely cystic and smaller than four inches in diameter, they are all benign (Herrmann 1987).

Age is on your side in this matter. Even when a cyst has particles within the fluid, is larger than a golf ball, or doesn't disappear on its own, it is rarely cancerous in perimenopause. In a study of 773 women under forty-five years of age with enlarged cystic ovaries, only eleven (or 1.4 percent) of the masses were ovarian cancers (Mecke 1992).

Nonfunctional Ovarian Cysts

Ovarian cysts larger than four inches are usually nonfunctional and won't be reduced with hormonal therapy or watchful waiting. They need to be removed. Whether a cyst is nonfunctional or not can only be determined by microscopic evaluation.

These cysts are rarely malignant. If the ovary is larger than a tennis ball and a nonfunctional cyst is suspected, removal of the ovary and sometimes the fallopian tube may be necessary. Again, age is on your side. In only 0.04 percent of 13,739 premenopausal women with apparently benign ovarian cysts did the result turn out to be ovarian cancer (Maiman 1995).

Endometriomas

Endometriomas result from endometriosis in the ovary, and they may prevent conception. As described earlier in the chapter, endometriosis tissue located in the pelvis bleeds during the menstrual period. When endometrial tissue is located in the ovary, bleeding results in an ovarian cyst that is full of old blood, which becomes very thick and turns brown. These cysts are nicknamed "chocolate cysts" because the fluid in them looks just like chocolate syrup.

Endometriomas are now removed routinely by laparoscopic surgery with a subsequent pregnancy rate approaching 40 percent (Marrs 1991). The advantage of laparoscopic removal over an open operation is a lower chance of adhesion formation and a much quicker recovery. If the accompanying pelvic endometriosis is already extreme, with dense adhesion formation, removal of endometriomas may require a larger open abdominal incision.

Summary of Ovarian Cysts

When smaller than a golf ball, ovarian cysts, including endometriomas, can be managed with a laparoscopic operation. When they are the size of a tennis ball or don't meet the clinical or ultrasound criteria for laparoscopic removal, they must be removed by a larger abdominal incision.

Ectopic (Tubal) Pregnancy

An ectopic pregnancy is a pregnancy that implants itself outside the uterus. The large majority of ectopic pregnancies occur in the fallopian tube, less frequently in the ovary, and very rarely in the abdomen.

When the fallopian tube has been damaged, the journey to the uterus can be interrupted; the fertilized egg nestles in the tube and results in a tubal, rather than a uterine pregnancy. The growing fetus strains the confines of the fallopian tube until it can stretch no further and ruptures, causing serious and potentially life-threatening internal hemorrhage. Without early diagnosis and medical treatment, tubal rupture and internal bleeding requiring emergency surgery occurs in approximately two-thirds of women who have ectopic pregnancies.

In the classic study of 215 consecutive ectopic pregnancies, 96 tubal pregnancies ruptured and required emergency surgery (Lund 1955). The other 120 women were simply observed. Forty-five percent of these 120 women eventually needed surgery to treat their ectopic pregnancies; but 68 out of the original 215, about one-third, resolved their ectopic pregnancies without an operation. Most doctors aren't willing to wait for an ectopic pregnancy to disappear, however, and will treat you as soon as the diagnosis is made, hoping to prevent tubal rupture. Treatment includes medication to terminate the pregnancy before the tube ruptures, or early laparoscopic surgery.

There has been a fourfold increase in the incidence of ectopic pregnancies over the last twenty-five years. Unfortunately, a high percentage of these occurred in perimenopause (Jaffe 1991). Following are contributing factors to this condition:

- **Endometriosis.** Women with endometriosis have gradually increasing damage to their tubes and ovaries. If they choose not to have children or to postpone pregnancy, they are more likely to have endometriosis in the fallopian tubes, resulting in an increased risk of ectopic pregnancy.

- **Early treatment of sexually transmitted diseases early in life.** When STDs are diagnosed and treated early, the result is damaged but not blocked fallopian tubes, causing a higher incidence of ectopic pregnancy. Perimenopausal women have had more years to contract an STD than have younger women, so the incidence of a previous STD and tubal damage is greater in perimenopause.

- **Corrective tubal surgery.** Today's fertility specialists are repairing previously damaged tubes, which results in an increased risk of tubal pregnancies.

Diagnosis of Ectopic Pregnancy

If you are at high risk for developing an ectopic pregnancy, you are encouraged to call your physician as soon as you miss your first period. Risk factors include a prior ectopic pregnancy, prior pelvic inflammatory disease (PID), a history of endometriosis, and previous tubal surgery. A series of blood tests will measure the exact amount of hCG (human chorionic gonadotropin), the hormone of pregnancy, in your blood. Your hCG rises 60 percent every two days and doubles every three days when you have a normal uterine pregnancy. If your hCG level hasn't risen by 100 percent in three days, a tubal pregnancy will be suspected. If the hCG levels continue to lag behind, an ultrasound scan of your uterus will determine if the pregnancy is in your uterus or not. If not, an ectopic pregnancy is diagnosed. Ectopic pregnancies earlier than six weeks' gestation can be treated with medication instead of surgery.

Medical Treatment of Ectopic Pregnancy

Methotrexate, an anticancer drug, effectively destroys ectopic pregnancy in the fallopian tube. After a methotrexate injection, hCG blood levels will be checked weekly until this test indicates the pregnancy is gone.

Methotrexate is almost always given in a single low dose with a high success rate (94 percent), but minimal side effects (Stovall 1995). In studies, only 4 percent needed a second dose to dissolve the pregnancy and only 6 percent required surgery (Gomel 1995; Stovall 1995). Women treated with methotrexate have a high subsequent successful pregnancy rate and a low recurrent ectopic pregnancy rate (Stovall 1991; Langer 1990; Silva 1993). When the diagnosis is made early, both patients and physicians prefer the medical treatment of ectopic pregnancy. Methotrexate doesn't work when the pregnancy is larger than 3.5 centimeters or when a heartbeat is detected in the fallopian tube; surgery then becomes the only treatment.

Surgical Treatment of Ectopic Pregnancy

Surgery remains the only method for treating women with ectopic pregnancies who are not candidates for medical therapy. Laparoscopic surgery has largely supplanted the larger abdominal incision except in life threatening emergencies. The type of tubal surgery is dependent on the extent of damage to the tube. Minor tubal damage may be repaired while greater damage may require removal of the entire tube or a portion of it. All three can be accomplished with a laparoscope or an open abdominal incision.

Urinary Incontinence

Significant urinary incontinence occurs in 25 percent of all women in their reproductive years and in 50 percent of all postmenopausal women. Some degree of incontinence occurs in 85 percent of women over age eighteen (Lyons 1995). Over $16 billion is spent annually on treatment of incontinence, including the cost of protective garments (Brown 1996). To help you understand the causes and treatment of incontinence, let's take another brief look at your anatomy.

The Genito-Urinary System

The reproductive organs (genitals) and the urinary organs form your genito-urinary system. Problems with both the genital and the urinary systems often coexist, so they are usually diagnosed and treated together. When urinary incontinence occurs, the following parts of your body are involved:

- **Kidneys:** Your kidneys filter wastes out of your blood and make urine, which is passed to the bladder by the **ureters.**

- **Bladder:** The bladder is simply a reservoir to store urine until it is convenient to empty it. When it fills to a certain amount, the detrusor (bladder muscle) contracts to expel the urine.

- **Urethra:** This is the tube connecting your bladder to the outside world. Your urethra is only about three inches long. It is surrounded by muscles that maintain their strength with the help of your estrogens. The urethra and the muscles around it lose tone with age and with estrogen depletion. In addition, the urethral muscles may have been damaged during childbirth. During perimenopause, when your tissues begin to lose their tensile strength, your damaged urethra may lose strength as well. The muscles may not be strong enough to keep urine from running out when you cough or sneeze. During and after menopause, prolonged estrogen depletion further damages the urethra and it may remain open, acting as a siphon from the bladder to the outside.

- **Bladder neck:** This is the area where your bladder joins the urethra. It is surrounded by muscles that automatically keep the bladder neck closed so urine stays in your bladder. When you urinate, the bladder neck opens, and urine enters the urethra. Age, estrogen depletion, and childbirth trauma cause these muscles to lose strength, resulting in urine loss.

- **External urethral sphincter:** Vaginal muscles support your bladder, bladder neck, and urethra. The external urethral sphincter is a portion of the vaginal muscles near the opening of your vagina. The sphincter prevents urine from escaping. It is under voluntary control. Unable to do the job alone, this sphincter needs help from its neighbors, the urethra and bladder neck. When your bladder neck and urethra cannot control urine loss, neither can your sphincter, no matter how tightly you squeeze it.

- **Pelvic floor muscles:** One of the pelvic floor muscles, the pubococcygeus or PC, circles your vagina and acts as a sling to suspend your uterus, bladder, bladder neck, and urethra. It is a voluntary muscle that helps the structures it supports to function correctly. Pregnancy, childbirth, and decreased estrogen states all cause the pelvic floor muscles to lose some of their strength. The organs it supports start sagging downward. If your bladder is one of these organs, incontinence results.

Continence—the Way It Ought to Be

When your bladder is full, it sends messages to your brain: "I have to go now!" Your brain sends a message back to your bladder giving it permission to empty, although it isn't always convenient to empty your bladder. If it isn't convenient, you send the message to "hold it." Your external sphincter tightens for all it's worth, the bladder muscles relax, the bladder neck remains closed, and your urge to urinate subsides. Once you *can* get to the bathroom, though, your bladder sends a more urgent message to your brain: "Are you folks up there aware that we have a problem down here?" Your brain answers, "Affirmative, detrusor. Let it go." Your external sphincter relaxes, your detrusor muscles contract, your bladder neck opens, and . . . RELIEF!

Types of Incontinence

Our description of normal continence may sound funny to you—but it's no fun when something goes wrong, causing you to lose urine when you don't want to. Depending upon which part of the body has a problem, you develop one (or more) types of incontinence: stress incontinence, urge incontinence, and urethral dysfunction siphon incontinence. More than 65 percent of all urinary incontinence is a mixture of these types (McGuire 1996).

Stress Incontinence

Stress incontinence is also called genuine stress incontinence (GUI). You can lose urine with any activity that increases the pressure (stress) on your bladder, including sneezing, laughing, coughing, jogging, lifting, and even sex. The increased pressure on the bladder puts added pressure on your bladder neck to open. If your external sphincter is not strong enough to compensate, urine escapes.

Stress incontinence occurs mainly in women who have had babies. Only 4 percent of childless women have stress incontinence (Brown 1996). (Note: Although women athletes sometimes lose urine with exercise, usually this is due to a bladder infection rather than true stress incontinence.)

For 22 to 32 percent of women, the first experience with incontinence is during pregnancy when the baby's head is pressing on the bladder (Brown 1996). Immediately after birth, 6 percent of these women are still incontinent, but by one year only 3 percent still lose urine. The time spent pushing a baby out in the second stage of labor is related to the development of incontinence: The longer a woman pushes during delivery, the greater her chance of developing incontinence when she reaches her mid- to late forties and beyond. The type of delivery also has an effect on how often stress incontinence occurs (Brown 1996). Forceps deliveries trigger a higher incidence of stress incontinence than do vacuum extraction deliveries. Still, women who have had a vacuum extraction have a higher incidence of incontinence than do women who had spontaneous vaginal deliveries. These results are deceiving, however, because women who have either forceps or vacuum deliveries have been pushing longer than women who have had spontaneous deliveries. Two large studies proved that the early intervention with forceps and episiotomy decreased the damage to the vaginal muscles and resultant incontinence

(Gainey 1955; Ranney 1990). Of all methods of delivery, Cesarean births have the lowest incidence of incontinence.

Knowing the cause of your incontinence may be interesting to you, but chances are you're more interested in fixing it. You've already had your last baby and you are dealing with incontinence now. You can't go back and change the way your children were delivered. What can you do today to help stop this embarrassing problem? Here are the medical treatments that work:

- **Kegel exercises:** Fifty percent of women can eliminate or decrease their incontinence by doing pelvic floor exercises called Kegel exercises. In a study of eighty women with documented anatomical stress incontinence who had been referred for corrective surgery, all were treated with Kegel exercises. By the end of one year, 50 percent didn't need the operation (Mouritsen 1991). Performing fifteen repetitions of Kegel exercises three or four times a day restores continence. The technique is to tighten the muscles that control urination. The way to identify these muscles is to place two fingers in your vagina and press on your rectum from inside the vagina. Try to tighten the muscles you can feel with your fingers. Kegel exercises also help urge incontinence (see the next section). In a study comparing Kegel exercises with electrical stimulation (we discuss this in a minute) and vaginal cones (also discussed below), 56 percent of women using Kegel exercise, 12 percent using electrical stimulus, and 10 percent using the vaginal cones were completely dry (Bø 1999). Unfortunately, at least 25 percent of women are unable to do Kegel exercises correctly. For them, electrical stimulation helped identify the correct muscles to exercise.

- **Electrical stimulation:** Low-voltage electrical current applied to the pelvic muscles treats both stress and urge incontinence. The stimulation is delivered either through the vagina or rectum and teaches you to recognize the contraction of your pelvic muscles and strengthen them. There is a 50 percent improvement in two-thirds of women who use this method, and 12 percent are cured (Bø 1999; Ostergard 1997).

- **Vaginal cones:** You can use gradually increasing weights to learn to contract your pelvic muscles. You place the 20-gram cone in your vagina and keep it in place by contracting your muscles. Once you are able to keep it there twice a day for fifteen minutes, you change to the next heavier cone. Fifty percent of women who use the cones improve their stress incontinence significantly, but only 10 percent become dry (Bø 1999).

- **Biofeedback:** With the help of biofeedback, women with stress and urge incontinence can learn to distinguish the contraction of their pelvic muscles from their abdominal muscles. This method requires one-hour sessions for four to eight weeks, but it achieves an 81 percent success rate (Ostergard 1997; Burgio 1998).

- **Weight loss:** Overweight women with large waists relative to their hips (apple shape) will get a 20 percent reduction in stress incontinence with weight loss. Women with defined hips (pear shape) do not get this benefit (Brown 1999).

- **Obstructing devices:** There are several devices in development that mechanically close off the urethra, stopping urine from leaking out (like a cork in a bottle). In studies, 50 to 80 percent of women using them were completely dry, though bladder infections were a frequent side effect (Versi 1998; Brubaker 1999; Singla 2000). Unfortunately none of these devices are commercially available.

- **Medication:** Pseudoephedrine and phenylpropanolamine (PPA) reduce or eliminate stress incontinence in 25 percent of women who use them (Brown 1999).

- **Bladder neck support prosthesis:** This silicon vaginal device supports the bladder neck and urethra, comes in sixteen different sizes, and prevents urine loss in 80 percent of the women who wear it. It must be removed and cleaned daily (Singla 2000).

- **Magnetic resonance therapy:** A magnet has been built into a special chair that aims at the pelvic floor. The resulting magnetic force causes contractions of the pelvic floor muscles. Unlike electrical stimulation, there are no vaginal or rectal probes. Early results show 56 percent of the women using it are dry. Seventy-seven percent had marked improvement in continence (Singla 2000).

- **Cough up:** Women who have mastered Kegel exercises can contract their pelvic floor muscles when they feel a sneeze or cough coming on. This method is very effective in women with mild to moderate stress incontinence (Brown 1999).

CAUTION! Some women are so afraid they will lose urine that they contract their vaginal muscles all the time. As a result, the muscles are in a state of constant fatigue. They can't tighten anymore because they are already tight. When the urge hits, these women lose urine anyway.

Urge Incontinence

Urge incontinence is also called detrusor instability (DI), or tiny bladder syndrome. In DI incontinence, your brain perceives the urge to urinate even though your bladder is only partially full, so your bladder contracts. Even when you can successfully keep your external sphincter closed and prevent passage of urine, your bladder continues to contract and the urge to void continues. You can lose urine when your bladder is full, or when you hear water running, or at any other time when your bladder thinks you have to urinate—your bladder has taken control!

If you give in to urge incontinence, the bladder contracts even sooner the next time, and then sooner again, until you are spending your day running from bathroom to bathroom. You may be up several times every night passing dribs and drabs of urine, ending up exhausted and upset about the loss of control. The good news is, you can fix this problem. The first step is to identify the cause.

There are many possible causes of urge incontinence:

- **Urinary tract infections.** Infections, both acute and chronic, keep the bladder inflamed and irritated, leading to spasms of the detrusor muscle. You need a full urological evaluation if you have frequent urinary tract infections, not just repeated antibiotic therapy.

- **Estrogen deficiency.** This leads to thinning (atrophy) of the lining of your urethra and bladder. In this situation, your resistance to infection is lowered.

- **Uterine enlargement.** This puts pressure on the bladder and can cause urge incontinence. Fibroids are the most common source of uterine enlargement in perimenopausal women. A simple pelvic exam will reveal this.

- **Hysterectomy.** Twenty percent of women who have had a hysterectomy will develop incontinence, a 50 percent greater incidence than in women who still have a uterus. Hopefully, the risk of incontinence will be reduced with the newer trend of leaving the cervix when performing a hysterectomy (Brown 1999).

- **Nerve damage.** Damage from a spinal cord injury or spinal nerve-root pressure from a ruptured disc can result in poor muscle control of the bladder wall.

- **Chemotherapy.** Such treatment may damage neurological control of the bladder or the muscles themselves.

- **Emotional stress.** This may increase your adrenaline (epinephrine) levels, causing your bladder to contract more frequently with smaller and smaller amounts of urine present each time. Counseling may help you deal with your stress, so your epinephrine levels will lower, as will the frequency of bladder spasms.

- **Cigarette smoke, alcohol, and caffeine.** These (even the amount of caffeine in decaffeinated coffee) all irritate the bladder and worsen the symptoms of urge incontinence.

- **Antihypertensive medications.** Some can cause urge incontinence.

If you have urge incontinence, an antispasmodic medicine may be pre-scribed, such as oxybutynin or propantheline to help you regain control. If these drugs don't work, a low dose of imipramine, a tricyclic antidepressant, can be tried (Appell 1997). You will also need to use an estrogen cream or estrogen-impregnated ring to increase your vaginal collagen strength (Fantl 1994).

The treatment of urge incontinence also involves behavior modification techniques to retrain your out-of-control bladder. Retraining is a very suc-cessful remedy but requires a great deal of effort of your part. Your retraining program should start with a regular schedule of urination every two hours, even if you don't need to go. In addition, it is most important that you do not give in to the urge to empty your bladder before the scheduled time. (It's okay to lose a little urine.) Once you can hold it for two hours, increase the time to two hours and ten minutes. Over a period of weeks, slowly increase the time between voidings until you can hold your urine for four hours. At this time you can usually go off the medication and retain control of your bladder.

Hypnosis can cure urge incontinence 58 percent of the time and improve it 30 percent of the time. Acupuncture can improve incontinence by 85 percent (Ostergard 1997).

TIP! When you feel you have to go, stop what you are doing, sit down if you can, and do six quick Kegel exercises. The Kegel exercises relax your blad-der's detrusor muscle so it stops contracting. You can then take a leisurely walk to the bathroom.

Gynecologists can cure stress incontinence in 80 percent with a variety of surgical procedures (Cosiski-Marana 1996). If you have a combination of urge incontinence and stress incontinence, however, you must acquire control of your urge incontinence before having surgery for stress incontinence (McGuire 1996). The stitches used to repair stress incontinence will make urge incontinence worse.

CAUTION! Since the stitches add an extra irritant to an already irritable bladder, it is important that you be completely evaluated before undergoing any bladder surgery. Many doctors use a trial of oxybutynin or imipramine before agreeing to do any surgery. These bladder relaxants help determine what portion of your incontinence, if any, is due to an irritable bladder. If urge incontinence is the only type of incontinence you have, medical treat-ment is the only way to cure your problem.

Intrinsic Sphincter Deficiency

Intrinsic sphincter deficiency (ISD) is due to a weak urethra. This condi-tion is also called "stove-pipe urethra" because the urethra has become a rigid, straight tube instead of a pliable structure. ISD incontinence is not common in perimenopausal women; it occurs as the result of multiple surgical repairs or prolonged estrogen depletion.

Surgical Options for Incontinence

When you need surgery, several diagnostic tests are needed to help your doctor decide which operation to perform. First your urine will be cultured to make sure incontinence is not due to a bladder infection. Then a urologist or gynecologist will insert a fiberoptic-equipped cystoscope inside the urethra and bladder to evaluate local causes of incontinence. During this procedure, water or gas is added to distend your bladder and allow visualization of your entire bladder and urethra. The distention pressure your bladder can withstand before it begins to contract is measured. This information helps determine which type of incontinence you have and what operation, if any, is best for you.

Stress (GSI) and ISD incontinence can be repaired by either a vaginal or abdominal operation, but surgery will not correct DI (urge) incontinence.

Vaginal Repair of Incontinence

Kelly described the first vaginal repair for incontinence in 1913 and it is still used today. The Kelly repair tightens the connective tissue beneath the urethra by suturing the tissue along the sides of the urethra, raising the bladder neck to its original position. The Kelly repair has an immediate success rate of 84 percent, but less than 50 percent remain continent five years after their surgery. A variety of vaginal suspension operations have since been designed but have proved no more successful over the long run than the original Kelly repair.

Still, a Kelly repair or another urethral suspension operation remains one of the treatments of choice for incontinence, in conjunction with extensive vaginal surgery to repair the bladder and rectum when they have ballooned into the vagina (these hernias are called, respectively, cystocele and rectocele).

Abdominal Surgery for Incontinence Repair

The original abdominal repair to correct stress incontinence was described by Marshall, Marchetti, and Krantz in 1949. The MMK operation suspends the bladder neck by stitching it to the covering of the pubic bone. The success rate with this operation is 85 percent, but the stitches may cause an infection in the bone, which is difficult to treat (Marshall 1949).

For this reason, the MMK has been largely replaced by the Burch procedure. In this operation, the stitches are attached to an abdominal ligament, rather than anchored to the pubic bone. The success rate with the Burch procedure is between 88 and 90 percent (Burch 1961; Bergman 1995; Kjolhede 1994).

Neither the Burch nor the MMK procedure restores the bladder to its original position. And when there is a large cystocele or rectocele present, the surgical success rate of these operations is reduced to 60 percent (Cosiski-Marana 1996). Seventeen to 50 percent of women who have had a Burch procedure may develop an intestinal hernia that drops into the vagina which may require future corrective surgery (Nichols 1991).

The Burch operation is also being done through the laparoscope, with success rates similar to those seen with an abdominal incision (Lyons 1995).

Fascial slings have become very popular for the treatment of GSI and ISD incontinence. A variety of tissues and synthetic materials are used with excellent results. The sling is placed under the urethra and attached to the abdominal wall. Two incisions are required; one through the abdomen, and the other in the vagina. Success rates are excellent: 90 to 92 percent of women remain dry (Singla 2000). Ten percent of women have difficulty voiding after this operation and may need to self-catheterize themselves to empty their bladders. For women with ISD, who were constantly wet prior to this operation, being dry is a welcome relief.

A tension-free vaginal tape (TVT) has recently been introduced for the treatment of GSI and ISD. A small incision is made in the vagina and the tape is placed under the urethra with the ends floating in the tissue next to the urethra and bladder. The surgery is performed with local anesthetic, so you may go home the same day. Long-term success rates are comparable to those of the fascia sling or Burch procedure (86 to 90 percent cure rate), but the surgery is quick with minimal postoperative discomfort (Wang 1998; Ulmsten 1999; Singla 2000).

Even if incontinence persists after Kegel exercises and the avoidance of caffeine and alcohol, your tissues will be in much better shape when you have a corrective operation (Brown 1996). Healing is improved, as are the chances of long-term success. And the retraining can do wonders for your continence and sex life even if your vaginal muscles have been seriously damaged in childbirth.

The Estrogen Connection

Estrogen deficiency contributes to urinary incontinence. Loss of estrogen translates to loss of collagen anywhere in your body where collagen exists: breasts, face, neck, abdomen, vagina, and bladder. Supplementation of estrogen during these years, in the form of pills or vaginal cream or both, can help avert these difficulties.

The vaginal estrogen ring (called Estring) delivers a slow, steady dose of estrogen to the vagina and bladder, with only small amounts getting into general circulation. Unfortunately, the ring is contraindicated when you have a cystocele, rectocele, or uterine prolapse, because the device will continually fall out or may cause a vaginal ulcer (Ayton 1996; Henriksson 1996). In women who can use this product, however, the ring will help prevent problems due to long-term estrogen deprivation.

Summary

Anatomic and functional changes in your gynecologic organs may never become a problem for you. If they do, though, these pages will serve as a guide to current thinking about surgical management and nonsurgical alternatives.

Pharmaceutical and technological advances continue to be made, offering welcome alternatives to traditional surgical intervention. Nevertheless, surgery is sometimes the only alternative. The primary goal is always to restore function and return you to a normal lifestyle.

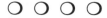

Conclusion

As your generation has moved through its various stages of life, it has made fundamental changes in many aspects of American culture. Because of your sheer size, you changed the number of schools in existence and even how they were built. Mickey Mouse Clubbers, Howdy Doody devotees, and Captain Kangaroo watchers changed children's television. Bell-bottom pants, miniskirts, and long hair became the norm for many years. Sexual liberation from long-held social standards of propriety was a mark of your generation, although this may not have been one of your best moves. You embraced Elvis and the Beatles to change contemporary music. As you began to marry, an enormous housing boom blossomed and so did suburbs with connecting freeways. You changed childbirthing with natural childbirth, and made it a family event with fathers in attendance. Two of you have been elected president. Yours is an energized and energizing group. Unlike your predecessors, you have always taken control of challenges and events facing you, rather than being controlled by them.

This book has been about another change facing you: perimenopause. It certainly isn't anything new in life's scheme, but it is new to you. It is the old age of your youth and the gateway to mid-life. The four or five decades of your life to this point have been blatantly oriented toward youthfulness. Look young, act young, stay young. Social bias and commercialism have favored your youth, and curried your favor every step of the way. You grew up thinking that youth is perpetual and that aging and death are only theoretical considerations. For that matter, so did we all. We aren't worried about you though. We have every faith in you and your peers that you will not fall into a "lost youth" funk. You have seized the moment in every other phase of your life, and perimenopause should be no exception.

We hope we have convinced you that perimenopause is a watershed time in your life. It is a transition from the wonderful years of the first half of life to the fantastic years of the second half. Our purpose has been to inform and educate you about certain changes you can expect, and to empower you to deal with them successfully. To do this, we have heaped a lot of good news–bad news concepts on you. Some of our advice may be welcome, and we regretfully acknowledge that some of it is probably not. Still, we hope you recognize that we are in your corner when it comes to things that can benefit you.

We do not want you to dwell on perimenopause and the changes it may impose on your body and in your life. Once you are aware of what is required to protect yourself from adverse changes, and once you have woven the protective techniques into the fabric of your life, move on. Life and living it are much too precious to be subverted by daily preoccupation with burdensome details of techniques, treatments, and menus. This isn't a dress rehearsal you are going through, it's an authentic life and we want you to live it that way. Our hope for you as our reader is that you have increased your fund of knowledge about perimenopause; but our fondest and most fundamental wish for you as a woman is that you stay focused on your journey.

O O O O

Appendix

Information Resources

Aging

National Council on the Aging
409 Third Street, Southwest
Washington, DC 20024
202-479-1200

National Institutes of Health
National Institute on Aging
31 Center Drive
Bethesda, MD 20892
301-496-1752

Alternative Medicine

National Institutes of Health
National Center of Complementary
   and Alternative Medicine
(NCCAM)
P.O. Box 8218
Silver Spring, MD 20901
888-644-6226
http://nccam.nih.gov/nccam/

Traditional Chinese Medicine

American College of Traditional
   Chinese Medicine
455 Arkansas Street
San Francisco, CA 94107
415-282-7600
Offers M.S. degree in traditional
Chinese medicine.

National Acupuncture and Oriental
   Medicine Alliance
14637 Starr Road, Southwest
Olalla, WA 98359
253-851-6896

National Commission for the
  Certification of Acupuncture and
  Oriental Medicine (NCCAOM)
11 Canal Center Plaza, Suite 300
Alexandria, VA 22314
703-548-9004
*Ensures minimal entry-level professional
competence.*

Naturopathy

American Association of
Naturopathic Physicians
8201 Greensboro Drive, Suite 300
McLean, VA 22102
703-610-9005
Referrals to naturopaths

National College of Naturopathic
  Medicine
049 Southwest Porter Street
Portland, OR 97201
503-499-4343
*Offers degrees in naturopathic medicine
and provides referrals.*

Homeopathy

National Center for Homeopathy
810 North Fairfax Street, Suite 306
Alexandria, VA 22314
703-548-7790
*Maintains directory of homeopaths with
a wide range of training and education.*

Cancer

American Cancer Society
1599 Clifton Road NE
Atlanta, GA 30329
800-227-2345
www.cancer.org

American Lung Association
1740 Broadway
New York, NY 10019
212-315-8700

American Gastroenterological
  Association
7910 Woodmont Avenue
Bethesda, MD 20814
301-654-2055

National Society of Genetic
  Counselors
233 Canterbury Drive
Wallingford, PA 19086
610-872-7608

National Cancer Institute
31 Center Drive
Bethesda, MD 20205
800-422-6237
www.nci.nih.gov

National Coalition for Cancer
  Survivorship
1010 Wayne Avenue, Suite 770
Silver Spring, MD 20910
877-622-7937

The Skin Cancer Foundation
P.O. Box 561
New York, NY 10156
800-754-6490

Society of Gynecologic Oncologists
401 North Michigan Avenue
Chicago, IL 60611
312-644-6610

Diet and Nutrition

American Dietetic Association
216 West Jackson Blvd
Chicago, IL 60606
312-899-0040

U.S. Department of Agriculture
Food and Nutrition Information
  Center
www.nal.usda.gov/fnic

Exercise

American College of Sports Medicine
401 West Michigan Street
Indianapolis, IN 46202
317-637-9200

Fertility and Pregnancy

The Alan Guttmacher Institute
120 Wall Street
New York, NY 10005
212-248-1111

American College of Obstetricians
and Gynecologists
Office of Public Information
409 Twelfth Street Southwest
P.O. Box 96920
Washington, DC 20090
202-484-3321

American Society for Reproductive
Medicine
1209 Montgomery Highway
Birmingham, AL 35216
205-978-5000

National Center for Education in
Maternal and Child Care
2000 Fifteenth Street, North, Suite 701
Arlington, VA 22201
703-524-7802

National Down Syndrome Society
666 Broadway
New York, NY 10012
800-221-4602

National Society of Genetic
Counselors
233 Canterbury Drive
Wallingford, PA 19086
610-872-7608

RESOLVE: The National Infertility
Association
1310 Broadway
Somerville, MA 02144
617-623-0744
www.resolve.org

Heart Disease

American Heart Association
7272 Greenville Avenue
Dallas, TX 75231
800-242-8721

National Heart, Lung and Blood
Institute Information Center
National Cholesterol Education
Program
P.O. Box 30105
Bethesda, MD 20824
301-592-8573

Medicines

American Pharmaceutical
Association
2215 Constitution Avenue
Washington, DC 20037
202-628-4410

Food and Drug Administration
Center for Drug Evaluation and
Research
www.fda.gov/cder

Menopause

American Menopause Foundation
350 Fifth Avenue
New York, NY 10118
212-714-2398

North American Menopause Society
P.O. Box 94527
Cleveland, OH 44101
440-442-7550

Mental Health

American Psychiatric Association
1400 K Street, Northwest
Washington, DC 20005
888-357-7924

American Psychological Association
750 First Street, Northwest
Washington, DC 20002
202-336-5500

Anxiety Disorders Association of
America
11900 Parklawn Drive, Suite 100
Rockville, MD 20852

National Alliance for the Mentally Ill
Colonial Place Three
2107 Wilson Boulevard, Suite 300
Arlington, VA 22201
800-950-6264

National Depressive and
Manic-Depressive Association
730 North Franklin Street, Suite 501
Chicago, IL 60610
800-826-3632

Mind/Body Medicine

Academy for Guided Imagery
P.O. Box 2070
Mill Valley, CA 94942
800-726-2070
*Training program; publishes directory of
practitioners.*

American Massage Therapy
Association
820 Davis Street, Suite 100
Evanston, IL 60201
847-864-0123
*Members must graduate from an
AMTA-accredited program or pass a
certification exam.*

American Society of Clinical
Hypnosis
130 East Elm Court, Suite 201
Roselle, IL 60172
630-980-4740
*Will provide list of medical doctors and
dentists who also do hypnosis.*

Association for Applied
Psychophysiology Biofeedback
10200 West Forty-fourth Avenue,
Suite 304
Wheat Ridge, CO 80033
303-422-8436
*Trains and certifies biofeedback
practitioners.*

Mind/Body Institute
Beth Israel Deaconess Hospital
110 Francis Street
Boston, MA 02215
617-632-9530
Tapes on relaxation available.

National Guild of Hypnotists, Inc.
P.O. Box 308
Merrimack, NH 03054
603-429-9438
Training and certification programs

Osteoporosis

National Osteoporosis Foundation
1232 Twenty-second Street,
Northwest
Washington, DC 20037
202-223-2226

Physicians' Organizations

American Board of Medical
Specialities
800-776-2378

American College of Obstetricians
and Gynecologists
Office of Public Information
409 Twelfth Street, Southwest
P.O. Box 96920
Washington, DC 20090
202-484-3321

American Medical Association
515 North State Street
Chicago, IL 60610
312-464-5000

American Society for Dermatologic
Surgery
930 North Meacham Road
Schaumburg, IL 60173
847-330-9830

American Society for Laser Medicine
and Surgery
2404 Stewart Square
Wausau, WI 54401
715-845-9283

American Society of Plastic Surgeons
444 East Algonquin Road
Arlington Heights, IL 60005
708-228-9900

Sexuality

American Association of Sex
Educators, Counselors, and
Therapists
P.O. Box 238
Mount Vernon, IA 52314
www.aasect.org
*Referral services for professionals in your
area*

Sexuality Information and Education
Council of the US
130 West Forty-second Street,
Suite 350
New York, NY 10036
212-819-9776
Information on a wide range of sex topics

Sexually Transmitted Diseases

American Social Health Association
P.O. Box 13827
Research Park Triangle, NC 27709
919-361-8400
Written educational information
800-230-6039

Centers for Disease Control and
Prevention
Division of STD Prevention
1600 Clifton Road, Northeast
Atlanta, GA 30333
404-639-3311

National STD and AIDS Hotline
800-342-2437

Specialty Pharmacies (for Natural Hormones)

International Academy of
Compounding Pharmacists
P.O. Box 1365
Sugar Land TX 77487
800-927-4227
*Referrals to compounding pharmacies in
your area*

Substance Abuse

Al-Anon Family Group
Headquarters
P.O. Box 862, Midtown Station
New York, NY 10018
800-356-9996 for free pamphlets
800-344-2666 for USA meeting dates
800-443-4525 for Canadian meeting
dates

Alcoholics Anonymous
General Service Office
475 Riverside Drive
New York, NY 10015
212-870-3400

Cocaine Anonymous
3740 Overland Avenue, Suite C
Los Angeles, CA 90034
310-559-5833

Narcotics Anonymous
World Services Office
P.O. Box 9999
Van Nuys, CA 91409
818-773-9999

Substance Abuse and Mental Health
   Services Administration
National Clearinghouse for Alcohol
   and Drug Information
P.O. Box 2345
Rockville, MD 20847
800-729-6686 or 301-468-2600

U.S. Department of Health and
   Human Services
National Drug and Alcohol
Treatment Referral Service
Center for Substance Abuse
Treatment
800-662-4357

Women for Sobriety
P.O. Box 618
Quakertown, PA 18951
215-536-8026

Urinary Incontinence

American Urological Association
1120 North Charles Street
Baltimore, MD 21201
401-727-1100

National Association for Continence
P.O. Box 8310
Spartanburg, SC 29305
800-252-3337
www.nafc.org

The Simon Foundation for
Continence
P.O. Box 835
Wilmette, IL 60097
(800) 2337-4666

Weight Control

American Dietetic Association
216 West Jackson Boulevard
Chicago, IL 60606
312-899-0040

Healthfinder
www.healthfinder.gov

Mayo Clinic Health Oasis
www.mayohealth.org

Shape Up America!
6707 Democracy Boulevard,
   Suite 306
Bethesda, MD 20817
www.shapeup.org

Weight-control Information
Network
   (WIN)
National Institutes of Health
1 WIN Way
Bethesda, MD 20892
877-946-4627
www.niddk.nih.gov/health/nutrit/
win

Women's Health

The Endometriosis Association
8585 North 76th Place
Milwaukee, WI 53223
800-962-3636

National Institutes of Health
Office of Research on Women's
   Health
Building 1, Room 201
9000 Rockville Pike
Bethesda, MD 20892
301-402-1770

National Self-Help Clearinghouse
365 Fifth Avenue, Suite 3300
New York, NY 10016
212-817-1822
Databank for self-help groups

National Women's Health Network
514 Tenth Street, Northwest
Washington, DC 20004
202-628-7814

Women's Health Initiative
Federal Building, Room 6A09
9000 Rockville Pike
Bethesda, MD 20892
800-548-6636

O O O O

References

Chapter 1: What Changes? An Overview

American Heart Association. 1997. *Heart and Stroke Statistical Update.* Dallas: American Heart Association.

Campbell, S., and M. Whitehead. 1977. Estrogen therapy and the menopausal syndrome. *Clinical Obstetrics and Gynecology* 4 (3):94–99.

Eskin, B., and L. Dumas. 1995. *Midlife Can Wait: How to Stay Young and Healthy After 35.* New York: Ballantine Books.

Graham, E. 1995. The Baby Boom Hits 50. *Wall Street Journal*, October 31.

Kronenberg, F. 1993. Menopausal hot flashes. Paper presented at annual meeting of the North American Menopause Society, May 21.

Kronenberg, F. 1994. Hot Flashes. In *Treatment of the Postmenopausal Woman: Basic and Clinical Aspects,* edited by R. E. Lobo. New York: Raven Press, 97–117.

Phillips, S.M., and B.B. Sherman. 1992. Effects of estrogen on memory function in surgically menopausal women. *Psychoneuroendocrinology* 17:485–495.

Sheehy, G. 1991. *The Silent Passage.* New York: Random House.

Sherwin, and B. B., 1996. Hormones, mood, and cognitive function in postmenopausal women. *Obstetrics and Gynecology* 87 (Suppl. 2):20S–26S.

Speroff, L., et al. 1989. *Clinical Gynecologic Endocrinology and Infertility.* Baltimore: Williams and Wilkins.

Tang, M.-X., et al. 1996. Effect of oestrogen during menopause on risk and age at onset of Alzheimer's disease. *Lancet* 348:429–432

Chapter 2: Changes in Fertility: Pregnancy, Infertility, and Contraception

American College of Obstetricians and Gynecologists. 1993. Folic acid for the prevention of recurrent neural tube defects. ACOG Committee Opinion, March 102:1–3.

American College of Obstetricians and Gynecologists. 1991. Alpha-Fetoprotein. *ACOG Guide to Preconception Care, Technical Bulletin,* April 154:28–30.

Asch, R. H., and R. P. Marrs. 1993. *Assisted Reproductive Technologies.* Serono Patient Education Library. Norwell, Mass.: Serono Laboratories, Inc.

Burkman, R. T., Jr., et al. 1992. Lipid and carbohydrate effects of a new triphasic oral contraceptive containing norgestimate. *Acta Obstetrica and Gynecologica Scandinavica* (Supplement)156:5–8.

Brown, J. R., et al. 1996. A defect in nurturing in mice lacking the immediate early gene fosB. *Cell* 86:297–309.

California Department of Health Services, Genetic Disease Branch. 1995. *Prenatal Testing Choices for Women 35 Years and Older* (monograph). Berkeley: California Department of Health Services.

Centers for Disease Control and Prevention. 1997. Knowledge and use of folic acid by women of child-bearing age—United States. *Morbidity and Mortality Weekly Report* 46:721–723.

Connolly, B. H., et al. 1993. A longitudinal study of children with Down syndrome who experienced early intervention programming. *Physical Therapy* 73 (3):170-181.

Croft, P., and P.C. Hannaford. 1989. Risk factors for acute myocardial infarction in women: Evidence from the royal college of general practitioners' oral contraception study. *British Medical Journal* 298: 165-168.

Cuckle, H. A., et al. 1987. Estimating a woman's risk of having a pregnancy associated with Down's syndrome using her age and serum alpha-fetoprotein level. *British Journal of Obstetrics and Gynaecology* 94:387.

Darney, P. D. 2000. Contraception for women with medical problems. *Audio Digest, Obstetrics and Gynecology* 47:(3).

———. 1996. Oral contraceptives and upcoming slow-release hormones. *Audio Digest, Obstetrics and Gynecology* 43:(16).

Dorris, M. 1990. *The Broken Cord.* New York: HarperCollins.

Edge, V. L., and R. K. Laros. 1993. Pregnancy outcomes in nulliparous women aged 35 or older. *American Journal of Obstetrics and Gynecology* 168 (6, Part 1):1881–1885.

Fortney, J. A., et al. 1999. Intrauterine devices: The optimal long-term contraceptive method? *Journal of Reproductive Medicine* 44 (3):269–274.

Fraser, I. S., and G. J. Dennerstein. 1994. Depo-Provera use in an Australian metropolitan practice. *The Medical Journal of Australia* 160:553–556.

Frayne, J., and L. Hall. 1999. The potential use of sperm antigens as targets for immunocontraception; past, present and future. *Journal of Reproductive Immunology* 43 (1):1–33.

Gilbert, W. M., et al. 1999. Childbearing beyond age 40: pregnancy outcome in 24,032 cases. *Obstetrics and Gynecology* 93 (1):9–14

Grimes, D. 1997. Sense and sensuality: contraceptives. *Audio Digest, Obstetrics and Gynecology* 44(2).

Grimes, D., et al. Task Force on Postovulatory Methods of Fertility Regulation: World Health Organization. 1998. Randomized controlled trial of levonorgestrel versus the Yuzpe regimen of combined oral contraceptives for emergency contraception. *Lancet* 352 :428–433.

Huber, J. 1991. Clinical experience with a new norgestimate-containing oral contraceptive. *International Journal of Fertility* 36 (Supplement):25–31.

Irvine, G. A., et al. 1998. Randomised comparative trial of the levonorgestrel intrauterine system and norethisterone for treatment of idiopathic menorrhagia. *British Journal of Obstetrics and Gynaecology* 105 (6):592–598.

Jaffe, S. B., and R. Jewelewicz. 1991. The basic infertility investigation. *Fertility and Sterility* 56:599–613.

Jauniaux, E., et al. 1999 Maternal tobacco exposure and cotinen levels in fetal fluids in the first half of pregnancy. *Obstetrics and Gynecology* 93 (1):25–29

John, E. M., et al. 1991. Prenatal exposure to parents' smoking and childhood cancer. *American Journal of Epidemiology* 133:123–132.

Kaunitz, A. M. 1996. Long-acting contraceptive options. *International Journal of Fertility and Menopausal Studies* 41:69–76.

Leventhal, J. 1997. Libido and Menopause. Lecture given to the Women's Health Department, Kaiser Permanente Medical Group, Walnut Creek, Calif., April 1.

Lurie, D., et al. 2000. Pregnancy rates per cycle similar for the first four transfers despite improved pregnancy rates. Paper presented at the forty-eighth annual meeting of the Pacific Coast Reproductive Society, Palm Springs, Calif., April 26–30.

Menken, J., et al. 1986. Age and infertility. *Science* 233:1389.

Nelson, A. L. 1996. Norplant and Depo-Provera. *Audio Digest, Obstetrics and Gynecology* 43:(16).

Oelkers, W., et al. 1995. Effects of a new oral contraceptive containing an antimineralocorticoid progestogen, Drospirenone, on the renin-aldosterone system, body weight, blood pressure, glucose tolerance, and lipid metabolism. *Journal of Clinical Endocrinology and Metabolism* 80 (6):1816–1821.

Ondrizek, R. R., et al. 1999. An alternative medicine study of herbal effects on the penetration of zona-free hamster oocytes and the integrity of sperm deoxyribonucleic acid. *Fertility and Sterility* 71 (3):517–522.

Palomali, G. E., et al. 1995. Risk-based prenatal screening for trisomy 18 using alpha-fetoprotein, unconjugated oestriol, and human chorionic gonadotropin. *Prenatal Diagnosis* 15:713–723.

Perlow, J. H. 1999. Education about folic acid: the ob-gyn's role in preventing neural tube defects. *Contemporary OB/GYN* March:39–53.

Physician's Desk Reference, 51st ed. 1997. Montvale, N.J.: Medical Economics.

Piccinino, L. J., and W. D. Mosher. 1998. Trends in contraceptive use in the United States: 1982–1995. *Family Planning Perspectives* 30 (4):4–10, 46.

Qureshi, M., and M. Attaran. 1999. Reviews of newer contraceptive agents. *Cleveland Clinic Journal of Medicine* 66 (6):358–366.

Reichman, J. 1996. *I'm Too Young to Get Old: Health Care for Women After Forty.* New York: Times Books.

Rose, N. C., et al. 1994. Maternal serum alpha-fetoprotein screening for chromosomal abnormalities: a prospective study in women aged 35 and older. *American Journal of Obstetrics and Gynecology* 170:1073–1080.

Scholes, D, et al. 1999. Bone mineral density in women using depot medroxyprogesterone acetate for contraception. *Obstetrics and Gynecology* 93 (2):233–238.

Scott, R. T., et al. 1995. Life table analysis of pregnancy rates in a general infertility population relative to ovarian reserve and patient age. *Human Reproduction* 10:1706–1710.

Shulman, L. P. 1999. Combined hormonal injectable contraceptive: A new option in birth control. Paper given at Continuing Medical Education symposium, Philadelphia, May 18.

Silberstein, S. D. 1992. The role of sex hormones in headache. *Neurology* 42 (2):37–42.

Silva, P. D., et al. 1999. Impact of lifestyle choices on female infertility. *Journals of Reproductive Medicine* 44 (3):288–296.

Soares, C. J. 1996. Learning in the fast lane: Making the most of your evolving brain. *Perspectives* May/June:33–41.

Society for Assisted Reproductive Technology and the American Society for Reproductive Medicine. 1996. Assisted reproductive technology in the United States and Canada: 1994 results generated from the American Society for Reproductive Medicine/Society for Assisted Reproductive Technology Registry. *Fertility and Sterility* 68:697–704.

Stjernfeldt, M., et al. 1986. Maternal smoking during pregnancy and risk of childhood cancer. *Lancet* 1 (8494):1350–1351.

U.S. Department of Health, Education and Welfare/Public Health Service. 1977. Immune globulins for the protection against viral hepatitis. *Morbidity and Mortality Weekly Report* 26:425–442.

University of Minnesota Office of Continuing Medical Education. 1997. New developments and practice guidelines: OCs and IUDs. Video satellite conference, San Francisco, April 19.

Chapter 3: PMS Can Change You: Premenstrual Syndrome in Your Transitional Years

American Psychiatric Association. 1994. *Diagnostic and Statistical Manual of Mental Disorders*, 4th ed. Washington, D.C.: American Psychiatric Association.

Bailey, J. W., and L. S. Cohen. 1999. Prevalence of mood and anxiety disorders in women who seek treatment for premenstrual syndrome. *Journal of Women's Health and Gender Based Medicine* 8 (9):1181–1184.

Barnhart, K. T., et al. 1995. A clinician's guide to the premenstrual syndrome. *Medical Clinics of North America* 79:1457–1473.

Condon, J. T. 1993. The premenstrual syndrome: a twin study. *British Journal of Psychiatry* 162:481–486.

Dalton, K., and M. J. Dalton. 1987. Characteristics of pyridoxine overdose neuropathy syndrome. *Acta Neurologica Scandinavica* 76:811.

Danjou, P., et al. 1999. A comparison of the residual effects of zaleplon and zolpidem following administration 5 to 2 hours before awakening. *British Journal of Clinical Pharmacology* 48:367–374.

Ekholm, U. B., and T. Backstrom. 1994. Influence of premenstrual syndrome on family, social life, and work performance. *International Journal of Health Services* 24:629–647.

Elie, R., et al. 1999 Sleep latency is shortened during 4 weeks of treatment with zaleplon, a novel nonbenzodiazepine hypnotic. *Journal of Clinical Psychiatry* 60 (8):536–544.

Epperson, C. N., et al. 1999 Gonadal steroids in the treatment of mood disorders. *Psychosomatic Medicine* 61 (5):676–697.

Eriksson, E. 1999. Serotonin reuptake inhibitors for the treatment of premenstrual dysphoria" *International Clinical Psychopharmacology* 14 (Suppl. 2):S27–33.

Facchinetti, F., et al. 1991. Oral magnesium successfully relieves premenstrual mood changes. *Obstetrics and Gynecology* 78:177.

Fava, M., et al. 1998. An open trial of oral sildenafil in antidepressant-induced sexual dysfunction. *Psychotherapy and Psychosomatics* 67:328–331

Forrest, A. R. W. 1979. Cyclical variations in mood in normal women taking oral contraceptives. *British Medical Journal* 1:1410–1410.

Frank, R. T. 1931. The hormonal causes of premenstrual tension. *Archives of Neurology and Psychiatry* 26:1053.

Freeman, E. K., et al. 1999. Full-or half-cycle treatment of severe premenstrual syndrome with a serotonergic antidepressant. *Journal of Clinical Psychopharmacology* 19(1):3–8

———. 1990. Ineffectiveness of progesterone suppository treatment for premenstrual syndrome. *Journal of the American Medical Association* 264:349.

Greene, R. and K. Dalton. 1953. The premenstrual syndrome. *British Medical Journal* 1 (4818):1007–1014.

Halbreich, U., et al. 1991. Elimination of ovulation and menstrual cyclicity (with Danazol) improves dysphoric premenstrual syndromes. *Fertility and Sterility* 56:1066–69.

Hendrix, S. 1998. The Evidence on Alternative Menopause Treatment Options. Lecture given at the sixth national conference on issues in women's health sponsored by Symposia Medicus, Playa Conchal, Costa Rica, November 7–14.

Jermain, D. M., et al. 1999. Luteal phase sertraline treatment for premenstrual dysphoric disorder. Results of a double-blind, placebo-controlled crossover study. *Archives of Family Medicine* 8 (4):328–332.

Kendler, K. S., et al. 1992. Genetic and environmental factors in the aetiology of menstrual, premenstrual and neurotic symptoms: A population-based twin study. *Psychological Medicine* 22:85–100.

Khoo, S. K., et al. 1990. Evening primrose oil and treatment of premenstrual syndrome. *The Medical Journal of Australia* 153:189–192.

Kirby, A. W., et al. 1999. Melatonin and the reduction or alleviation of stress. *Journal of Pineal Research* 27 (2):78-85.

Kleijnen, J. 1994. Evening primrose oil: Currently used in many conditions with little justification. *British Medical Journal* 309:824–825.

Labbate, L. A., and M. H. Pollack. 1994 Treatment of fluoxetine-induced sexual dysfunction with bupropion: A case study. *Annals of Clinical Psychiatry* 6:13–15.

Lam, R. W., et al. 1999. A controlled study of light therapy in women with late luteal phase dysphoric disorder. *Psychiatry Research* 86 (3):185–92.

Lanka, L. D., and J. Klingman. Research in progress on ongoing evaluation of the use of testosterone pellets in the treatment of recalcitrant menstrual migraines. Kaiser Foundation Hospital, Walnut Creek, Calif.

Leather, A. T., et al. 1999 The treatment of severe premenstrual syndrome with goserelin with and without "add-back" estrogen therapy: A placebo-controlled trial. *Gynecological Endocrinology* 13(1):48–55.

Lee, J. R., and V. Hopkins. 1996. *What Your Doctor May Not Tell You About Menopause*. New York: Warner Books.

Leventhal, J. 1997. Libido and Menopause. Lecture given to the Women's Health Department, Kaiser Permanente Medical Group, Walnut Creek, Calif., April 1.

———. 1996. Premenstrual Dysphoric Disorder. Lecture given to the Women's Health Department, Kaiser Permenente Medical Group, Walnut Creek, Calif., October 15.

Modell, J. G., et al. 1997. Comparative sexual side effects of bupropion, fluoxetine, paroxetine, and sertraline. *Clinical Pharmacology & Therapeutics* 61 (4):476–487.

Moline, L. 1993. Pharmacological strategies for managing premenstrual syndrome. *Clinical Pharmacology* 12:181–196.

Mortola, J. F. 1992. Issues in the diagnosis and research of premenstrual syndrome. *Clinics of Obstetrics and Gynecology* 35:587–598.

———. 1994. A risk-benefit appraisal of drugs used in the management of premenstrual syndrome. *Drug Safety* 10:160–169.

O'Brien, P. M., and I. E. Abukhalil. 1999. Randomized controlled trial of the management of premenstrual syndrome and premenstrual mastalgia using luteal phase-only danazol. *American Journal of Obstetrics and Gynecology* 189 (1, part 1):18–23.

Pallanti, S., and L. M. Koran. 1999. Citalopram and sexual side effects of selective serotonin reuptake inhibitors. *American Journal of Psychiatry* 156 (5):796.

Parker, P. D. 1994. Premenstrual syndrome. *American Family Physician* 50:1309–1317.

Parry, G., and D. Bredesen. 1985. Sensory neuropathy with low dose pyridoxine. *Neurology* 35:1466–1468.

Revlin, M. E., et al. 1990. *Manual of Clinical Problems in Obstetrics and Gynecology*, 3rd ed. Boston: Little, Brown.

Riggs, L., and L. J. Melton. 1986. Involutional osteoporosis. *New England Journal of Medicine* 314:1676–1686.

Rubinow, D. 1992. The premenstrual syndrome: New views. *Journal of the American Medical Association* 268:1908.

Sarno, A. P., Jr., et al. 1987. Premenstrual syndrome: Beneficial effects of periodic, low-dose danazol for the treatment of premenstrual tension. *Obstetrics and Gynecology* 70:30–36.

Schagen van Leeuwen, J. H., et al. 1993. Is premenstrual syndrome an endocrine disorder? *Journal of Psychosomatic Obstetrics and Gynaecology* 14:91–109.

Schmidt, P. J., et al. 1993. Alprazolam in the treatment of premenstrual syndrome. A double-blind, placebo-controlled trial. *Archives of General Psychiatry* 50:467–73.

Severino, S. K., and M. L. Moline. 1995. Premenstrual syndrome. Identification and management. *Drugs. Practical Therapeutics* 49 (1):71–82.

Sildberstein, S. D. 1990. Advance in the understanding of the pathology of headaches. *Neurology.* 42 (2):6–10.

Smith, S., and I. Schiff. 1993. *Modern Management of Premenstrual Syndrome.* New York: Norton.

Steinberg, S., et al. 1999. A placebo-controlled clinical trail of L-tryptophan in premenstural dysphoria. *Biological Psychiatry* 45 (3):313–320.

Steiner, M., et al. 1995. Fluoxetine in the treatment of premenstrual dysphoria. *New England Journal of Medicine* 332:1529–34.

Stone A. B., et al. 1990. Fluoxetine in the treatment of premenstrual syndrome. *Psychopharmacology Bulletin* 26:331–335.

Taylor, D. 1999. Effectiveness of professional-peer group treatment: Symptom management for women with PMS. *Res. Nurs. Health* 22(6):496–511.

Thy-Jacobs, S., et al.1998. Calcium carbonate and the premenstrual syndrome: Effects on premenstrual and menstrual symptoms. *American Journal of Obstetrics and Gynecology* 178 (2):444–452.

Vermeeren, A., et al. 1999. Residual effects of evening and middle-of-the-night administration of zaleplon 10 and 20 mg on memory and actual driving performance. *Human Psychopharmacology and Clinical Experimentation* 13:S98–S107.

Wilson, C. A., et al. 1991. Firstborn adolescent daughters and mothers with and without premenstrual syndrome: A comparison. *Journal of Adolescent Health* 12:130–137.

Wyatt, K. M., et al. 1999. Efficacy of vitamin B_6 in the treatment of premenstrual syndrome: Systematic review. *British Medical Journal* 318 (7195):1375–1381.

Chapter 4: Serious Changes: Cardiovascular Disease and Osteoporosis

Agnusdei, D., and L. Bufalino. 1997. Efficacy of ipriflavone in established osteoporosis and long-term safety. *Calcif. Tissue Int.* 61 (Suppl. 1):S23–S27.

American Heart Association. 1997. *Heart and Stroke Statistical Update.* Dallas: American Heart Association.

Bass, K. M., et al. 1993. Plasma lipoprotein levels as predictors of cardiovascular deaths in women. *Circulation* 153:2209.

Black D. M., et al. 1996. Randomised trial of effect of alendronate on risk of fracture in women with existing vertebral fractures. *Lancet* 348:1535–1541.

Blair, H. 1996. Action of genistein and other tyrosine kinase inhibitors in preventing osteoporosis. In: *Program and Abstracts* of second international symposium on the role of soy in preventing and treating chronic disease, Brussells, Belgium, September. Available at http:soyfoods.com/symposium.

Campodarve, I., et al. 1994. Intranasal salmon calcitonin (INSC), 50–200 IU, does not prevent bone loss in early menopause. *Journal of Bone and Mineral Research* 9 (Suppl. 1):S391.

Cauley, J. A., D. G. Seeley, K. Ensrud, B. E. Hinger, and D. Black. 1995. Prevention of fractures requires long-term estrogen treatment. *Annals of Internal Medicine* 122:9-16.

Civitelli, R., 1997. In vitro and in vivo effects of ipriflavone on bone formation and bone biomechanics. *Calcif. Tissue Int.* 61 (Suppl. 1):S12–S14.

Clarkson, T. B., and M. S. Anthony., 1997. Effects on the cardiovascular system: Basic aspects. In *Estrogens and Antiestrogens,* edited by R. Lindsay, et al. Philadelphia: Lippincott-Raven Publishers.

Cohen, F. J., et al. 2000. Uterine effects of 3-year raloxifene therapy in postmenopausal women younger than age 60. *Obstetrics & Gynecology* 95 (1):111–114.

Cooper, C., and L. J. Melton, III. 1992. Epidemiology of osteoporosis. *Trends in Endocrinology and Metabolism* 3:224–229.

Cummings, S. R., et al. 1998. Effect of alendronate on risk of fracture in women with low bone density but without vertebral fractures. *Journal of the American Medical Association* 280:2077–2082.

Cushman M. 1999. Effect of postmenopausal hormones on inflammation-sensitive proteins—the Postmenopausal Estrogen/Progestin Interventions (PEPI) study. *Circulation* 100:717–722.

Darling, G. M., et al. 1997. Estrogen and progestin compared with simvistatin for hypercholesterolemia in postmenopausal women. *New England Journal of Medicine* 337:595.

Davidson, M. H., et al. 1997. A comparison of ERT, pravistatin and combined treatment for management of hypercholesterolemia in postmenopausal women. *Archives of Internal Medicine* 157:1186–1192.

Downs, J. R., et al. 1998. Primary prevention of acute coronary events with lovostatin in men and women with average cholesterol levels: Results of AFCAPS/TexCaps—Air Force/Texas Coronary Prevention Study. *Journal of the American Medical Association* 279:1615–1622.

Eastman, P. 1997. Osteoporosis: New treatment. *AARP Bulletin* 38(3).

Ettinger, B. 1999. Reduction of vertebral fracture risk in postmenopausal women with osteoporosis treated with raloxifene: Results from a three-year randomized clinical trial. *Journal of the American Medical Association* 282:637–645.

Feskanich, D. 1999. Moderate alcohol consumption and bone density among postmenopausal women. *Journal of Women's Health* 8:65–73.

Food and Drug Administration. 1997. Proceedings of FDA Advisory Committee Meeting. November 20, 1997.

Hammond, C. B. 1998. *Therapeutic Options for Menopausal Health.* Durham, N.C.: Duke University Medical Center, Office of Continuing Medical Education, Department of Obstetrics/Gynecology.

Harvard Heart Letter. 2000. Women and heart disease. *Harvard Heart Letter* 10 (5):1

Harvard Women's Health Watch. 1999. Coronary heart disease: New guidelines for prevention. 6 (12):2–3.

Hosking, D., et al. 1998. Prevention of bone loss with alendronate in postmenopausal women under 60 years of age. *New England Journal of Medicine* 338:485–492.

Hully, S., et al. for the Heart and Estrogen/Progestin Replacement Study (HERS) Research Group. 1998. Randomized trial of estrogen plus progestin for secondary prevention of coronary heart disease in postmenopausal women. *Journal of the American Medical Association* 280:605–613.

Institute of Medicine, Standing Committee on the Scientific Evaluation of Dietary Reference Intakes. 1997. *Dietary Reference Intakes: Calcium, Phosphorus, Magnesium, Vitamin D, and Fluoride.* Washington, D.C.: National Academy Press.

Kawachi, I., et al. 1997. A prospective study of passive smoking and coronary heart disease. *Circulation* 95:2374–2379.

Lane, N. E., S. Sanchez, G. W. Modin, H. K. Genant, E. Pierini, and C. D. Arnaud. 2000. Bone mass continues to increase at the hip after parathyroid hormone treatment is discontinued in glucacorticoid-induced osteoporosis: Results of a randomized controlled trial. *Journal of Bone and Mineral Research* 15 (5):944-951.

Leonetti, H. B., et al. 1999. Transdermal progesterone cream for vasomotor symptoms and postmenopausal bone loss. *Obstetrics and Gynecology* 94:225–228.

Lindsay, R., et al. 1999. Addition of alendronate to ongoing hormone replacement therapy in treatment of osteoporosis: A randomized, controlled clinical trial. *Journal of Clinical Endocrinology and Metabolism* 84:3076–3081.

Lukkin, E. 2000. Personal communication. 18th Annual Hawaii Obstetrics-Gynecology Conference, sponsored by Kaiser Permanente of San Francisco, July 15–22.

Melton, L. J., III, et al. 1997. Fractures attributable to osteoporisis: Report from the National Osteoporosis Foundation. *Journal of Bone and Mineral Research* 12:16–23.

Michelson, D. 1996. Bone mineral density in women with depression. *New England Journal of Medicine* 335:1176–1181.

Nachtigall, L. E., and J. Rattner Heilman. 1995. *Estrogen: The Facts Can Change Your Life*. New York: HarperCollins.

National Osteoporosis Foundation. 1998. Statistics published by National Osteoporosis Foundation, Washington, D.C.

Nisly, N., and T. Klepser. 1999. Phytoestrogens for the prevention and treatment of osteoporosis. *Alternative Medicine Alert* 2 (12):138–142.

Paganini-Hill, A. 1995. The benefits of estrogen replacement therapy on oral health. *Archives of Internal Medicine* 155:2325–2329.

Prince, R. 1995. The effects of calcium supplementation (milk powder or tablets) and exercise on bone density in postmenopausal women. *Journal of Bone and Mineral Research* 10:1068–1075.

Raisz, L. G. 1996. Bone formation and resorption in menopausal women using estrogen and androgen. *Journal of Endocrinology and Metabolism* 81:37–43.

Ray, N. F., et al. 1997. Medical expenditures for the treatment of osteoporotic fractures in the United States in 1995: Report from the National Osteoporosis Foundation. *Journal of Bone Mineral Research* 12:24–35.

Ridker, P. M. 1999. Hormone replacement therapy and increased plasma concentration of C-reactive protein. *Circulation* 100:713–716.

Ridker, P. M., et al. 2000. C-reactive protein and other markers of inflammation in the prediction of cardiovascular disease in women. *New England Journal of Medicine* 342:836–843.

Rimm, E. B., et al. 1998. Folate and vitamin B from diet and supplements in relation to risk of coronary heart disease among women. *Journal of the American Medical Association* 279(5):359–364.

Silverman, S. L., et al., for the PROOF Study Group. 1998. Salmon calcitonin nasal spray (NS-CT) reduces the rate of new vertebral fractures independently of known major pre-treatment risk factors. *Bone* 23S:S177.

Speroff, L. 1999. Treatment options for the prevention of osteoporosis. *Ob/Gyn Clinical Alert* 16 (6):45–48.

————. Estrogen and cardiovascular disease. *Ob/Gyn Clinical Alert* 10:86–88.

Taechakraichana, N., et al. 2000. A randomized trial of oral contraceptive and hormone replacement therapy on bone mineral density and coronary heart disease risk factors in postmenopausal women. *Obstetrics & Gynecology* 95 (1):87–94.

Theistz, G. 1992. Bone mass accumulation in adolescent and young adult women. *Journal of Clinical Endocrinology and Metabolism* 75:1060–65.

Wellness Letter 2000. Eat fat, get thin? *UC Berkeley Wellness Letter* 16 (7):1–3.

Wellness Letter 1999. Progress against heart disease: An advance you can live with. *UC Berkeley Wellness Letter* 16 (2):2.

Wenger, N. K., et al. 1993. Cardiovascular health and disease in women. *New England Journal of Medicine* 329:72–75.

Wilson, R., 1999. Dade Behring gets approval for test tied to heart risk. *Wall Street Journal*, November 10.

Windham, G. C. 1999. Cigarette smoking and effects on menstrual function. *Obstetrics and Gynecology* 93:59–65.

Chapter 5: The Great Imitator: Thyroid Change Can Fool You

Danese, M. 1996. Screening for mild thyroid failure at the periodic health exam. *Journal of the American Medical Association* 276:285–92.

Dyan, C. M., and G. H. Daniels. 1996. Chronic autoimmune thyroiditis. *New England Journal of Medicine* 335 (2):99–107.

Eskin, B. A., and L. S. Dumas. 1995. *Midlife Can Wait.* New York: Ballantine Books.

Franklin, J. A., et al. 1998. The management of hyperthyroidism. *New England Journal of Medicine* 330:1731–1738.

Hayslip, C. C. 1988. The value of serum antimicrosomal antibody testing in screening for symptomatic postpartum thyroid dysfunction. *American Journal of Obstetrics and Gynecology* 159:203–9.

Klee, G. G., and I. D. Hay. 1994. Biochemical thyroid function testing. *Mayo Clinic Proceedings* 69 (5):469–470.

Chapter 6: Frightening Changes—Cancer

Agency for Health Care Policy and Research. 1999. Evaluation of cervical cytology. *Evidence Report/Technology Assessment #5*, AHCPR Publication 99-E010. Washington, D.C.

American Cancer Society. 1998. Cancer facts and figures—1998 www.cancer.org/stastics.html.

———. 1997. Cancer facts and figures—1997. http://www.cancer.org/statistics.

American College of Obstetricians and Gynecologists, 1999. Federal study shows conventional Pap test remains most effective way to diagnose cervical cancer. *ACOG Today*. March.

———. 1997. ACOG Maintains Mammography Screening Guidelines for Women Ages 40–49. *ACOG Newsletter* 41 (3):8.

———. 1993. Routine cancer screening. *ACOG Committee Opinion* No. 128. Washington, D.C.: ACOG.

———. 1993. Cervical cytology: Evaluation and management of abnormalities. *ACOG Technical Bulletin* No. 183. Washington, D.C.: ACOG.

Antman, K., S. Shea. 1999. Screening mammography under age 50. *Journal of the American Medical Association* 281:1470–1472.

Bennicke, K., et al. 1995. Cigarette smoking and breast cancer. *British Medical Journal* 310:1431–1433.

Bernstein, L. 1999. Tamoxifen therapy for breast cancer and endometrial cancer risk. *Journal of the National Cancer Institute* 91:1654-1662.

Braly, P. S. 1997. The NIH Consensus Conference on Cervical Cancer: Implications for Practice. Presentation at 45th annual clinical meeting of the American College of Obstetricians and Gynecologists, May.

Brown, A. D., and A. M. Garber. 1999. Cost-effectiveness of 3 methods to enhance the sensitivity of Papanicolaou testing. *Journal of the American Medical Association* 281 (4):347–352.

Bruning, P. F., et al. 1992. Insulin resistance and breast-cancer risk. *International Journal of Cancer* 52:511–516.

Calle, E. E., and M. J. Thun. 1997. The epidemiology of the effects of estrogen and aspirin on colorectal cancer. *Menopausal Medicine* 5 (1):9–12.

Celentano, D. D., and G. deLissovoy. 1989. Assessment of cancer screening and follow-up programs. *Public Health Review* 17:173–240.

Colditz, G. A., et al. 1993. Family history, age and the risk of breast cancer. Prospective data from the Nurses' Health Study. *Journal of the American Medical Association* 270:338–343.

Collaborative Group on Hormonal Factors in Breast Cancer. 1996. Breast cancer and hormonal contraception: Collaborative reanalysis of individual data on 53,297 women with breast cancer and 100,239 women without breast cancer from 54 epidemiologic studies. *Lancet* 347:1713–1717.

Cummings, S. R. 1999. The effect of raloxifene on risk of breast cancer in postmenopausal women. *Journal of the American Medical Association* 281:2189–2197.

Darney, P. 2000. Contraception for women with medical problems. *Audio Digest, Obstetrics and Gynecology* 47(3).

Fisher, B. 1998. Tamoxifen cuts risk of breast cancer in half. *Journal of the National Cancer Institute* 90:1371–1388.

Fuchs, C.S., et al. 1999. Dietary fiber and the risk of colorectal cancer and adenoma in women. *New England Journal of Medicine* 340 (3):169–176.

Gemmell, J., et al. 1990. How frequently need vaginal smears be taken after hysterectomy for cervical intraepithelial neoplasia? *British Journal of Obstetrics and Gynaecology* 91:67–72.

Gershenson, D. 1997. ERT in patients with a history of endometrial cancer. *Ob/Gyn Clinical Alert* 13 (10):79–80.

———. 1996. Genetic testing for cancer susceptibility. *Ob/Gyn Clinical Alert* 13 (4):31–32.

Giovannucci, E. 1998. Multivitamin use, folate, and colon cancer in women in the Nurses' Health Study. *Annals of Internal Medicine* 129:517–524.

Greendale, G. A., et al. for the Postmenopausal Estrogen/Progestin Interventions (PEPI) investigators. 1999. Effects of estrogen and estrogen-progestin on mammographic parenchymal density. *Annals of Internal Medicine* 130:262–269.

Grodstein, F., and E. Martinez. 1999. Postmenopausal hormone therapy reduces risk of colorectal cancer. *American Journal of Medicine* 106:574–582.

Guidos, B. J., and S. M. Selvaggi. 1999. Use of the ThinPrep Pap Test in clinical practice. *Diagnostic Cytopathology* 20:70–73.

Hartmann, L. C., et al. 1999. Efficacy of bilateral prophylactic mastectomy in women with a family history of breast cancer. *New England Journal of Medicine* 340 (2):389–397.

Harvard Women's Health Watch 2000. Tobacco smoke and women: A special vulnerability? *Harvard Women's Health Watch;* 7 (9):1.

Harvard Women's Health Watch 2000. Breast imaging: Mammograms still rule. *Harvard Women's Health Watch* 7 (10):5–6.

Harvard Women's Health Watch 2000. Progress report on ovarian cancer. *Harvard Women's Health Watch* 7 (9):2–4.

Holmberg, L. 1994. Effect of hormonal contraception on breast cancer and benign breast conditions. *European Journal of Cancer* 30A:351.

Hoskins, K. F., et al. 1995. Assessment and counseling for women with a family history of breast cancer: A guide for clinicians. *Journal of the American Medical Association* 273:577–85.

Jacobs, E. J. 1999. Hormone replacement therapy and colon cancer among members of a health maintainance organization. *Epidemiology* 10:445–451.

Ji, B., et al. 1997. Green tea consumption and the risk of pancreatic and colorectal cancers. *International Journal of Cancer* 70:255–258.

Kavanagh, A. M., et al. 2000. Hormone replacement therapy and accuracy of mammographic screening. *Lancet* 355:270–274.

Kerlikowske, K., et al. 1999. Continuing screening mammography in women aged 70 to 79. *Journal of the American Medical Association* 282 (22):2156–2163.

Kinney, W., 1997. Gynecologic oncologist, Kaiser Permanente of Northern California. Personal communication.

Koutsky, L. A., et al. 1992. A cohort study of the risk of cervical intraepithelial neoplasia grade 2 or 3 in relation to papillomavirus infection. *New England Journal of Medicine* 327:1272–78.

Krainer, M., et al. 1997. Differential contributions of BRCA1 and BRCA2 to early onset breast cancer. *New England Journal of Medicine* 336:1416–1420.

Linder, J., and D. Zahniser. 1997. The ThinPrep Paptest: A review of clinical studies. *Acta Cytologica* 47:30–38.

Lu, L.-J. W., et al. 1996. Effects of soya consumption for one month on steroid hormones in premenopausal women: Implications for breast cancer risk reduction. *Cancer Epidemiology, Biomarkers and Prevention* 5:63–70.

Malone, K. E. 1998. BRCA1 mutations and breast cancer in the general population: Analyses in women before age 45 years with first-degree family history. *Journal of the American Medical Association* 279:922.

Mandel, J. S., et al. 1993. Reducing mortality from colorectal cancer by screening for fecal occult blood. *New England Journal of Medicine* 328:1365–1371.

Manos, M. M., et al. 1999. Identifying women with cervical neoplasia using human papillomavirus DNA testing for equivocal Papanicolaou results. *Journal of the American Medical Association* 281:1605–1610.

Michels, K. B. 1996. Birth weight as a risk factor for breast cancer. *Lancet* 348:1542–46.

Moss, S. M., 1999. Decreased breast cancer mortality with mammography compared to breast self examination. *Lancet* 353 (9168):1909–1914.

Nawa, A., et al. 1995. Association of human leukocyte antigen-B1*03 with cervical cancer in Japanese women aged 35 years and younger. *Cancer* 75:518–21.

Newman, B. 1998. Frequency of breast cancer attributable to BRCA1 in a population-based series of American women. *Journal of the American Medical Association* 279:915.

Notelovitz, M., and D. Tonnessen. 1993. *Menopause and Midlife Health*. New York: St. Martin's Press.

Paavonen, R. 1999. Four serotypes of C. trachomatis have been shown to increase risk of cervical cancer. *OB/GYN News* 34 (16):14.

Parham, G. et al. 1999 Computer-assisted screening using Pap plus speculopathy (Papsure). Proceedings of the Second Annual International Conference on Lower Genital Tract Infections and Disorders for Clinicians, October 15.

Potischman, N., et al. 1996. Reversal of relation between body mass and endogenous estrogen concentrations with menopausal status. *Journal of the National Cancer Institute* 88:756–758.

Reichman, J. 1996. *I'm Too Young to Get Old: Health Care for Women After Forty*. New York: Times Books.

Rockhill, B., et al. 1999. A prospective study of recreational physical activity and breast cancer risk. *Archives of Internal Medicine* 159:2290–2296.

Sankaranarayanan, R., et al. 1999. Visual inspection of the uterine cervix after application of acetic acid in the detection of cervical carcinoma and its precursors. *Lancet* 83 (10):2150–2156.

Seltzer, V. L. 1996. Presentation on breast cancer at ACOG 44th Annual Clinical Meeting.

Shattuck-Eidens et al. 1997. A collaborative survey of 80 mutations in BRCA1 breast and ovarian cancer susceptibility gene. *Journal of the American Medical Association* 273:535–41.

Sheehan, K. M., et al. 1999. The relationship between cyclooxygenase-2 expression and colorectal cancer. *Journal of the American Medical Association* 282 (13):1254–1257.

Shoff, S., and P. A. Newcomb. 1998. Diabetes, body size, and risk of endometrial cancer. *American Journal of Epidemiology* 148 (3):234–240.

Smith-Warner, S. A., et al. 1998. Alcohol and breast cancer in women: A pooled analysis of cohort studies. *Journal of the American Medical Association* 279:535–540.

Speroff, L. 1998. Hormones and breast cancer: Part 1, a clinician's formulation. *Ob/Gyn Clinical Alert* (Suppl.): 15(5).

Struewing, J. P., et al. 1997. The risk of cancer associated with specific mutations of BRCA1 and BRCA2 among Ashkenazi Jews. *New England Journal of Medicine* 336:1401–1404.

Suneja, A., et al. 1998. Comparison of magnified chemiluminescent examination with incandescent light examination and colposcopy for detection of cervical neoplasia. *Indian Journal of Cancer* 35(2):81–87.

Tarone, R. 1996. Breast cancer death rate continues to decline. *News from the National Cancer Institute,* July.

Vetto, J., et al. 1995. Use of the "Triple Test" for palpable breast lesions yields high diagnostic accuracy and cost savings. *American Journal of Surgery* 169:519–522.

Wellness Letter. 2000. A cancer-causing virus: Should you be tested? *UC Berkeley Wellness Letter* 16 (7):4.

———. 1999. Can this drug prevent breast cancer? *UC Berkeley Wellness Letter* 16 (3):1–3.

Willett, W. 1994. Diet and health: What should we eat? *Science* 264:532–37.

Winawer, S. J., et al. 1997. Colorectal cancer screening: Clinical guidelines and rationale. *Gastroenterology* 112:594–642.

Xu, Y. 1998. Lysophosphatidic acid as a potential biomarker for ovarian and other gynecologic cancers. *Journal of the American Medical Association* 280:719–723.

Zhang, S. 1999. A propective study of folate intake and the risk of breast cancer. *Journal of the American Medical Association* 281:1632–1637.

Zheng, W. 1998. Well-done meat intake and the risk of breast cancer. *Journal of the National Cancer Institute* 90:1724–1729.

Ziegler, R. G., et al. 1996. Relative weight, weight change, height, and breast cancer in Asian-American women. *Journal of the National Cancer Institute* 88:650.

Chapter 7: You Can Change Your Hormones: The Case for Hormone Replacement Therapy

Adams, M. R., and M. L. Golden. 1995. Atheroprotective effects of estrogen replacement therapy are antagonized by medroxyprogesterone acetate in monkeys. *Circulation* 92:I-627.

American College of Obstetricians and Gynecologists. 2000. ACOG releases statement on recent studies of HRT and breast cancer. *ACOG Today* 44 (4):9.

Araneo, B. A., et al. 1995. DHEAS as an effective adjuvant in elderly humans: Proof-of-principle studies. *Annals of the New York Academy of Science* 774:232–248.

Arlt, W., et al. 1999. Dehydroepiandrosterone replacement in women with adrenal insufficiency. *New England Journal of Medicine* 341:1013–1020.

Ayton, R., et al. 1996. A comparative study of safety and efficacy of continuous low dose oestradiol released from a vaginal ring compared with conjugated oestrogen vaginal cream in the treatment of menopausal urogenital atrophy. *British Journal of Obstetrics and Gynecology* 103:291–92.

Barton, D. L. 1998. Prospective evaluation of vitamin E for hot flashes in breast cancer survivors. *Journal of Clinical Oncology* 16:495–500.

Bates, G. W., et al. 1995. Dehydroepiandrosterone attenuates study-induced declines in insulin sensitivity in postmenopausal women. *Annals of the New York Academy of Science* 774:291–93.

Baulieu, E. 1995. Dehydroepiandrosterone (DHEA) is a neuroactive neurosteroid. *Annals of the New York Academy of Science* 774:82–110.

Baxter, L. R., et al. 1987. Cerebral glucose metabolic rates in normal human females vs. normal males. *Psychiatry Research* 21 (3):137–145.

Berga, S. 2000. Menopausal estrogen and estrogen-progestin replacement therapy and breast cancer risk. *OB/GYN Clinical Alert* 16 (11):81–82.

———. 1999. HRT and risk of breast cancer with a favorable histology. *OB/GYN Clinical Alert* 16 (4):25–26.

Berman, J. S., et al. 1996. Compliance with postmenopausal hormone therapy. *Journal of Women's Health* 5:213–20.

Casson, P. R. 1998. Postmenopausal dehydroepiandrosterone administration increases free insulin-like growth factor-I and decreases high-density lipoproteins: A six-month trial. *Fertility and Sterility* 70:107–110.

Cauley, J. A., et al. 1995. Prevention of fractures requires long-term estrogen treatment. *Annals of Internal Medicine* 122:9–16.

Colditz, G. A., et al. 1995. The use of estrogens and progestins and the risk of breast cancer. *New England Journal of Medicine* 332:1589–93.

Collaborative Group on Hormonal Factors in Breast Cancer. 1997. *Lancet* 350:1047.

Cutler, W. 1990. *Hysterectomy: Before and After.* New York: Harper & Row.

Cutler, W., and C. R. Garcia. 1992. *Menopause: A Guide for Women and the Men Who Love Them.* New York: W. W. Norton.

Cummings, S. R., et al. 1989. Lifetime risk of hip, colles', or vertebral fracture and coronary heart disease among white postmenopausal women. *Archives of Internal Medicine* 149:94–98.

Darney, P. 2000. Contraception for women with medical problems. *Audio Digest, Obstetrics and Gynecology* 47(3).

de Lignieres B. 1999. Oral, micronized progesterone. *Clinical Therapeutics* 21 (1):41–60.

Elkind-Hirsch, K. E. , et al. 1993. Hormone replacement therapy alters insulin sensitivity in young women with premature ovarian failure. *Journal of Clinical Endocrinology and Metabolism* 76:472–475.

Ettinger, B. 1999. Reduction of vertebral fracture risk in postmenopausal women with osteoporosis treated with raloxifene: Results from a three-year randomized clinical trial. *Journal of the American Medical Association* 282:637–645.

———. 1999. Personal perspective on low-dosage estrogen therapy for postmenopausal women. *Menopause* 6:273–276.

———. 1996. Continuation rates with postmenopausal hormone therapy. *Menopause* 3:185–89.

Ettinger, B., et al. 1994. Cyclic hormone replacement therapy using quarterly progestin. *Obstetrics and Gynecology* 83:693–700.

Eye-Disease Case-Control Study Group. 1992. Risk factors for neovascular age-related macular degeneration. *Archives of Ophthalmology* 110:1701–1708.

Gambrell, R. et al. 1983. Decreased incidence of breast cancer in postmenopausal women. *Obstetrics and Gynecology* 62:435–43.

Gapstur, S. M. 1999. Hormone replacement therapy and risk of breast cancer with a favorable histology: Results of the Iowa Women's Health Study. *Journal of the American Medical Association* 281:2091–2097.

Gershenson, D. 1996. Genetic testing for cancer susceptibility. *Ob/Gyn Clinical Alert* 13 (4):31–32.

Grady, D., et al. 1995. Hormone replacement and endometrial cancer risk: A meta-analysis. *Obstetrics and Gynecology* 85:304.

Greene, R. A., et al. 1998. Comparison between cerebral blood flow in hypoestrogenic women and patients with Alzheimer's disease—a descriptive study. *Neurobiology of Aging* 19 (4):S180.

Grodstein, F. 1999. Postmenopausal hormone therapy reduces risk of colorectal cancer. *American Journal of Medicine* 106:574–582.

Grodstein, F., et al. 1997. Postmenopausal hormone therapy and mortality. *New England Journal of Medicine* 336:1769–75.

———. 1996. Postmenopausal estrogen and progestin use and the risk of cardiovascular disease. *New England Journal of Medicine* 335:453–461.

Harvard Heart Letter. 2000. Women and heart disease. *Harvard Heart Letter* 10 (5):1–4.

Harvard Women's Health Watch. 2000. Women's health in the next millennium: The future of women's health. *Harvard Women's Health Watch* 7 (5):4–5.

Henderson, V. 1995. Alzheimer's disease in women: Is there a role for estrogen replacement therapy? *Menopausal Management* 4 (6):10–13.

Jackson, S. 1999. The effect of oestrogen supplementation on post-menopausal urinary stress incontinence: A double-blind placebo-controlled trial. *British Medical Journal* 106:711-718.

Judd, H. J. 1996. The impact of ovarian hormone replacement on selected risk factors of coronary heart disease. *Menopausal Medicine* 4 (1):9–11.

Kaplan, H. S., and T. Owett. 1993. The female androgen deficiency syndrome. *Journal of Sex and Marital Therapy* 19:3–24.

Keating, N. L. 1999. Use of hormone replacement therapy by postmenopausal women in the United States. *Annals of Internal Medicine* 6:545–553.

Klein, B. E., et al. 1994. Are sex hormones associated with age-related maculopathy in women? The Beaver Dam Eye Study. *Trans American Ophthalmology Society* 92:289–295.

Leventhal, J. 1997. Libido and Menopause. Lecture given to the Women's Health Department, Kaiser Permanente Medical Group, Walnut Creek, Calif., April 1.

Luthold W. 1993. Serum testosterone fractions in women: Normal and abnormal clinical states. *Metabolism* 42 (5):638–643.

Miygawa, K., et al. 1997. Medroxyprogesterone interferes with ovarian steroid protection against coronary vaspspasm. *Natural Medicine* 3:324–327.

Mulnard, R. A., et al. 2000. Estrogen replacement therapy for treatment of mild to moderate Alzheimer's disease. *Journal of the American Medical Association* 283:1007–1015.

Nestel, P. J. 1999. Isoflavones from red clover improve systemic arterial compliance but not plasma lipids in menopausal women. *Journal of Clinical Endocrinology and Metabolism* 84:895–898.

Nestler, J. E. 1995. Regulation of human dehydroepiandrosterone metabolism by insulin. *Annals of the New York Academy of Science* 774:ix–xi.

Nieto, J. J., et al. 2000. Lipid effects of hormone replacement therapy with sequential transdermal 17-beta-estradiol and oral dydrogesterone. *Obstetrics & Gynecology* 95 (1):111–114.

Notelovitz, M., and D. Tonnessen. 1993. *Menopause and Midlife Health.* New York: St. Martin's Press.

Pike, M. C., et al. 1997. Estrogen-progestin replacement therapy and endometrial cancer. *Journal of the National Cancer Institute* 89:1110–1116.

Reichman, J. 1996. *I'm Too Young to Get Old: Health Care for Women After Forty.* New York: Times Books.

Rosenberg, S., et al. 1988. Serum levels of gonadotropins and steroid hormones in post-menopause and later life. *Maturitas* 10:215–24.

Ross, R. K., et al. 2000. Effect of hormone replacement therapy on breast cancer risk: Estrogen vs. estrogen plus progestin. *Journal of the National Cancer Institute* 92:328–332.

Santen, R., and J. V. Pinkerton. 1999. Alternatives to estrogen use in postmenopausal women. *Menopausal Medicine* 7 (4):1–7.

Schairer, C., et al. 2000. Menopausal estrogen and estrogen-progestin replacement therapy and breast cancer risk. *Journal of the American Medical Association* 283 (4):485–489.

Sellers, T. A., et al. 1997. The role of hormone replacement therapy in the risk for breast cancer and total mortality in women with a family history of breast cancer. *Annals of Internal Medicine* 127:973–980.

Sherwin, B. B. 1996. In *Progress in the Management of Menopause,* edited by B. G. Wren. New York: Pantheon Publishing Group.

Skolnick, A. 1996. Scientific verdict still out on DHEA. *Journal of the American Medical Association* 276:1365–67.

Speroff L. 2000. Postmenopausal estrogen-progestin therapy and breast cancer. *OB/GYN Clinical Alert* 16 (12):89–91.

———. 1999. Post-menopausal hormone therapy and breast cancer. *Contraceptive Technology Update* 20 (Suppl. 1): 1–2.

———. 1994. Estrogen and cardiovascular disease. *Ob/Gyn Clinical Alert* 10 (11):86–88.

———. 1994. Managing therapy-related postmenopausal bleeding. *Ob/Gyn Clinical Alert* 11 (8):62–64.

Sorensen, K., et al. 1998. Combined hormone replacement therapy does not protect women against age-related decline in endothelium-dependent vasomotor function. *Circulation* 97:1234–1238.

Sourander, L. 1998. A reduction in cardiovascular mortality with postmenopausal estrogen therapy. *Lancet* 352:1965–1969.

Stanford, J., et al. 1995. Combined estrogen and progesterone replacement therapy in relation to risk of breast cancer in middle-aged women. *Journal of the American Medical Association* 274:137–42.

Vingerling, J. R., et al. 1995. Macular degeneration and early menopause: A case-control study. *British Medical Journal* 310:1570–1571.

Walsh, B. W. 1998. Effects of raloxifene on serum lipids and coagulation factors in healthy postmenopausal women. *Journal of the American Medical Association* 279:1445–1451.

Washburn, S. 1999. Effect of soy protein supplementation on serum lipoproteins, blood pressure, and menopausal symptoms in postmenopausal women. *Menopause* 6:7–13.

Wild, R. A. 1996. Estrogen effects on the cardiovascular tree. *Obstetrics and Gynecology* 87:275–355.

Wolkowitz, O. M., et al. 1995. Antidepressant and cognition-enhancing effects of DHEA in major depression. Presentation to the New York Academy of Science. *Annals of the New York Academy of Science* 774:337–39.

Woodruff, J. D., and J. H. Pickar. 1994. Incidence of endometrial hyperplasia in postmenopausal women taking conjugated estrogen (Premarin) with medroxyprogesterone acetate or conjugated estrogens alone. *American Journal of Obstetrics and Gynecology* 170:1213.

Writing Group for the PEPI Trials. 1995. Effects of estrogen or estrogen/progestin on heart disease risk factors on postmenopausal women. *Journal of the American Medical Association* 273:199–08.

Yaffe, K. Y. 1998. Serum estrogen levels, cognitive performance, and risk of cognitive decline in older community women. *Journal of the American Geriatric Society* 46:918–919.

Zhang, Y., et al. 1997. Bone density and risk of breast cancer in postmenopausal women. *New England Journal of Medicine* 336:611–17.

Chapter 8: Integrative (Alternative) Medical Disciplines: Are They a Good Choice for You?

Aldercreutz, H., et al. 1991. Urinary excretion of lignans and isoflavonoids: Phytoestrogens in Japanese men and women consuming a traditional diet. *American Journal of Clinical Nutrition* 54:1093–1100.

Baber, R. J. 1999. Randomized placebo-controlled trial of an isoflavone supplement and menopausal symptoms. *Climacteric* 2:85–92.

Baker, B. 1999. Dong quai, black cohosh unproven for menopause. *Internal Medicine News* March 1:p 42.

Barsoum, G., et al. 1990. Postoperative nausea is relieved by acupressure. *Journal of the Royal Society of Medicine* 83:86–89.

Bienfield, H., and E. Korngold. 1991. *Between Heaven and Earth: A Guide to Chinese Medicine.* New York: Ballantine Books.

Brevcort, P. 1998. The booming US botanical market: A new overview. *HerbalGram* 44:33–48.

Brewington, V., et al. 1994. Acupuncture as a detoxification treatment: An analysis of controlled research. *Journal of Substance Abuse* 11 (4):289–307.

Chopra, D. 1990. *Quantum Healing: Exploring the Frontiers of Mind/Body Medicine.* New York: Bantam.

Coan, R. M., et al. 1980. The acupuncture treatment of low back pain: A randomized controlled study. *American Journal of Chinese Medicine* 9:326–332.

Collinge, W. 1996. *The American Holistic Association Complete Guide to Alternative Medicine.* New York: Warner.

De Aloysio, D., and P. Penacchioni. 1992. Morning sickness control in early pregnancy by Neiguan point acupressure. *Obstetrics and Gynecology* 80:852–854.

Ehrlich, D., and P. Haber. 1992. Influence of acupuncture on physical performance capacity and haemodynamic parameters. *Internatioal Journal of Sports Medicine* 13:486–491.

Eisenberg, D. M., et al. 1998. Trends in alternative medicine use in the United States, 1990-1997: Results of a follow-up national survey. *Journal of the American Medical Association* 280 (18):1569–1575.

Ernst, E. 1995. St. Johnswort, an antidepressant? A systematic, criteria-based review. *Phytomedicine* 2 (1):67–71.

Fugh-Berman, A. 1997. *Alternative Medicine: What Works.* Baltimore: Lippincott, Williams & Wilkins.

Hardy, M. L. 1999. Valerian root for insomnia. *Alternative Medicine Alert* 2 (8):85–88.

Harvard Women's Health Watch 2000. Echinacea vs. the common cold. *Harvard Women's Health Watch* 7 (6):1.

Hornig, M. 1998. Ginkgo biloba for attention and memory disorders. *Alternative Medicine Alert* 1 (12):137–139.

Hu, H. H., et al. 1993. A randomized controlled trial on the treatment for acute partial ischemic stroke with acupuncture. *Neuroepidemiology* 12:106–113.

Integrative Medicine 2000. Background sheet: Obesity. *Integrative Medicine Consult* 2 (6):69.

Jacobs, J., et al. 1994. Alternative systems of medical practice. In *Alternative Medicine: Expanding Medical Horizons.* A report to the NIH on alternative medical systems and practices in the U.S., Workshop on Alternative Medicine, Chantilly, Va.

Khoo, S. K., et al. 1990. Evening primrose oil and treatment of PMS. *Medical Journal of Australia* 153:189–92.

Kleijmen, J. 1994. Evening primrose oil currently used in many conditions with little justification. *British Medical Journal* 309:824–825. Also see comment of the editor, 309:1437.

Knight, D. C. 1999. The effect of Promensil, an isoflavone extract, on menopausal symptoms. *Climacteric* 2:79–84.

Nisly, N., and T. Klepser. 1999 Phytoestrogens for the prevention and treatment of osteoporosis. *Alternative Medicine Alert* 2 (12):138–142.

Ojeda, L. 1995. *Menopause without Medicine.* Alameda, Calif.: Hunter House.

Ondrizek, R. R. 1999. An alternative medicine study of herbal effects on the penetration of zona-free hamster oocytes and the integrity of sperm deoxyribonucleic acid. *Fertility and Sterility* 71 (3):517–522.

Philipp, M. 1999. Hypericum extract versus imipramine or placebo in patients with moderate depression: Randomised multicentre study of treatment for eight weeks. *British Medical Journal* 319:1534–1538.

Physicians' Desk Reference for Herbal Medicines. 1998. Montvale, N. J.: Medical Economics Company, Inc.

Reichman, J. 1996. *I'm Too Young to Get Old: Health Care for Women After Forty.* New York: Times Books.

Robbers, J. E., and V. E. Tyler. 1999. *Tyler's Herbs of Choice: The Therapeutic Use of Phytomedicinals.* Binghamton, N.Y.: Haworth Press.

Scheidermeyer, D. 1998. Little evidence for ginseng as treatment for menopausal symptoms. *Alternative Medicine Alert* 1 (7):77–78.

Shao, Z. M. 1998. Genistein exerts multiple suppressive effects on human carcinoma cells. *Cancer Research* 58 (21):4851–4857.

Tyler, V. E. 1997. The bright side of black cohosh. *Prevention* 4:76–79.

Ullman, D. 1991. *Discovering Homeopathic Medicine for the 21st Century.* Berkeley: North Atlantic Books.

Vincent, C. A. 1990. The treatment of tension headache by acupuncture: A controlled single case design with time series analysis. *Journal of Psychosomatic Research* 34 (5):553–561.

―――. 1989. A controlled trial of the treatment of migraine by acupuncture. *Clinical Journal of Pain* 5(4):305-312.

Warwick-Evans, L. A., et al. 1991. A double-blind placebo controlled evaluation of acupressure in the treatment of motion sickness. *Aviation, Space, and Environmental Medicine* 62:776–778.

Washburn, S. 1999. Effect of soy protein supplementation on serum lipoproteins, blood pressure, and menopausal symptoms in postmenopausal women. *Menopause* 6:7–13.

Wellness Letter 2000. Wellness made easy. *UC Berkeley Wellness Letter* 16 (4):8.

Wellness Letter 2000. Worry wort. *UC Berkeley Wellness Letter* 16 (8):7.

Wellness Letter 2000. The herb with a thousand faces. *UC Berkeley Wellness Letter* 16 (10):2–3.

Women's HealthSource 2000. Herbs and surgery don't mix. *Mayo Clinic Women's HealthSource* 4 (3):8.

Wynon, Y., et al. 1995. Effects of acupuncture on climacteric vasomotor symptoms, quality of life, and urinary excretion of neuropeptides among postmenopausal women. *Menopause: Journal of the North American Menopausal Society* 2 (1):3–12.

Yang, L. C., et al. 1993. Comparison of P-6 acupoint injection with 50% glucose in water and intravenous droperidol for prevention of vomiting after gynecologic laparoscopy. *Acta Anaesthesiologica Scandinavia* 37 (2):192–194.

Zava, D. T. 1998. Estrogen and progestin bioactivity of foods, herbs and spices. *Proceedings of the Society for Experimental Biological Medicine* 217:369–378.

Chapter 9: Wellness for a Change: Good Nutrition and Exercise

Albert, C. M., et al. 1998. Fish consumption and the risk of sudden cardiac death. *Journal of the American Medical Association* 279 (1):23–28.

American College of Obstetricians and Gynecologists. 1992. *Planning for Pregnancy, Birth and Beyond.* New York: Dutton.

Bellerson, K. 1993. *The Complete Fat Book.* Garden City, N.Y.: Avery Publishing.

Benson, H., and E. Stuart. 1993. *The Wellness Book: A Comprehensive Guide to Maintaining Health and Treating Stress-Related Illness.* New York: Fireside.

Blair, S. N., et al. 1989. Physical fitness and all-cause mortality: A prospective study of healthy men and women. *Journal of the American Medical Association* 262:2395–2401.

Bland, J. S. 1999. *Genetic Nutritioneering.* Los Angeles: Keats Publishing.

Block, G. 1991. Dietary guidelines: The results of food consumption surveys. *American Journal of Clinical Nutrition* 53:356(S)–357(S).

Brink, S. 1995. Health Guide, 1995. Interview with R. Rikli, co-director, Lifespan Wellness Clinic at California State University, Fullerton. *U.S. News and World Report* May 15:76–84.

Cutler, W., and C. R. Garcia. 1992. *Menopause: A Guide for Women and the Men Who Love Them.* New York: W. W. Norton.

Daoust, J., and G. Daoust. 1996. *Fat Burning Nutrition.* Del Mar, Calif.: Wharton Publishing.

Davis, R. 1996. Yoga and you. *Weight Watchers* 29 (11):55–61.

Diaz, M. N., et al. 1997. Antioxidants and atherosclerotic heart disease." *New England Journal of Medicine* 337:408–409.

Dreon, D. M., et al. 1990. The effects of polyunsaturated fat vs. monounsaturated fat on plasma lipoproteins. *Journal of the American Medical Association* 263:2461–66.

Duke, J. A. 2000. Beans to soy. *Alternative Therapies in Women's Health* 2 (5):36–38.

Eikelboom, J. W., et al. 1999. Homocysteine and cardiovascular disease: A critical review of the epidemiological evidence. *Annals of Internal Medicine* 131 (5):363–375.

Frisch, R. E., et al. 1987. Lower prevalence of reproductive system cancers among former college athletes. *Medical Science in Sports and Exercise* 21:83–90.

Hallfrisch, J., et al. 1994. High plasma vitamin C associated with high plasma HDL and LDL-2 cholesterol. *American Journal of Clinical Nutrition* 60:100–105.

Hallikainen, M. A., and M. I. Uusitupa. 1999. Effects of two low-fat stanol ester-containing margarines on serum cholesterol concentrations as part of a low-fat diet in hypercholesterolemic subjects. *American Journal of Clinical Nutrition* 69:403–410.

Harvard Heart Letter. 2000. Women and heart disease. *Harvard Heart Letter* 10 (5):1–4.

Harvard Women's Health Watch 1999. Vitamin D update. *Harvard Women's Health Watch* 6 (11):6.

Hu, F. B. 1999. A prospective study of egg consumption and risk of cardiovascular disease in men and women. *Journal of the American Medical Association* 281:1384–1394.

Hu, F. B., et al. 1999. Dietary fat intake and the risk of coronary heart disease in women. *New England Journal of Medicine* 337 (21):1491–2004.

Hunter, D., et al. 1993. A prospective study of the intake of vitamins C, E, and A and the risk of breast cancer. *New England Journal of Medicine* 329:234–40.

Jandak, J., and S. Richardson. 1989. Alpha-tocopherol and effective inhibition of platelet adhesion. *American Journal of Clinical Nutrition* 60:100–05.

Kardinaal, A., et al. 1994. Antioxidants in adipose tissue and risk of myocardial infarction: The EURAMIC Study. *Lancet* 342:1379–84.

Krasinski, A., et al. 1989. Relationship of vitamin A and vitamin E intake to fasting plasma retinol, retinol-binding protein, retinyl esters, carotene, tocopherol, and cholesterol among elderly people and young adults: Increased plasma retinyl esters among vitamin A users. *American Journal of Clinical Nutrition* 49:112–20.

Kromhaut, D., et al. 1985. The inverse relation between fish consumption and 20 year mortality from coronary heart disease. *New England Journal of Medicine* 312:1205–09.

Landau, C., et al. 1994. *The Complete Book of Menopause: Every Woman's Guide to Good Health.* New York: G. P. Putnam's Sons.

Lapidus, L. 1986. Ischemic heart disease, stroke, and mortality in women: Results from a prospective population study in Gothenburg, Sweden. *Acta Medicus Scandinavia* 219 (Supplement):1–42.

Leibel, R. L., et al. 1995. Changes in energy expenditure resulting from altered body weight. *New England Journal of Medicine* 332:621–628.

Levine, M. 1987. Vitamin C utilization with stress. *Annals of the New York Academy of Science* 498:424–44.

Lohman, W. 1987. Ascorbic acid and cancer. Third Conference on Vitamin C. *Annals of the New York Academy of Science* 498:402–17.

McDowell, M. A., et al. 1994. Third National Health and Nutrition Examination Survey with Data from National Center for Health Statistics. Washington, D.C: Government Printing Office.

Medical Research Council Vitamin Study Research Group. 1991. Prevention of neural tube defects: Results of the Medical Research Council vitamin study. *Lancet* 338:131–37.

Melbus, H. 1998. Excessive dietary intake of vitamin A is associated with reduced bone mineral density and increased risk for hip fracture. *Annals of Internal Medicine* 129:770–778.

Notelovitz, M., and D. Tonnessen. 1993. *Menopause and Midlife Health.* New York: St. Martin's Press.

Nutrition and Your Health: Dietary Guidelines for Americans. 1995. *Home and Garden Bulletin* no. 232. Washington, D.C: U.S. Department of Agriculture and U.S. Department of Health and Human Services.

Ojeda, L. 1995. *Menopause without Medicine.* Alameda, Calif.: Hunter House.

Pauling, L. 1986. *How to Live Long and Feel Better.* New York: Freeman.

Pollack, M., and V. Froelicher. 1990. Position stand of the American college of sports medicine: The recommended quantity and quality of exercise for development and maintaining cardiorespiratory and muscular fitness in healthy adults. *Journal of Cardiopulmonary Rehabilitation* 10:235–45.

Reichman, J. 1996. *I'm Too Young to Get Old: Health Care for Women After Forty.* New York: Times Books.

Rexrode, K. M., and J. E. Manson. 1996. Antioxidants in cardiovascular disease prevention: Fact or fiction? *Menopausal Medicine* 4 (3):8–12.

Schmidt, R. 1998. Plasma antioxidants and cognitive performance in middle-aged and older adults: Results of the Austrian Stroke Prevention Study. *Journal of the American Geriatric Society* 46:1407–1410.

Schwarzbein, D. 1999. *The Schwartzbein Principle*. Deerfield Beach, Fla.: Health Communications, Inc.

Selhub, J. 1999. Serum total homocysteine concentrations in the third national health and nutrition survey (1991–1994): Population reference ranges and contribution of vitamin status to high serum concentrations. *Annals of Internal Medicine* 131:331–339.

Stampfer, M., et al. 1993. Vitamin E consumption and the risk of coronary disease in women. *New England Journal of Medicine* 328:1444–49.

Stampfer. M., and W. Willett. 1993. Homocysteine and marginal vitamin D deficiency: The importance of adequate vitamin intake. *Journal of the American Medical Association* 270:2726–27.

Szapary, P. O., and M. D. Cirigliano. 2000. Plant stanols in the treatment of hypercholesterolemia. *Alternative Medicine Alert* 3 (1):6–10.

Tribble, D. L. 1999. Antioxidant consumption and risk of coronary heart disease: Emphasis on vitamin C, vitamin E, and beta-carotene. *Circulation* 99:591–595.

Wellness Letter. 2000. Beta carotene pills: Might help, might hurt. *UC Berkeley Wellness Letter* 16 (6):4.

Wellness Letter. 2000 Vitamin C: We still take it, and so should you. *UC Berkeley Wellness Letter* 16 (8):1.

Wellness Letter 2000 Low-fat foods: The numbers game. *UC Berkeley Wellness Letter* 16 (8):3.

Wellness Letter 2000 Does this mineral prevent cancer? *UC Berkeley Wellness Letter* 16 (9):1–2.

Wallace, J. P., et al. 1982. Changes in menstrual function, climacteric syndrome, and serum concentrations of sex hormone in pre- and postmenopausal women following a moderate intensity training program. *Modern Science in Sports and Exercise* 14:154.

Willett, W. 1994. Diet and health: What should we eat? *Science* 264:532–37.

Willett, W., et al. 1993. Intake of trans fatty acids and risks of coronary heart disease among women. *Lancet* 341:581–85.

Wolever, T. M. 1997. The glycemic index: Flogging a dead horse? *Diabetes Care* 20:452–456.

Wolk, A., et al. 1999. Long-term intake of fiber and increased risk of coronary heart disease among women. *Journal of the American Medical Association* 281 (21):1998–2004.

Yosuf, S., et al. 2000. Vitamin E supplementation and cardiovascular events in high-risk patients: The Heart Outcomes Prevention Evaluation (HOPE) Study. *New England Journal of Medicine* 342:154–160.

Zannoni, T. 1987. Ascorbic acid, alcohol, and environmental chemicals. Third Conference on Vitamin C. *Annals of the New York Academy of Sciences* 498:364–88.

Chapter 10: Wellness from Lifestyle Changes: Weight Control, Plus Detoxifying Your Body and Mind

Abenheim, J., et al. 1996. Appetite suppressant drugs and the risk of pulmonary hypertension. *New England Journal of Medicine* 335:609–15.

Autti-Ramo, I., et al. 1992. Dysmorphic features in offspring of alcoholic mothers. *Archives of Diseases in Children* 67:712–16.

Baron, R. B. 1997. Treating obesity: Diet, exercise, and Phen-Fen. *Audio Digest, Obstetrics and Gynecology* 44 (5).

Barrette, E. P. 2000. Metabolife 356 for weight loss. *Alternative Medicine Alert* 3 (1):1–6.

Bland, J. S. 1999. *Genetic Nutritioneering*. Los Angeles: Keats Publishing.

Brody, J. 1990. *Jane Brody's Good Food Gourmet*. New York: W. W. Norton.

Centers for Disease Control and Prevention. 2000. Prevalence of overweight and obesity among adults: United States, 1999. www.cdc.gov.nchs.

Connor, S. L., and W. E. Connor. 1991. *The New American Diet System*. New York: Simon & Schuster.

Butts, N. K., and S. Price. 1994. Effects of a 12-week weight training program on the body composition of women over 30 years of age. *Journal of Strength Conditioning Research* 8:265–69.

Daoust, J., and G. Daoust. 1996. *Fat Burning Nutrition*. Del Mar, Calif: Wharton Publishing.

Davidson, M. H., et al. 1999. Weight control and risk factor reduction in obese subjects treated 2 years with Orlistat. *Journal of the American Medical Association* 281 (3):235–242.

Fontham, E. T. H. 1994. Environmental tobacco smoke and lung cancer in nonsmoking women. *Journal of the American Medical Association* 271:1752–59.

Frezza, M. 1990. The role of gastric alcohol dehydrogenase activity and first pass metabolism. *New England Journal of Medicine* 322:967–76.

Ginsburg, E. S., et al. 1995. The effects of ethanol on the clearance of estradiol in postmenopausal women. *Fertility and Sterility* 63:1227–1230.

Glantz, S. A., and W. W. Parmley. 1995. Passive smoking and heart disease: Mechanisms and risk. *Journal of the American Medical Association* 273:1047–1053.

Gold, M. 1991. *The Good News about Drugs and Alcohol.* New York: Random House.

Goldring, L. A., et al., eds. 1989. *Y's Ways to Physical Fitness,* 3rd ed. Chicago: Human Kinetics.

Horm, J., and K. Anderson. 1993. Who in America is trying to lose weight? *Annals of Internal Medicine* 119:672–76.

Institute of Medicine. 1995. *Weighing the Options: Criteria for Evaluating Weight-Management Programs.* Washington, D.C.: National Academy Press.

Johannessen, S., and H. Liu. 1986. High-frequency, moderate-intensity training in sedentary middle-aged women. *Physician Sports Medicine* 14:99–102.

Kayman, S., et al. 1990. Maintenance and relapse after weight loss in women: Behavioral aspects. *American Journal of Clinical Nutrition* 52:800–07.

Kuczmarski, R. J., et al. 1994. Increasing prevalence of overweight among U.S. adults. *Journal of the American Medical Association* 272:205–11.

Landau, C., et al. 1994. *The Complete Book of Menopause: Every Woman's Guide to Good Health.* New York: G. P. Putnam's Sons.

Langreth, R. 1997. Alternatives to Redux still are years away. *Wall Street Journal,* September 16.

Larson, J. 1993. *Seven Weeks to Sobriety: The Proven Program to Fight Alcoholism Through Nutrition.* New York: Columbine Fawcett.

Notelovitz, M., and D. Tonnessen. 1993. *Menopause and Midlife Health.* New York: St. Martin's Press.

Ojeda, L. 1995. *Menopause without Medicine.* Alameda, Calif.: Hunter House.

O'Mathuna, D. P. 1999. Pyruvate for the treatment of obesity. *Alternative Medicine Alert* 2 (3):31–33.

Physicians' Desk Reference (PDR). 1997. Montvale, N.J.: Medical Economics Company.

Prochaska, J. P., et al. 1992. In search of how people change: Applications to addictive behavior. *American Psychologist* 47: 1102–14.

Reichman, J. 1996. *I'm Too Young to Get Old: Health Care for Women Aftre Forty.* New York: Times Books.

Rexrode, K. M., et al. 1998. Abdominal adiposity and coronary heart disease in women. *Journal of the American Medical Association* 280 (21):1843–1848.

Rigotti, N. 1992. Smoking Cessation Strategies for Women. Paper presented on primary care of women, Harvard Medical School.

Roubenoff, R., et al. 1995. Predicting body fatness: The body mass index vs. estimation by bioelectrical impedance. *American Journal of Public Health* 85:726–28.

Sears B. 1995. *The Zone: A Dietary Roadmap.* New York: HarperCollins.

Schwarzbein, D. 1999. *The Schwarzbein Principle.* Deerfield Beach, Fla.: Health Communications, Inc.

Sjostrom, L., et al. 1998. Randomised placebo-controlled trial of Orlistat for weight loss and prevention of weight gain in obese patients. *Lancet* 352 (9123):167–173.

Smith-Warner, S., et al. 1998. Alcohol and breast cancer in women. *Journal of the American Medical Association* 279 (2):399–403.

Stampfer, M. J., and W. Willet. 1988. A prospective study of moderate alcohol consumption and the risk of coronary disease and stroke in women. *New England Journal of Medicine* 318:267–73.

Warner, K. E. 1991. Health and economic implications of a tobacco free society. *Journal of American Medical Association* 258:2080–88.

Wellness Letter 2000. Not Kool or Lucky. *UC Berkeley Wellness Letter* 16 (5):8.

Women's HealthSource 1999. Weight Control, Special Report. *Mayo Clinic Women's Health Source.* Rochester, Minn.

Chapter 11: Relax for a Change: Management of Stress and Depression

American College of Obstetricians and Gynecologists. 1993. Depression in Women. *Technical Bulletin,* no. 182. Washington, D.C.: ACOG.

Benson, H., and E. Stuart. 1993. *The Wellness Book: The Comprehensive Guide to Maintaining and Treating Stress-Related Illness.* New York: Fireside.

Consensus treatment guidelines for bipolar disorder: A guide for patients and families. 1996. *Journal of Clinical Psychiatry* 57 (Suppl. 12A):237.

Depression Guideline Panel. 1993. Depression in Primary Care: Detection, Diagnosis, and Treatment. AHCPR Publication No. 93-0552. Rockville, Md.: U.S. Department of Health and Human Services, Public Health Service, Agency for Health Care Policy and Research.

Diagnostic and Statistical Manual of Mental Disorders, 4th ed. 1994. Washington, D.C.: American Psychiatric Association.

Eikelboom, J. W., et al. 1999. Homocysteine and cardiovascular disease: A critical review of the epidemilogical evidence. *Annals of Internal Medicine* 131 (5):363–375.

Gaster, B. 1999. S-adenosylmethionine (SAMe) for treatment of depression. *Alternative Medicine Alert* 2 (12):133–135.

Gise, L. H. 1996. What you can do about depression at menopause. *Menopausal Medicine* 4 (1):1–5.

Harvard Women's Health Watch. 1999. Gender and stress. *Harvard Women's Health Watch* 7 (2):1.

Hauri, P., and S. Linde. 1990. *No More Sleepless Nights.* New York: John Wiley and Sons.

Kaplan, A. G. 1986. The "self in relation": Implications for depression in women. *Psychotherapy: Theory, Research, and Practice* 23:235–42.

Kiecolt-Glaser, J., and R. Glaser. 1991. Stress and immune function in humans. In *Psychoneuroimmunology,* 2nd ed., edited by R. Ader et al. San Diego: Academic Press.

Kiecolt-Glaser, J. 1996. The negative influence of stress on the immune system. Presentation at the annual meeting of the International Society of Neuroimmunomodulation.

Kobasa, S., et al. 1982. Hardiness and health: A prospective study. *Journal of Personality and Social Psychology* 42:168–177.

Landau, C., et al. 1994. *The Complete Book of Menopause: Every Woman's Guide to Good Health.* New York: G. P. Putnam's Sons.

McGrath, E., et al. 1990. Women and depression: Risk factors and treatment issues. Washington, D.C.: American Psychological Association.

McKinley, J., et al. 1987. The relative contributions of endocrine changes and social circumstances to depression in mid-aged women. *Journal of Health and Social Behavior* 28:345–63.

Moyers, B. 1993. *Healing and the Mind.* New York: Bantam Doubleday Dell.

Nolen-Hoeksema, S. 1987. Sex differences in unipolar depression: Evidence and theory. *Psychological Bulletin* 101:259–82.

Notelovitz, M., and D. Tonnessen. 1993. *Menopause and Midlife Health.* New York: St. Martin's Press.

O'Hara, M. W. 1991. Postpartum mental disorders. In *Gynecology and Obstetrics,* vol. 6, edited by J. J. Sciarra. Philadelphia: J. B. Lippincott.

Ojeda, L. 1995. *Menopause without Medicine.* Alameda, Calif.: Hunter House.

Sherwin, B. 1993. Menopausal Depression: Myth or Reality? Chair of symposium at fourth annual Meeting of the North American Menopausal Society, San Diego.

Somer, E. 1993. *Nutrition for Women.* New York: Henry Holt

Weissman, M. M., et al. 1996. Cross-national epidemiology of major depression and bipolar disorder. *Journal of the American Medical Association* 276:293–299.

Wellness Letter 2000. A "natural" treatment of depression? *UC Berkeley Wellness Letter* 16 (4):1–2.

Wilde, L. 1997. Humor: Rx for Healing, Health, and Happiness. Presentation at Rogue Valley Medical Center, Medford, Oregon, April 22.

Yerkes, R. M., and J. D. Dodson. 1989. The relation of strength of stimulus to rapidity of habit formation. *Journal of Comparative Neurology* 18:459–82.

Chapter 12: Sexuality: Good Sex Doesn't Need to Change

Arlt, W., et al. 1999. Dehydroepiandrotserone replacement in women with adrenal insufficiency. *New England Journal of Medicine* 341:1013–1020.

Azar, B. 1998. Communicating through pheromones. *American Psychological Association Monitor* 29 (1):1–12.

Bachman, G. A., and S. R. Leiblum. 1991. Sexuality in sexagenarian women. *Maturitas* 13:43–50.

Beck, J. 1995. Hypoactive sexual desire disorder: An overview. *Journal of Consulting and Clinical Psychology* 63 (6):919–923.

Cone, F. K. 1993. *Making Sense of Menopause.* New York: Simon & Schuster.

Edelman, D. 1992. *Sex in the Golden Years.* New York: Donald I. Fine.

Harvard Women's Health Watch. 2000. It takes two: Coping with erectile dysfunction. *Harvard Women's Health Watch* 7 (7):2–3.

Helstrom, L. 1994. Sexuality after hysterectomy: A model based on quantitative and qualitative analysis of 104 women before and after subtotal hysterectomy. *Journal of Psychosomatic Obstetrics and Gynecology* 4:219–29.

Hirsch, A. 1995. *Scentsational Sex: The Secret to Using Aroma for Arousal.* Rockport, Mass.: Element Books.

Kaverne, E., et al. 1989. Beta-endorphin concentration in cerebrospinal fluid of monkeys are influenced by grooming relationships. *Psychoneuroendocrinology* 14 (1–2):155–61.

Kegel, A. M. 1951. Physiologic therapy for urinary stress incontinence. *Journal of the American Medical Association* 146:915–17.

Labbate, L. A., and M. H. Pollack. 1994. Treatment of fluoxitine-induced sexual dysfunction with buprop ion: A case study. *Annals of Clinical Psychiatry* 6:13–15.

Lechner, M. E., et al. 1993. Self-reported medical problems of adult female survivors of childhood sexual abuse. *Journal of Family Practice* 36 (6):633–37.

Masters, W., and V. Johnson. 1970. *Human Sexual Inadequacy.* Boston: Little, Brown.

———. 1966. *Human Sexual Response.* Boston: Little, Brown.

Meana, M. 1997. Dyspareunia: Sexual dysfunction or pain syndrome. *Journal of Nervous and Mental Disease* 185 (9):561–569.

Medical Letter. 1992. Drugs that cause sexual dysfunction: An update. *Medical Letter: Drug Therapy* 34:74–77.

Meston, C., and B. Gorzalka. 1996. Differential effects of sympathetic activation on sexual arousal in women. *Journal of Abnormal Psychology* 104 (4):582–591.

Mitchell, D. 2000. FDA OKs first female sex device. *Wall Street Journal*, May 4.

Morales, A. J., et al. 1994. Effects of replacement dose of dehydroepiandrosterone in men and women of advancing age. *Journal of Clinical Endocrinology and Metabolism* 78:1360–1367.

North American Menopause Society Roundtable Highlights. 1998. Physiologic androgen replacement in menopausal women. *Menopause Management* March/April:26-28.

Nurnberg, H. G. 1999. Sildenafil for women patients with antidepressant-induced sexual dysfunction. *Psychiatric Serices* 50:1076–1078.

Reichman, J. 1998. *I'm Not in the Mood.* New York: William Morrow and Company.

————. *I'm Too Young to Get Old: Health Care for Women After Forty.* New York: Times Books.

Rhodes, J. C., et al. 1999. Hysterectomy and sexual functioning. *Journal of the American Medical Association* 282:1934–1941.

Russell, D. 1986. *The Secret Trauma.* New York: Basic Books.

Sachs, J. 1991. *What Women Should Know About Menopause.* New York: Bantam Doubleday Dell.

Sarrel, P. M. 1990. Sexuality and menopause. *Obstetrics and Gynecology* 75 (4):26S–30S.

Sherwin, B., and M. Gelfand. 1985. Sex steroids and affect in the surgical menopause: A double blind, cross-over study. *Psychoneouroendocrinology* 3:325–35.

Sherwin, B. B. 1996. The use of androgens in the postmenopause: Evidence from clinical studies. In *Progress in the Management of Menopause*, edited by B. G. Wren. New York: Pantheon.

Chapter 13: Looking Good While Changing: Skin Care, Hair Care, and Cosmetic Surgery

Alster, T. S., and S. Garg. 1996. Treatment of facial rhytides with a high-energy pulsed carbon dioxide laser. *Plastic and Reconstructive Surgery* 98 (5):791–94.

American Society for Dermatological Surgery. 1994. *Chemical Peeling.* Brochure no. 003. Schaumberg, Ill.: American Society for Dermatologic Surgery.

Atillasoy, E. S., et al. 1998 UVB induces melanocytic lesions and melanoma in human skin. *American Journal of Pathology* 152 (5):1179–1186

Autier, P., et al. 1997. Melanoma and sunscreen use: Need for studies representative of actual behaviors. Melanoma Research 7 (Suppl. 2): S115–120

Baumann, L. S. 1999 The effects of topical vitamin E on he cosmetic appearance of scars. *Dermatologic Surgery* 25 (4):311–315

Brumberg, E. 1997. *Ageless: What Every Woman Needs to Know to Look Good and Feel Good*. New York: HarperCollins.

Epps, R. P., and S. C. Stuart. 1995. *Women's Complete Health Book*. New York: Delacorte.

Eskin, B. A., and L. S. Dumas. 1995. *Midlife Can Wait: How to Stay Young and Healthy After 35*. New York: Ballantine.

Fisher, A. A. 1995. *Contact Dermatitis*, 3rd ed. Philadelphia: Lea and Febiger.

Fruzzetti, F., 1999. Treatment of hirsutism: Comparisons between different antiandrogens with central and peripheral effects. *Fertility and Sterility* 71:445–451.

Fulton, J. E., et al. 1996. Effect of chocolate on acne vulgaris. *Journal of the American Medical Association* 210:2071–74.

Green, A., et al. 1999. Daily sunscreen application and betacarotene supplementation in prevention of basal-cell and squamous-cell carcinoma of the skin: A randomized controlled trial. *Lancet* 354 (180):723–729.

Gorgu, M. 2000. Comparison of alexandrite laser and electrolysis for hair removal. *Dermatologic Surgery* 26:37–41.

Hayman, G. 1996. *How Do I Look?* New York: Random House.

Leenutaphong, V. 1992. Evaluating the UVA protection of commercially available sunscreens (abstract). *Journal of the Medical Association of Thailand* 75 (11):619–24.

Leverette, K. 1991. The glycololic bandwagon: Fact and fiction. *Dermascope* 4:50–51.

McCallion, R., and A. Li Wan Po. 1993. Dry and photo-aged skin: Manifestations and management. *Journal of Clinical Pharmaceutical Therapeutics* 18:15–32.

Mitchell, D. L., et al. 1999. Effect of chronic low-dose ultraviolet B radiation on DNA damage and repair in mouse skin. *Cancer Research* 59 (12):2875–2884.

Moy, L. S. 1995. Glycolic Acid: A Safe Alternative for Chemical Peel. Presentation at Orlando, Fla., meeting on Cosmetic Dermatology, sponsored by Northwestern University School of Medicine.

Notelovitz, M., and D. Tonnessen. 1993. *Menopause and Midlife Health.* New York: St. Martin's Press.

Paige, T. 2000. Personal communication, May 15.

Podolsky, D., and B. Streisand. 1996. The price of vanity. *U.S. News and World Report* October 14:72–80.

Reichman, J. 1996. *I'm Too Young to Get Old: Health Care for Women After Forty.* New York: Times Books.

Stiller, M., et al. 1996. Topical 8% glycolic acid and 8% L-lactic acid creams in the treatment of photo-damaged skin. *Archives of Dermatology* 132:631–36.

Takeuchi, T., et al. 1998. A novel in vitro model for evaluating agents that protect against ultraviolet-A photoaging. *Journal of Investigative Dermatology* 110 (4):343–347.

Wikonkal, N. M., and D. E. Brash. 1999. Ultraviolet radiation induced signature mutations in photocarcinogenesis. *Journal of Investigative Dermatology Symposia and Procedures* 4 (1):6–10.

Women's HealthSource. 2000. Skin cancer: Discovering and treating trouble spots. *Mayo Clinic Women's HealthSource* 4 (5):4–6.

Chapter 14: Gynecologic Surgery and Medical Treatment: When the Unexpected Happens

Alexander, D. et al. 1996. Randomized trial comparing hysterectomy with endometrial ablation for dysfunctional uterine bleeding: Psychiatric and psychosocial aspect. *British Medical Journal* 312 (7026):280–284.

Amso, N. N., et al., for the International Collaborative Uterine Thermal Balloon Working Group. 1998. Uterine balloon therapy for the treatment of menorrhagia: The first 300 patients from a multi-centre study. *British Journal of Obstetrics and Gynecology* 105 (95):517–523.

Appell, R. A. 1997. Medications for urge incontinence. *Audio Digest Obstetrics and Gynecology* 44 (4).

Ayton, R. A., et al. 1996. A comparative study of safety and efficacy of continuous low dose oestradiol released from a vaginal ring compared with conjugated equine oestrogen vaginal cream in the treatment of postmenopausal urogenital atrophy. *British Journal of Obstetrics and Gynaecology* 103:351–358.

Barrington, J. W., et al. 1997. The levonorgesterel intrauterine system in the management of menorrhagia. *British journal of Obstetrics and Gynaecology* 103:351–358.

Bergman, A., and G. Elia. 1995. Three surgical procedures for genuine stress incontinence: Five-year follow-up of a prospective randomized study. *American Journal of Obstetrics and Gynecology* 173:66–71.

Bø, K., et al. 1999. Single blind randomised controlled trial of pelvic floor exercises, electrical stimulation, vaginal cones and no treament in management of genuine stress incontinenece in women. *British Medical Journal* 318:487–493.

Brill, A. I. 1995. What is the role of hysteroscopy in the management of abnormal uterine bleeding? *Clinical Obstetrics and Gynecology* 38:319–45.

Brown, J. 1999. Understanding Urinary Incontinence. Lecture presented at the Essentials of Women's Health course. UCSF Department of OB/GYN. Hapuna Prince Hotel, Hawaii, July.

————. 1996. Episiotomy and pelvic floor exercise for incontinence. *Audio Digest, Obstetrics and Gynecology* 43 (21).

Brubaker, L., et al. 1999. The external urethral barrier for stress incontinence: A multicenter trial of safety and efficacy. *Obstetrics and Gynecology* 93 (6):932–942.

Burch, J. C. 1961. Urethrovaginal fixation to Cooper's ligament for correction of stress incontinence, cystocele, and prolapse. *American Journal of Obstetrics and Gynecology* 81:281–86.

Burgio, K. L., et al. 1998. Behavioral vs. drug treatment for urge urinary incontinence in older women: A randomized controlled trial. *Journal of the American Medical Association* 280 (23):1995-2000.

Cameron, I. T., et al. 1990. The effects of mefenamic acid and norethisterone on measured menstrual blood loss. *Obstetrics and Gynecology* 76:85–8.

Carlson, K. J. 1993. Indications for hysterectomy. *New England Journal of Medicine* 328:856–60.

Casper, R. F., and M. T. Hearn. 1990. The effect of hysterectomy and bilateral oophorectomy in women with severe premenstrual syndrome. *American Journal of Obstetrics and Gynecology* 162:105–09.

Coleman, M., et al. 1997. The levonorgesterel-releasing intrauterine device: A wider role than contraception. *Australian and New Zealand Journal of Obstetrics and Gynecology* 37 (2):195–201.

Cooper, G. S., and J. M. Thorp. 1999. FSH levels in relation to hysterectomy and to unilateral oophorectomy. *Obstetrics and Gynecology* 94:969–972.

Cosiski-Marana, H.R., et al. 1996. Evaluation of long-term results of surgical correction of stress urinary incontinence. *Gynecologic and Obstetric Investigation* 41:214–19.

Cramer, D. W. 1994. Epidemiology and biostatistics. In *Practical Gynecologic Oncology*, 2nd ed. Baltimore: Williams and Wilkins.

Creasman, W. T. 1997. Ovarian cancer screening. *ACOG Clinical Review* 2 (2):1–2,14–15.

Dieden, J. D. 2000. Fibroids: Update on Embolization. Lecture given at New Comcepts in Reproductive Gynecology and Fertility, sponsored by Kaiser Permanente. Claremont Hotel, Oakland, Calif., October 14.

Dubuisson, J. B., and C. Chapron. 1996. Debate: Laparoscopic myomectomy today a good technique when correctly indicated. *Human Reproduction* 11 (5):934–937.

Dwyer, N., et al. 1993. Randomized controlled trial comparing endometrial resection with abdominal hysterectomy for the treatment of menorrhagia. *British Journal of Obstetrics and Gynaecology* 100:237–243.

Fairbanks, V. F., and E. Bentler. 1995. Iron deficiency. In *William's Hematology*, 5th ed., edited by E. Bentler et al. New York: McGraw-Hill.

Fantl, J. et al. 1994. Estrogen therapy for urinary incontinence in post menopausal women. *Journal of Obstetrics and Gynecology* 83:12–18.

Fedele, L., et al. 1997. Treatment of adenomyosis-associated menorrhagia with a levonorgestral-releasing intruterine device. *Fertility and Sterility* 68 (3):426–429.

Fong, Y. F., and K. Singh. 1999. Effect of the levonorgestral-releasing intrauterine system of uterine myomas in a renal transplant patient. *Contraception* 60:51–53.

Gainey, H. L. 1955. Postpartum observation of pelvic tissue damage: Further studies. *American Journal of Obstetrics and Gynecology* 70:800–807.

Gambone, J., et al. 1992. Short-term outcome of incidental hysterectomy at the time of adnexectomy for benign disease. *Journal of Women's Health* 1:197–200.

Garnet, J. 1964. Uterine rupture during pregnancy. *Obstetrics and Gynecology* 23:898–905.

Goldrath, M. H., et al. 1981. Laser photovaporization of endometrium for the treatment of menorrhagia. *American Journal of Obstetrics and Gynecology* 40 (1):14–19.

Goldrath, M. H. 1990. Use of danazol in hysteroscopic surgery for menorrhagia. *Journal of Reproductive Medicine* 35 (1, Suppl. 1):91–96

Gomel, V. 1995. For tubal pregnancy, surgical treatment is usually best. *Clinical Obstetrics and Gynecology* 38:353–61.

Goodwin, S., and B. McLucas. 1998. Uterine artery embolization for uterine fibroids. *Obstetrics and Gynecology* 45(17).

Goodwin, S. C., et al. 1999. Uterine artery embolization for the treatment of uterine leiomyomata midterm results. *Journal of Interventional Radiology* 10:1159–1165.

Goodwin, S. C., et al. 2000. Opportunity and responsibility: SCVIR's role with uterine artery embolization. Society of Cardiovascular & Interventional Radiology. *Journal of Vascular Interventional Radiology* 11(4): 409-410.

Grimes, D. A. 1982. Diagnostic dilation and curettage: A reappraisal. *American Journal of Obstetrics and Gynecology* 142:1–6.

Harris, W. J. 1992. Uterine dehiscence following laparoscopic myomectomy. *Obstetrics and Gynecology* 80:545–46.

Harvard Women's Health Watch. 2000. Progress report on ovarian cancer. *Harvard Women's Health Watch* 7 (9):2–4.

Hendricks-Matthews, M. K. 1991. The importance of assessing a woman's history of sexual abuse before hysterectomy. *Journal of Family Practice* 32:631–32.

Henriksson, L., et al. 1996. A one-year multicenter study of efficacy and safety of a continuous, low-dose, estradiol-releasing vaginal ring (Estring) in postmenopausal women with symptoms and signs of urogenital aging. *American Journal of Obstetrics and Gynecology* 174:85–92.

Herrmann, U. J., Jr., et al. 1987. Sonographic patterns of ovarian tumors: Prediction of malignancy. *Obstetrics and Gynecology* 69:777–81.

Jaffe, S. B., and R. Jewelewicz. 1991 The basic infertility investigation. *Fertility and Sterility* 56:599–613.

Kelly, H. A. 1913. Incontinence of urine in women. *Urologic and Cutaneous Review* 17:291–99.

Kjolhede, P., and G. Ryden. 1994. Prognostic factors and long-term results of the Burch colposuspension: A retrospective study. *Acta Obstetrics Gynecology Scandinavia* 73:642–47.

Langer, R., et al. 1990. Reproductive outcome after conservative surgery for unruptured tubal pregnancies—a 15-year experience. *Fertility and Sterility* 53:227–31.

Lefler, H. T., et al. 1991. Modified endometrial ablation: Electrocoagulation with vasopressin and suction curettage preparation. *Obstetrics and Gynecology* 77:949–56.

Leventhal, J. 1996. Premenstrual Dysphoric Disorder. Lecture given to the Women's Health Department, Kaiser Permanente Medical Group, Walnut Creek, Calif. October.

Liapis, A., et al. 1996. Genuine stress incontinence: Prospective randomized comparison of two operative methods. *European Journal of Obstetric and Gynecological Reproductive Biology* 64 (1):69–72.

Liu, C. Y. 1992. Laparoscopic hysterectomy: A review of 72 cases. *Journal of Reproductive Medicine.* 37:351–354.

Lund, J. J. 1955. Early ectopic pregnancy. *Journal of Obstetrics and Gynaecology of the British Empire* 62:70–76.

Lyons, T. L. 1995. Minimally invasive treatment of urinary stress incontinence and laparoscopically directed repair of pelvic floor defects. *Clinical Obstetrics and Gynecology* 38:380–91.

Lyons, T. L., and W. Parker. 1996. Highlights from the International Congress of Gynecologic Endoscopy. *Audio Digest, Obstetrics and Gynecology* 43 (17).

Magos, A. L., et al. 1991. Experience with the first 250 endometrial resections for menorrhagia. *Lancet* 337:1074–1078.

Maiman, M. 1995. Laparoscopic removal of the adnexal mass: The case for caution. *Clinical Obstetrics and Gynecology* 38:370–379.

Malone, L. 1969. Myomectomy: Recurrence after removal of solitary and multiple myomas. *Obstetrics and Gynecology* 34:200–03.

Mancuso, A., et al. 1991. The residual ovary after hysterectomy. *Clinical Experimental Obstetrics and Gynecology* 18 (2):117–19.

Mann, G. B., and P. I. Berger. 1998. Breast cancer genes and the surgeon. *Journal of Surgical Oncology* 67 (4):267–274.

Marshall, V. E., et al. 1949. The correction of stress incontinence by simple vesicourethral suspension surgery. *Obstetrics and Gynecology* 88:509–14.

Marrs, R. 1991. The use of potassium-titanyl-phosphate laser for laparoscopic removal of ovarian endometriomas. *American Journal of Obstetrics and Gynecology* 164:1622–28.

McGuire, E. J., and R. D. Cespedes. 1996. Proper diagnosis: A must before surgery for stress incontinence. *Journal of Endourology* 10:201–205.

Mecke, H., et al. 1992. Pelviscopic treatment of ovarian cysts in premenopausal women. *Gynecologic and Obstetric Investigations* 34 (1):36–42.

Medical Letter. 1995. Antimicrobial prophylaxis in surgery. *Medical Letter* 37 (957):79–82.

Miller, J. M., et al. 1998. A pelvic muscle precontraction can reduce cough-related urine loss in selected women with mild SUI. *Journal of the American Geriatric Society* 46:870–874.

Montz, F. J., and J. B. Schlaerth. 1995. Laparoscopic surgery: Does it have a role in the management of gynecologic malignancies? *Clinical Obstetrics and Gynecology* 38:426–433.

Mouritsen, L., et al. 1991. Long-term effect of pelvic floor exercises on female urinary incontinence. *British Journal of Urology* 68 (1):32–37.

Munro, M. G., and J. Neprest. 1995. Laparoscopic hysterectomy: Does it work? A bicontinental review of the literature and clinical commentary. *Clinical Obstetrics and Gynecology* 38:401–25.

Nezhat, C. 1999. Complications of Laparascopy. Lecture given at New Concepts in Reproductive Gynecology and Fertility, presented by the Fertility Group of the Permanente Medical Group, Northern California Region, Oakland, Calif., October 30.

Nezhat, C. H., et al. 1996. Vaginal vault evisceration after total laparoscopic hysterectomy. *Obstetrics and Gynecology* 87 (5, part 2):868–870.

Nezhat, F., et al. 1996. Debate: Laparoscopic myomectomy today—Why, when, and for whom. *Human Reproduction* 11 (5):933–934.

Nichols, D. H. 1991. Surgery for pelvic floor disorders. *Surgical Clinics of North America* 71 (5):927–946.

Oliver, D. I. 2000. Surgical and nonsurgical treatment of abnormal uterine bleeding. *Audio Digest, Obstetrics and Gynecology* 47 (12).

Ostergard, D. R. 1997. Biofeedback and other treatments for incontinence. *Audio Digest, Obstetrics and Gynecology* 44 (4).

Parker, W. H. 1995. The case for laparoscopic management of adnexal mass. *Clinical Obstetrics and Gynecology* 38:362–369.

———. 1995. Myomectomy: Laparoscopy or laparotomy? *Clinical Obstetrics and Gynecology* 38:392–400.

Ranney, B. 1990. Decreasing numbers of patients for vaginal hysterectomy and plasty. *South Dakota Journal of Medicine* 43 (1):7–12.

Ravina, J. et al. 1995. Arterial embolisation to treat uterine myomata. *Lancet* 346 (8976):671–672.

Reggiori, A., et al. 1996. Randomized study of antibiotic prophylaxis for general and gynaecological surgery from a single centre in rural Africa. *British Journal of Surgery* 83:356–59.

Schildkraut, J., et al. 1997. Relationship between lifetime ovulatory cycles and overexpression of mutant N epithelial ovarian cancer. *Journal of the National Cancer Institute* 89 (13):932–938

Silva, P. D., et al. 1993. Reproductive outcomes after 143 laparoscopic procedures for ectopic pregnancy. *Obstetrics and Gynecology* 81:710–15.

Silvin, I., and J. Stern. 1994. Health during prolonged use of levenogestral 20mcg/D and copper Tcu 380 Ag intrauterine contraceptive devices: A multicenter study. *Fertility and Sterility* 61:70–77.

Simon, N. V., at al. 1999. Laparascopic supracervical hysterectomy vs. abdominal hysterectomy in a community hospital. *Journal of Reproductive Medicine* 44 (4):339–345.

Singer, A., and A. Ikomi. 1994. Successful treatment of fibroids using an intrauterine progresterone device (abstract). *International Journal of Gynecology and Obstetrics* 46:55.

Singla, A. 2000. An update on the management of SUI. *Contemporary OB/GYN* January:68–85.

Storm, H. H., et al. 1992. Supravaginal uterine amputation in Denmark 1978-1988 and the risk of cancer. *Gynecologic Oncology* 45:198–201.

Stovall, T. G. 1995. Medical management should be routinely used as primary therapy for ectopic pregnancy. *Clinical Obstetrics and Gynecology* 38:346–352.

Stovall, T. G., et al. 1991. Methotrexate treatment of unruptured ectopic pregnancy: A report of 100 cases. *Obstetrics and Gynecology* 77:749–53.

Tanos, V., and N. Rojansky. 1994. Prophylactic antibiotics in abdominal hysterectomy. *Journal of the American College of Surgeons* 179:593–600.

Tulandi, T., et al. 1993. Adhesion formation and reproductive outcome after myomectomy and second-look laparoscopy. *Obstetrics and Gynecology* 82:213–15.

Van Den Eeden, S. K., et al. 1997. Quality of life: Health care utilization and costs among women undergoing hysterectomy in a managed care setting. *American Journal of Obstetrics and Gynecology* 178 (1, part 1):91–100.

Vashisht, A., at al. 1999. Fatal septicaemia after fibroid embolization. *Lancet* 354:307–308.

Versi, E., and M. A. Harvery. 1998. Efficacy of an external urethral device in women with genuine stress urinary incontinence and pelvic floor dysfunction. *International Urogynecology Journal* 9 (5): 271-274.

Ulmsten, U., et al. 1999. A three year follow-up tension free vaginal tape for surgical treatment of female stress urinary incontinence. *British Journal of Obstetrics and Gynaecology* 106:345–350.

Wang, A. C., and T. S. Lo. 1998. Tension-free vaginal tape. *Journal of Reproductive Medicine* 43 (5):429–434.

West, S., and P. Dranov. 1994. *The Hysterectomy Hoax: A Leading Surgeon Explains Why 90% of All Hysterectomies Are Unnecessary and Describes All the Treatment Options Available to Every Women, No Matter What Age.* New York: Doubleday.

Wong, G. C., et al. 2000. Uterine artery embolization: A minimally invasive technique for the treatment of uterine fibroids. *Journal of Women's Health & Gender Based Medicine* 9 (4):357–362.

Index

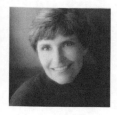 L. Darlene Lanka, M.D., has been a practicing obstetrician and gynecologist for thirty years with Kaiser Permanente in Northern California and is an assistant clinical professor at the University of California, San Francisco. She is the former Director of Women's Health for Kaiser-Permanente Medical Center in Walnut Creek, California and two times president of the East Bay GYN Society. She is a frequent lecturer and has been interviewed on numerous radio and television programs discussing women's health issues and by KPIX on women's health legislation in California. Dr. Lanka was awarded the Diablo Soroptimist Societies' Women Helping Women Award.

James E. Huston, M.D., specialized in obstetrics and gynecology before his retirement. He lives in Medford, Oregon. He is a frequent author and speaker on women's health topics.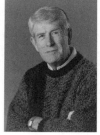

Both Dr. Lanka and Dr. Huston have visited Guatemala as participating doctors with the Hospital de la Familia in Guatemala, donating much-needed medical aid for indigenous families.

Some Other
New Harbinger Titles

Watercooler Wisdom, Item 4364 $14.95

The Juicy Tomato Guide to Ripe Living After 50, Item 4321 $16.95

What's Right With Me, Item 4429 $16.95

The Balanced Mom, Item 4534 $14.95

Women Who Worry Too Much, Item 4127 $13.95

In Harm's Way, Item 4003 $14.95

Breastfeeding Made Simple, Item 4046 $16.95

The Well-Ordered Office, Item 3856 $13.95

Talk to Me, Item 3317 $12.95

Romantic Intelligence, Item 3309 $15.95

Transformational Divorce, Item 3414 $13.95

The Rape Recovery Handbook, Item 3376 $15.95

Eating Mindfully, Item 3503 $13.95

Sex Talk, Item 2868 $12.95

Everyday Adventures for the Soul, Item 2981 $11.95

A Woman's Addiction Workbook, Item 2973 $19.95

The Daughter-In-Law's Survival Guide, Item 2817 $12.95

PMDD, Item 2833 $13.95

The Vulvodynia Survival Guide, Item 2914 $16.95

Love Tune-Ups, Item 2744 $10.95

Brave New You, Item 2590 $13.95

The Woman's Book of Sleep, Item 2418 $14.95

Pregnancy Stories, Item 2361 $14.95

The Women's Guide to Total Self-Esteem, Item 2418 $14.95

The Conscious Bride, Item 2132 $12.95

Call **toll free, 1-800-748-6273,** or log on to our online bookstore **www.newharbinger.com** to order. Have your Visa or Mastercard numb ready. Or send a check for the titles you want to New Harbinger Publi tions, Inc., 5674 Shattuck Ave., Oakland, CA 94609. Include $4.50 for first book and 75¢ for each additional book, to cover shipping and h dling. (California residents please include appropriate sales tax.) All two to five weeks for delivery.

Prices subject to change without notice.

More New Harbinger Titles

THE TAKING CHARGE OF MENOPAUSE WORKBOOK
Helps you ease the transition through this major life change by becoming an active member of your health care team.
Item PAUS Paperback $17.95

PMS
Women Tell Women How to Control Premenstrual Syndrome
Draws on the experiences of more than 1,000 women to show how to break the vicious PMS cycle of anger, guilt, denial, and depression.
Item PRE $13.95

NATURAL WOMEN'S HEALTH
New Zealand naturopath and acupuncturist Lynda Wharton brings together the best of traditional and alternative approaches to living well and staying well.
Item HLTH $13.95

THE DAILY RELAXER
Presents the most effective and popular techniques for learning how to relax—simple, tension-relieving exercises that you can learn in five minutes and practice with positive results right away.
Item DALY Paperback, $12.95

THE CHRONIC PAIN CONTROL WORKBOOK
A team of specialists in all areas of pain management detail the treatment strategies for managing and recovering from chronic pain.
Item PN2 Paperback $19.95

FIBROMYALGIA & CHRONIC MYOFASCIAL PAIN SYNDROME
This survival manual is the first comprehensive patient guide for managing these conditions. Readers learn how to identify trigger points, cope with chronic pain and sleep problems, and deal with the numbing effects of "fibrofog."
Item FMS Paperback, $19.95

Call **toll-free 1-800-748-6273** to order. Have your Visa or Mastercard number ready. Or send a check for the titles you want to New Harbinger Publications, 5674 Shattuck Avenue, Oakland, CA 94609. Include $4.50 for the first book and 75¢ for each additional book to cover shipping and handling. (California residents please include appropriate sales tax.) Allow four to six weeks for delivery.

Prices subject to change without notice.